Plasmodium Species and Drug Resistance

Edited by Rajeev K. Tyagi

Published in London, United Kingdom

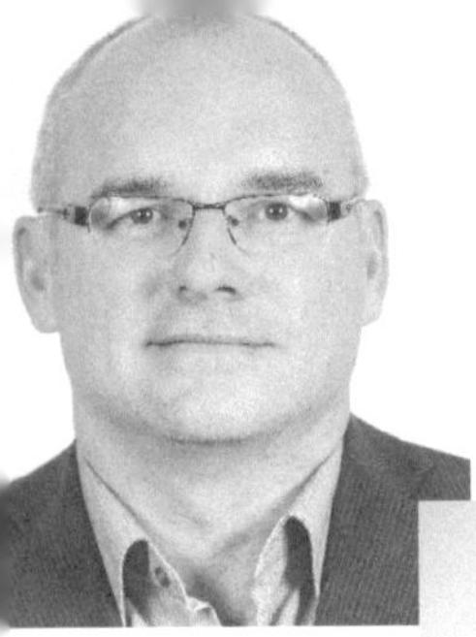
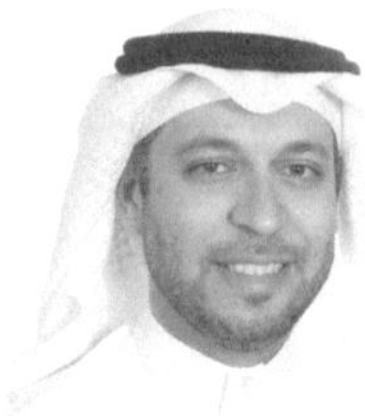
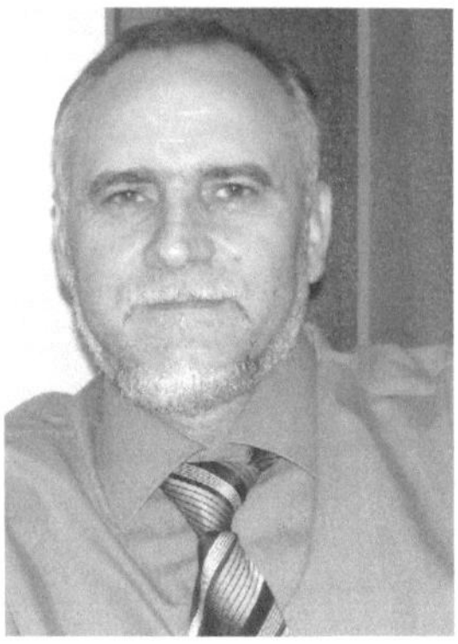
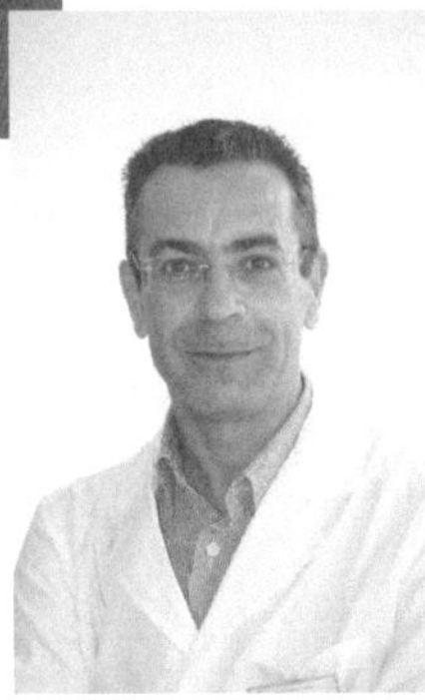
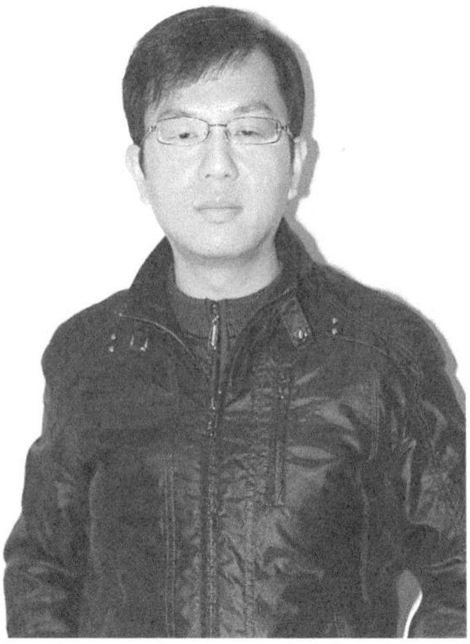
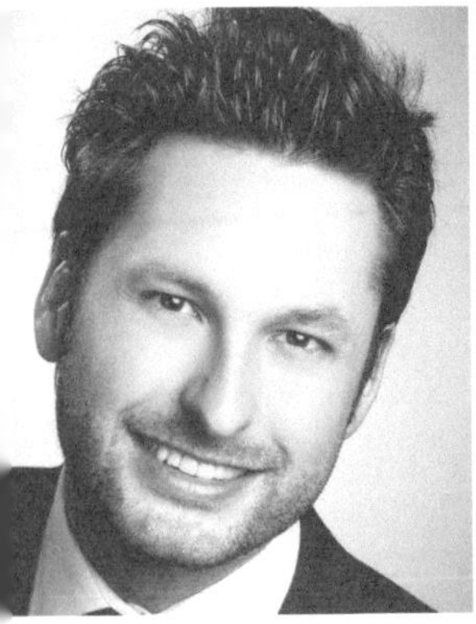
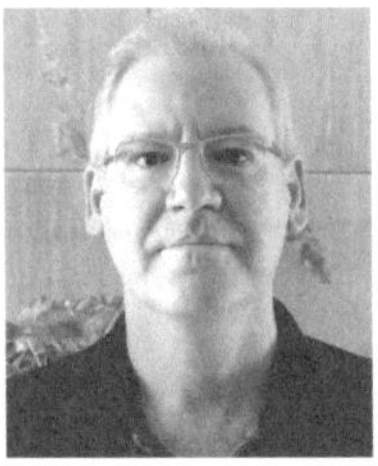

IntechOpen

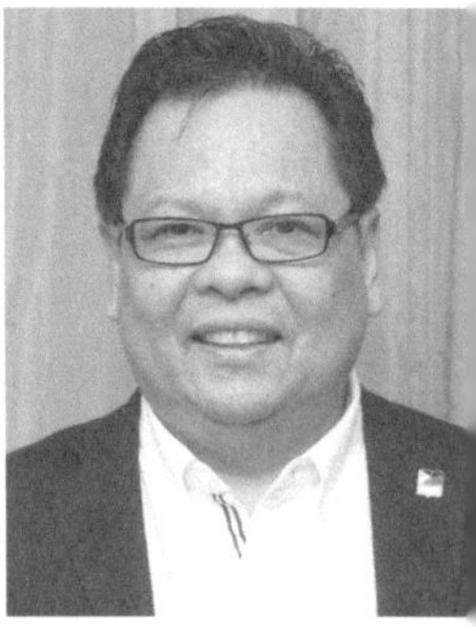
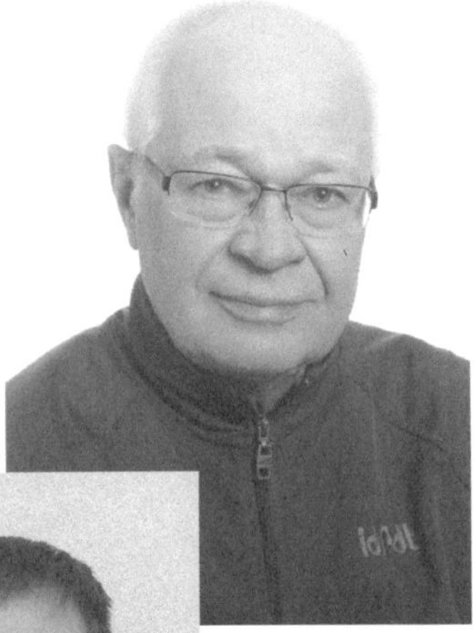
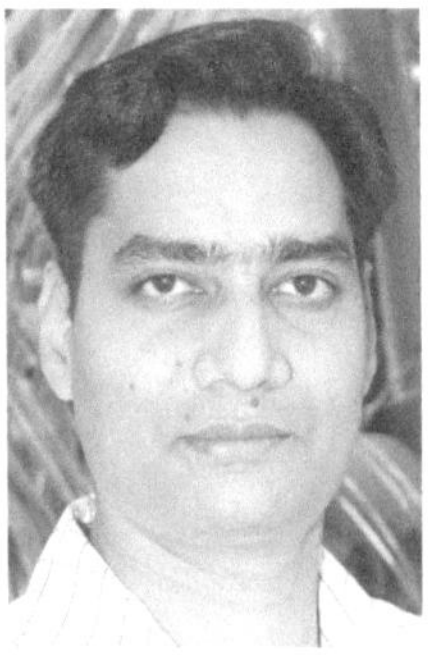
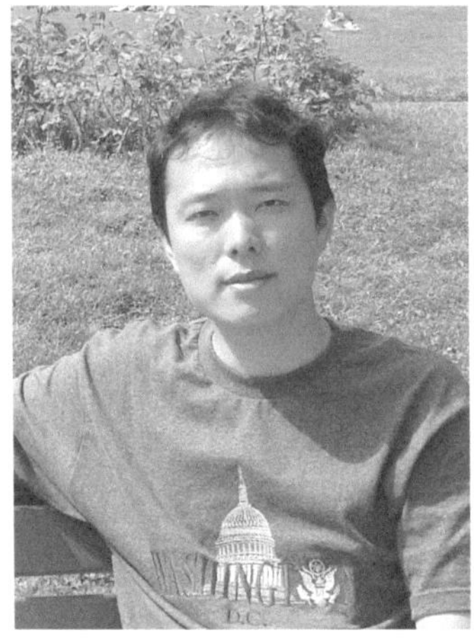
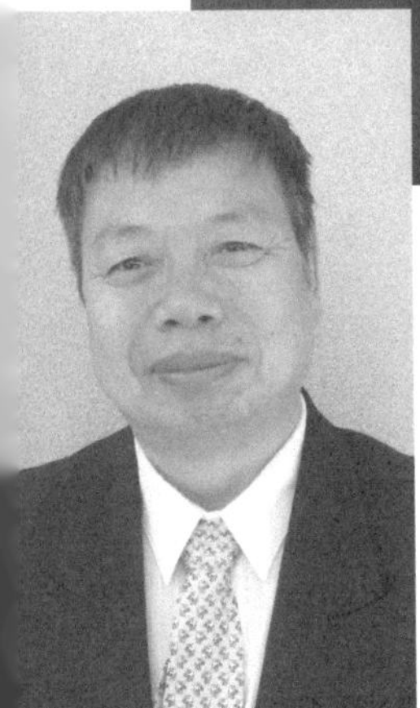
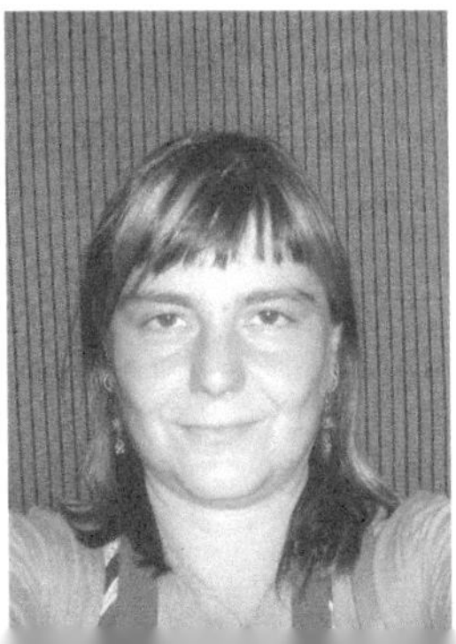

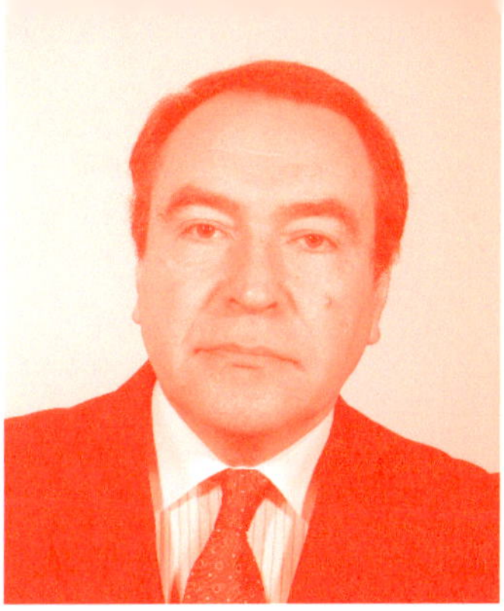

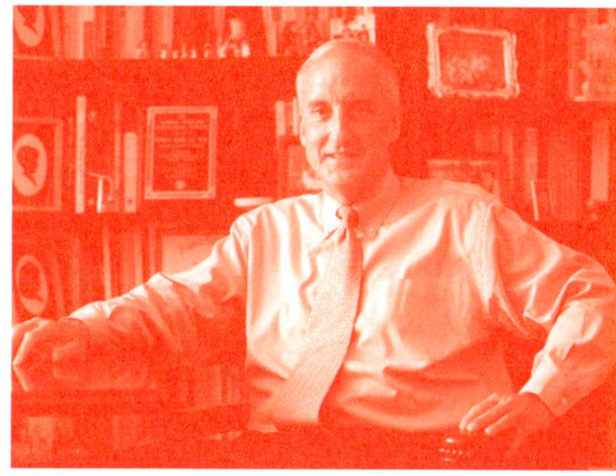

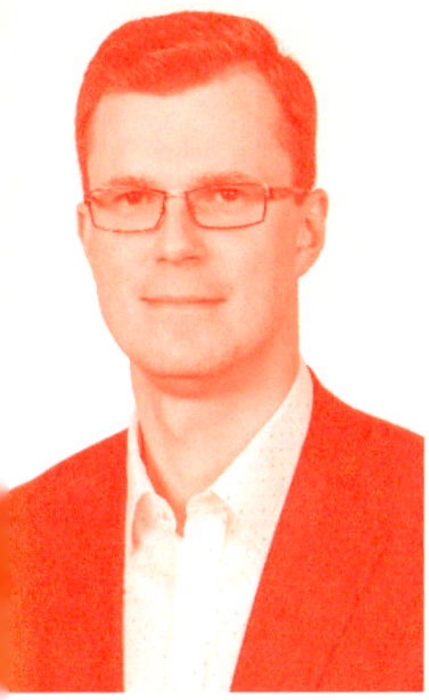

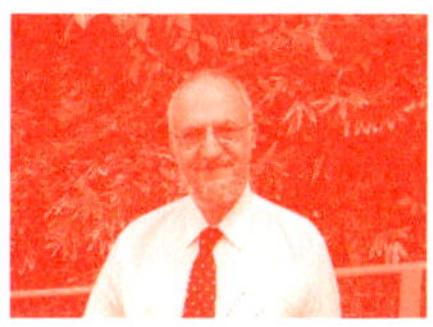

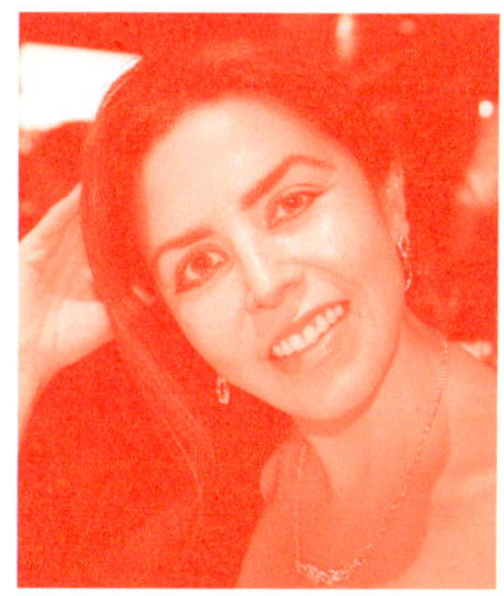

Supporting open minds since 2005

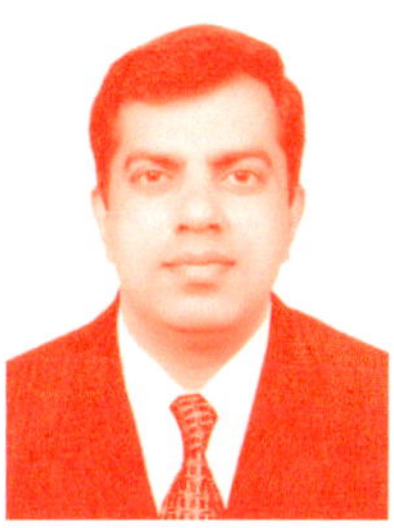

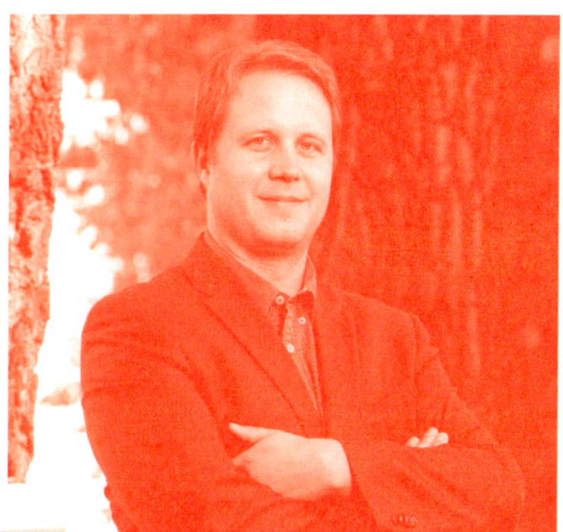

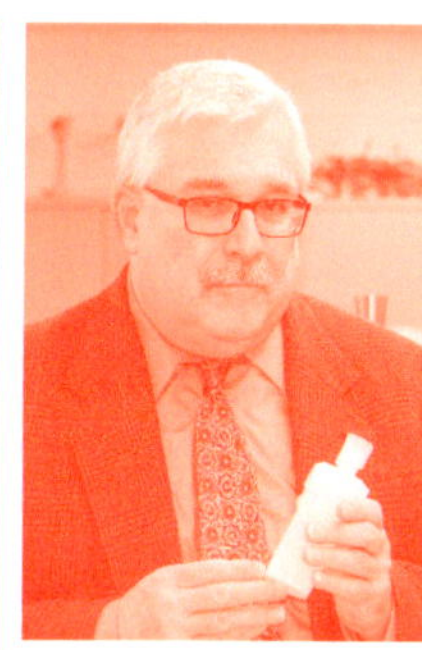

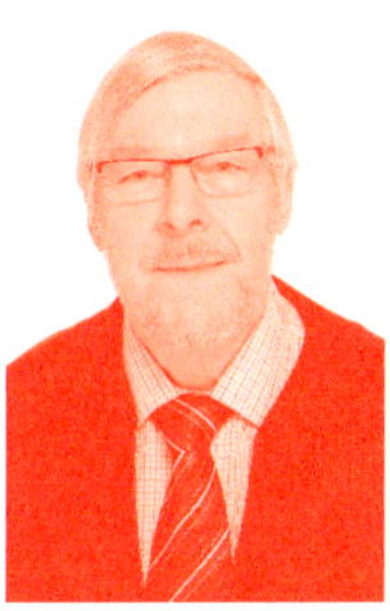

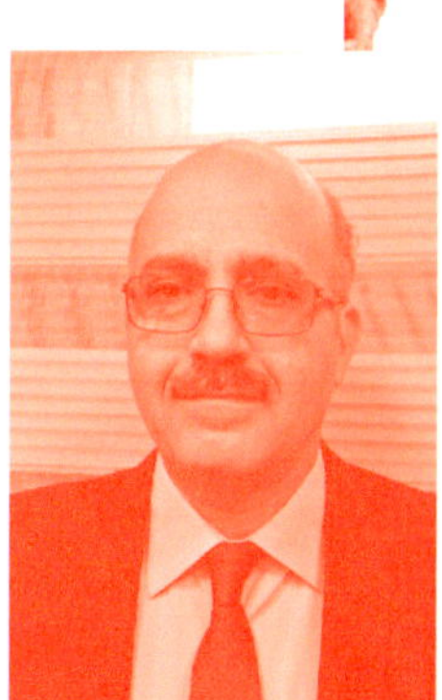

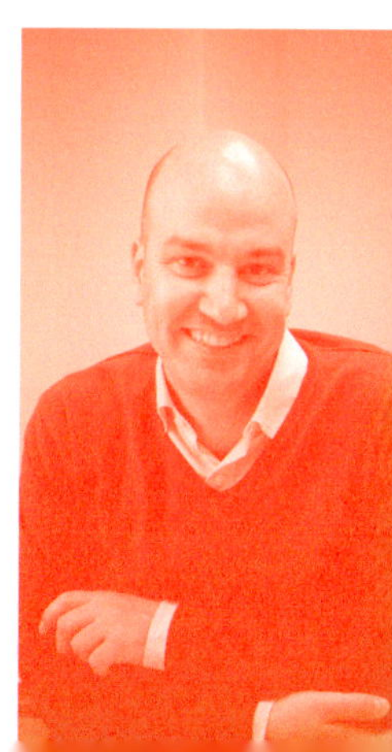

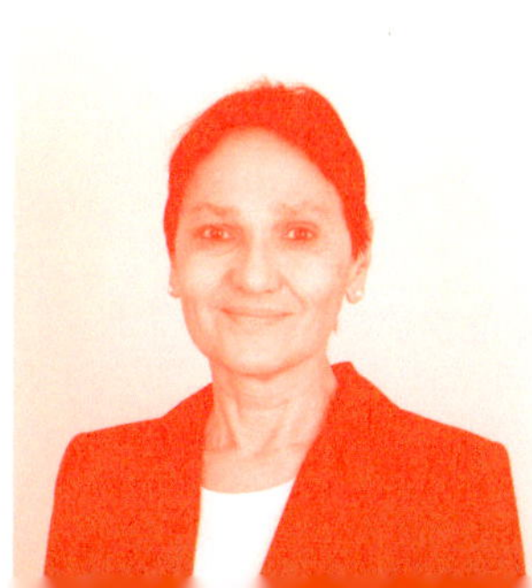

Plasmodium Species and Drug Resistance
http://dx.doi.org/10.5772/intechopen.91077
Edited by Rajeev K. Tyagi

Assistant to the Editor: Nikunj Tandel

Contributors
Benjamin Jr Fouda Abougou, Pooja Mina, Imrat, Ajeet Kumar Verma, Bernard Kofi Turkson, Michael Frimpong Baidoo, Alred Ofori Agyemang, Desmond Nkrumah, Reinhard Isaac Nketia, Merlin Lincoln Kwao Mensah, Xolani Henry Makhoba, Francis Jackim Mulaa, Harrison Ndung'u Mwangi, Arindam Bhattacharyya, Soubhik Ghosh, Saikat Mukherjee, Soham Choudhri, Bhaswar Ghosh, Dejen Nureye, Sintayehu Tsegaye Tseha, Moses Okpeku, Peter Hodoameda, Din Syafruddin, Puji Budi Setia Asih, Sushil Kumar Kashaw, Vikash Mishra, Mitali Mishra, Varsha Kashaw, Roman Manetsch, Ami H. Asakawa, Rajeev K. Tyagi, Sheetal Saini, Rajinder Kumar

First published in London, United Kingdom, 2021 by IntechOpen
IntechOpen is the global imprint of INTECHOPEN LIMITED, registered in England and Wales, registration number: 11086078, 5 Princes Gate Court, London, SW7 2QJ, United Kingdom
Printed in Croatia

British Library Cataloguing-in-Publication Data
A catalogue record for this book is available from the British Library

Additional hard and PDF copies can be obtained from orders@intechopen.com

Plasmodium Species and Drug Resistance
Edited by Rajeev K. Tyagi
p. cm.
Print ISBN 978-1-83969-255-0
Online ISBN 978-1-83969-256-7
eBook (PDF) ISBN 978-1-83969-257-4

Meet the editor

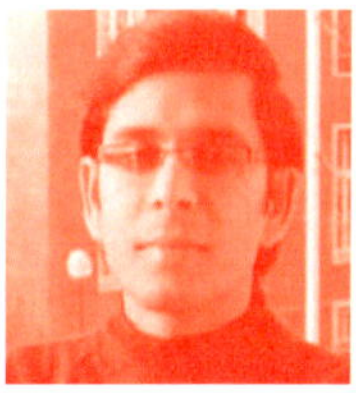

Dr. Rajeev K. Tyagi earned a Ph.D. in Malaria Immunology/Parasitology from the Biomedical Parasitology Unit, Institute Pasteur, Paris, France. He developed a long-lasting, stable, and straightforward laboratory animal model (humanized mouse) to study *Plasmodium falciparum*. Dr. Tyagi has worked as a post-doctoral scientist at the University of South Florida; Augusta University, Georgia; and Vanderbilt University Medical Center (VUMC), Tennessee. He had developed human blood and liver chimeric mice (reconstituted with human hepatocytes) in immunodeficient, NOD.*Prkdc*^{scid}*Il2rg*$^{-/-}$ (NSG) and transgenic/immunodeficient mice (TK/NOG) to study asexual blood and exoerythrocytic liver-stage infection of *P. falciparum*. Dr. Tyagi discovered a novel cell population called "pathogen differentiated dendritic cells (PDDCs)," upon incubation with *P. gingivalis* and tracking of DCs in reconstituted immunodeficient (NSG) mice to understand the host-pathogen interactions. Dr. Tyagi deployed his efforts at VUMC to understand the role of humanized mice to study the pathogenesis and immunobiology of colitis. Currently, Dr. Tyagi is leading a group at CSIR-Institute of Microbial Technology, Chandigarh, India to develop human liver chimeric mice to study liver-stage infection and transition to asexual blood-stage infection of *P. falciparum* to test antimalarial drugs and vaccine candidates. His lab is funded by DST-SERB, DBT and ICMR, CSIR, New Delhi.

Contents

Preface

As teachers of parasite biology, we are becoming increasingly aware of the lack of detailed information and experimental approaches about drugs and drug resistance in many medical schools and undergraduate courses. Therefore, this book provides much-needed detail about parasite biology, antimalarial drugs and their mechanism of action, and the dynamic situation of evolving drug resistance of parasites, which has become a pressing issue.

This book addresses the perceived needs of both medical school and undergraduate curricula by synthesizing key concepts in the rapidly advancing and dynamic field of parasite biology and drug resistance. The choice of what is most important is based on what is most clearly established by experimentation, what our students find puzzling, and what explains the efficiency of drugs to clear parasites without the risk of them gaining resistance to antimalarials. In vitro and animal models are used to study the mechanism of action of existing and novel drugs. These studies hold immense relevance in the wake of antimalaria drug resistance to develop mechanisms to stop the evolution and spread of resistance. Mouse models grafted with human immune systems (HIS) or reconstituted with human blood cells (human RBCs) are crucial to deciphering the mechanisms responsible for antimalarial drug resistance. If resistance to artesunate and artemisinin continues to evolve at a rapid rate, along with co-resistance to quinine and other antimalarials, we will be left with no satisfactory option for treating severe malaria and a compromised choice of treatments for uncomplicated malaria.

This book provides insight into the plasmodium species, the role of cytokines in activating immune response during malaria infection, the importance of antimalarials as a therapeutic option, issues of drug resistance and co-resistance, and validation of evolved resistance in humanized mouse models. It is a timely addition to the existing literature on malaria parasite biology and a useful resource for those working in the field of parasite biology, drugs, drug resistance of infectious diseases in general, and human malaria parasites in particular and beyond.

Rajeev K. Tyagi, Ph.D.
Division of Cell Biology and Immunology,
Biomedical Parasitology and Nano-immunology Lab,
CSIR-Institute of Microbial Technology (IMTECH),
Chandigarh, India

Section 1

Drug Resistance and Novel Approaches for Malaria Treatment

Chapter 1

Finding Novel Strategies to Overcome the Impact of Malaria Vector Resistance in Limited-Resources Settings. The Case of Cameroon as a Basis for Reflection

Benjamin Jr Fouda Abougou

Abstract

Malaria remains one of the most important and deadliest diseases in many countries in Africa, in the Americas, in South-East Asia, in the Eastern Mediterranean and in the Western Pacific regions, with high morbidity and mortality, despite important successes for the control of this disease borne by the vector *Anopheles* mosquitoes. Malaria elimination relies on different strategies including early diagnosis, improved drug therapies and better health infrastructure, and mainly the use of long-lasting insecticidal nets (LLINs) and indoor residual sprayings (IRS) of insecticide. In Cameroon, a country composed of several ethnic groups, malaria transmission is endemic in some regions, while it is seasonal in others; children and pregnant women are most vulnerable. Progress has been made towards malaria control, considering these specificities, and led to a reduction in both morbidity and mortality, but these accomplishments are under threat, mainly due to the development of resistance to insecticides among mosquitoes, targeting the 4 commonly used insecticide classes. To continue our route towards malaria control and elimination, it is urgent to have more knowledge about resistance mechanisms, in the objective of elaborating new strategies with the involvement of the community; these strategies should take into consideration socio-ecological factors such as the young age of the population, low literacy rate especially among women, population's beliefs, traditions, and customs. Forest ecosystems with abundant rains, humidity and hot temperature, lower access to water for populations living in rural areas, and poverty level are other factors to consider when elaborating malaria control approaches.

Keywords: Malaria, Anopheles, vector resistance, sociology, novel strategies, insecticides, community, research, social change

1. Introduction

Malaria is one of the most important and deadliest diseases in many countries in Africa, in the Americas, in South-East Asia, in the Eastern Mediterranean and in the Western Pacific regions. Malaria related morbidity and mortality remain high, despite important successes for the control of this disease borne by the vector *Anopheles* mosquitoes. In 2019, 229 million people suffered from malaria, with around 409,000 deaths, mainly in sub-Saharan Africa [1].

Important efforts have been made throughout the world to eliminate malaria leading to significant reduction in malaria cases and mortality in Africa by 44% and 67% respectively for the period 2000–2019, thanks to different strategies including early diagnosis, improved drug therapies and better health infrastructure, and mainly the use of long-lasting insecticidal nets (LLINs) and indoor residual sprayings (IRS) of insecticide [1].

In Cameroon, progresses have been made towards malaria control, and the number of deaths has been reduced from 1 million in 2000 to less than 450.000 in 2017. In parallel, morbidity was reduced from 41–26% in 2018 [2]. However, these accomplishments are under threat, mainly due to development of resistance to insecticides among mosquitoes, and this resistance targets the 4 commonly used insecticide classes – pyrethroids, organochlorines, carbamates, and organophosphates [3, 4].

Cameroon's population is composed of several ethnic groups, living in different regions with important diversity. In some regions, malaria transmission is endemic, while it is seasonal in others [2]. Children and pregnant women are the most affected and therefore most vulnerable.

To prevent the development of resistance, it is urgent to have more insight into resistance mechanisms and factors, intending to elaborate innovative strategies and to continue our path towards malaria control and elimination.

For this article, we reviewed official statistics from known public health agencies (WHO, CDC, UNICEF, etc.) and from Cameroon National Malaria Control Program, the coordinating body in charge of defining and implementing malaria control strategies and interventions. We also read various studies conducted not only in Cameroon, but also in other parts of the world, that could serve as benchmark to design and/or adjust intervention strategies besides vector control using indoor residual spraying (IRS) and the use of impregnated bed nets (ITN) [5].

This article intends to assess antimalarial drug resistance as well as insecticide resistance, especially for the Anopheles species found in Cameroon, and to suggest other strategies such as the use of new insecticides, and other vector control interventions that should be population-based, using specific communication strategies, and advocating for policies to improve the health of a given population. [6, 7].

By performing within interprofessional teams, one will be able to assess the positive social change impact that will occur because of this type of intervention [8].

2. Overview of malaria control and sociodemographic description of Cameroon regions

2.1 Description and organization of National Malaria Control Program (NMCP)

Cameroon National Malaria Control Program (NMCP) is the coordinating body in charge of defining and implementing malaria control strategies and interventions. In 2002, the minister of Public Health signed a decision reorganizing malaria control in Cameroun, highlighting the priority role of NMCP [9].

At national level, management of NMCP is ensured by the National Committee Roll Back Malaria (CRBM) presided over by the minister of Public Health (MINSANTE). Vice-President is a medical personality named by the MINSANTE, and CRBM is composed of several members among them representatives from the

Presidency, Prime Ministry, Ministry of Public Health and almost all other ministries, along with representatives from private sector, charity organizations, Non-Governmental Organizations, Donors involved, and Development Partners.

The Central Technical Group of NMCP is the executive body of CRBM, led by a Permanent Secretary. It is composed of 6 sections: 1) Management, 2) Prevention, 3) Information/Communication/Social Mobilization & Partnership, 4) Training and Research, 5) Administration & Finances, 6) Surveillance, Monitoring & Evaluation. At regional level, there are Regional Units for malaria control, with Cost Accountant and Statistics cells [9].

NMCP has also an important number of Technical and Financial Partners (PTF) that are involved in research, communication, social mobilization, case management and prevention namely [2]. Therefore, to conduct any malaria-related project, given the high-level management involved in National malaria control in Cameroon, there is a need for approvals from Permanent Secretary of NMCP.

Cameroon National Malaria Control program (NMCP) vision is to have "an emerging Cameroon without malaria", and its mission is related to universal and equitable access to the most efficient interventions in terms of prevention and case management, in an affordable cost for the whole Cameroonian population, including the most vulnerable and the most in need [2].

NMCP guiding principles are health equity and human / gender promotion, community participation, optimal management of the health information and stratification of interventions, quality of care and services, good governance, decentralization, leadership, partnership, multi sectorial collaboration, and result-based management [2].

In order to reach the goal to have a malaria-free Cameroon, NCMP has defined 4 pillars and strategic axes among which training and research; several interventions are necessary and include prevention, using insecticide-treated nets and indoor residual spraying; case management; monitoring & evaluation, epidemiological surveillance and response, communication for development, training and operational research, among which entomologic studies including observing insecticide resistance management [2, 10, 11]. Other activities consist of elaboration of cartography on malaria transmission, and study on the evolution of antimalarial (drugs) resistance molecular markers [2, 12].

In its Strategic Plan, NMCP has also foreseen to elaborate mapping of partners intervening in research, and cartography of malaria transmission to detect areas with high resistance towards specific insecticides or antimalarial drugs. Other axes of research include the assessment of the therapeutic efficiency of antimalarial drugs. Finally, there is a plan to create review committees with partners and to have a platform where research results would be shared [2].

2.2 Sociological factors affecting the health of the population in Cameroon

According to demographic projections from the Ministry of Public health, Cameroon population is around 25.5 million inhabitants in 2019, with children under 5 years and pregnant women representing respectively 15% and 3.6%, and considered as the most vulnerable categories, though the whole population is at risk of developing malaria [2]. Social determinants of health include the young age of the population: median age is 17.7 years; average age is 22.1 years; people less than 15 years and under 25 years represent 43.6% and 64.2% respectively. Mortality is still high among children under 5 years, around 60‰ [13].

Other elements consist of low literacy rate especially among women, which is around 64.7%. Cameroon is composed of Christians, Muslims, and Animists with more than 250 ethnic groups having their specific and diverse traditions and customs, all of them influencing their participation in health interventions. The Center region is concentrating more than 20% of the population, and is part of the south forest ecosystem, with abundant rains, humidity, and hot temperature, allowing the development of malaria vector. In addition, and according to regions, between 20% and 65% of the population is living below the poverty level. Households are directly financing health care, which is an important load especially for malaria that is increasing dramatically family expenses [2].

Finally, access to water is lower for populations living in rural areas compared to those living in cities; gender approach is not well considered, due to the low literacy rate among women, and their low presence at management position.

Beside official or conventional communication and social Medias, other means are available such as drama, role playing, with the involvement of community health workers [2].

3. Malaria resistance status: synthesis of literature review

Malaria elimination is based on several strategies among which the use of long-lasting insecticidal nets (LLINs) and indoor residual sprayings (IRS) of insecticide. However, a majority of mosquitoes' species vector of malaria and found in the African continent develop resistance towards the main insecticides used, thus hindering the efforts to control this disease.

While it is important to have an overview of the current resistance status, it is also crucial to understand resistance mechanisms to develop novel approaches.

A study aiming at investigating the relationship between malaria insecticide resistance and effectiveness of impregnated bed nets was conducted in five African countries that were using Pyrethroids as the main insecticide for bed nets or indoor residual spraying (IRS) [14]. During 4 years and 5 months between 2012 and 2016, 1.4 million follow up visits were carried out, and in each of the selected clusters, community health workers (CHWs) monitored 40.000 children and measured clinical malaria and prevalence of this infection; in parallel, 80.000 mosquitoes were tested for resistance using the WHO bioassay test.

The authors found that children using insecticidal bed nets had lower prevalence and malaria incidence, even though they were exposed to high malaria infection risk. To the contrary, they found no correlation between insecticide resistance and malaria incidence or prevalence, indicating that the use of long-lasting insecticidal nets remains important to reduce the risk of infection. However, with a limited protection provided by bed nets, there is a need for supplementary vector control tools to reduce malaria burden.

This study is somehow representative of the situation found in many African countries and could be used to support the necessity of alternative ways of controlling malaria and to support the usefulness of impregnated mosquito's nets.

Another study conducted had the objective of defining resistance and understanding resistance mechanisms, types, and impact of resistance along with resistance status in African malaria vectors [15].

While they reminded the causes of resistance and stated the limited number of studies related to the epidemiological impact of resistance on current malaria control activities, the authors highlighted the need for further research and prompt response to resistance management to avoid jeopardizing current interventions. Despite the alarming observation that resistance is reported to all four classes of insecticides, there are few initiatives such as The Innovative Vector Control Consortium (IVCC), a partnership to stimulate research related to better makings of insecticides [16].

Even though this review is quite old, it is still useful as the authors proposed the development of non-insecticidal methods to help reduce the dependence on pyrethroid insecticides and given the long process to have new chemicals for malaria control programs.

In an article presenting the evolution of insecticide resistance over the last 30 years in the main malaria vectors in Cameroon, other authors reviewed 33 scientific publications and found that resistance was widespread in the two main Anopheles species, and concerned mostly DDT, permethrin, deltamethrin and bendiocarb insecticides [17]. They also noticed the different mechanisms involved in resistance towards each of the insecticide.

The review is of interest since it provides an update of insecticide resistance status in malaria vector populations in Cameroon, while insisting on the necessity to implement additional interventions to reinforce malaria control strategies in the future.

Some researchers categorized insecticide resistance of 2 anopheles' species to assess its impact on malaria control in the main city of Democratic Republic of Congo (DRC) [18]. They collected mosquitoes and sent them to London with their eggs for analysis, which reveals high and multiple insecticide resistance patterns, along with a low efficacy of mosquito nets impregnated with conventional insecticides.

Although it was limited to the city capital of DRC, this study highlights the urgent need for actions to better manage the issue of insecticide resistance and could be useful for other countries with a similar resistance pattern. In this respect, malaria control programs would remain effective.

In another study, Riveron et al. [19] monitored the aggravation of resistance and assessed its impact on the usefulness of control methods based on insecticides in Mozambique. They collected indoor female Anopheles mosquitoes in a village of farmers where most families had impregnated bed nets, and where indoor residual spraying (IRS) with dichlorodiphenyltrichloroethane (DDT) was applied. The authors observed an important loss of effectiveness of impregnated bed nets, even those using the new insecticide piperonyl butoxide (PBO). They manage to determine the main mechanisms involved in this insecticide resistance.

Despite the fact that it was conducted in a village of the Southern part of Mozambique, this study is important as it reveals multiple resistance of malaria vectors to insecticides, associated or not with PBO; the consequences of this could be the abandon of PBO if immediate action are not taken, provided that PBO-based nets be further assessed.

Other authors tested the hypothesis that female-driven auto dissemination of insect growth regulators (IGRs) that are used to reduce population of some insect species could be also efficient to reduce Anopheles population [20]. They exposed female Anopheles to three substances namely novaluron, pyriproxyfen and triflumuron for 4 hours immediately after blood feeding, and observed that larval survivability and adult development were meaningfully reduced in habitats that were visited by novaluron treated adults; to the contrary, there was no statistical differences with pyriproxyfen or triflumuron, suggesting that novaluron was horizontally transferred from the adult mosquito to the larval habitat during oviposition.

The study suggested that autodissemination method with novaluron could be useful as a novel approach to manage Anopheles populations, with regards to the need for a method that is cost efficient, sustainable, and requires minimal human intervention. However, there is a need to perform more experiences in the field to ensure the reproducibility of such study.

In another article, the dynamics of deltamethrin resistance in Anopheles populations found in the North Cameroon was explored [21], and researchers collected mosquito larvae from 24 locations of three Health Districts between 2011 and 2015. The authors tested female mosquitoes for deltamethrin resistance and observed that resistance was mostly found in urban settings compared with semi-urban and rural settings, and that there was a rapid increase and widespread deltamethrin resistance.

Even though the study was carried out in few areas, it is reproducible in other parts of the country and it highlights the urgent need for vector surveillance and insecticide resistance management strategies adapted to the context.

Meanwhile, the vulnerability of major malaria vectors towards insecticides used for IRS and bed nets in Tanzania was screened [22]. The authors collected mosquito larvae in 20 sites of Tanzania mainland in 2015 and determined resistance and distribution of *Anopheles gambiae* sub-species. Results showed that almost all sub-species presented resistance to the four main insecticides, reinforcing the need to implement resistance management strategies.

This is another study confirming the high level of insecticide resistance in an African country, showing the necessity of collaborative efforts to find rapid response to this worrying topic.

Finally, some authors compared the efficacy of non-pyrethroid insecticide-treated, durable wall lining (ITWL), long-lasting insecticidal nets (LLIN), and non-pyrethroid ITWL + LLIN [23]. This novel ITWL was developed to control vectors when fixed to the inner walls of houses, and this product is responsible for a low mortality among Anopheles species, despite high mortality in bioassays.

Results on mosquitoes mortality were below expectations, even though it was evaluated for only two months, but insecticide resistance and low efficacy are probably responsible for this situation, since the ceiling of the hut was left uncovered, allowing some mosquitoes to find refuge on this untreated surface.

This is a promising study even though there is a need for further experiences on the use of this new non-pyrethroid insecticide, comparable to a long-lasting indoor residual spraying, when fixed to the inner walls and ceiling of houses.

4. Success factors and prerequisites for malaria resistance management

4.1 Sustainability

In contexts where various resources are limited there is a need for sustainability plan that will include several components, starting with interventions that could have an important public health impact especially on morbidity and mortality rates among children. Political support and partnerships with many International Organizations and Public Health agencies should be ensured, to have a funding stability [24].

Besides NMCP, there are several institutions dealing with malaria in Cameroon, for instance the Coordination for the Fight Against Endemics in Central Africa (OCEAC), which coordinates research on epidemics and endemics in Central Africa, and where many researchers are working. Any study absolutely needs their support and complete appropriation, unless at risk of failing. Other partner's organizations include WHO, UNICEF, and some other United Nations Agencies, as well as Associations working on social mobilization and fundraising.

All these stakeholders will work in close collaboration and under the supervision of the Training & Research Unit of NMCP, and its Technical and Financial Partners (PTF) that are involved in research [2].

4.2 Partnerships

Funding or financial capacity are essential to conduct interventions in the field of malaria vector resistance, along with the collaboration of specialized and experienced staff to perform evaluation [25].

A combination of literature review and field work is required in order to verify resistance status and mechanisms in the defined regions of a given country, for instance Cameroon. Some studies have already been conducted in some African countries, and it is important that the situation be assessed precisely in the chosen region to ensure its adequacy and its specificity, having other studies serving as benchmark [5, 7]. In addition, the World Health Organization (WHO) has elaborated several guidelines and procedures related to insecticide resistance monitoring in malaria vector mosquitoes.

In order to propose novel strategies, referring to existing studies conducted in other places, and assessing their reproducibility and feasibility will be important.

4.3 Program evaluation

Insecticide resistance is an important issue that needs to be well understood and tackled in the best way. There is a need to understand its mechanisms and to have a broad picture of its status in the area where interventions are planned.

Therefore, it is crucial to evaluate if a project is conducted appropriately and if there are positive results to influence decision-making process [26]. Evaluation methods will include process evaluation, outcome evaluation and impact evaluation.

Process evaluation will assess how well insecticide resistance studies are working, and whether they are being implemented as designed; it will allow researchers to monitor their intervention and will serve for staff and program managers to apply corrective measures.

Outcome evaluation will assess effectiveness in identifying resistance mechanisms and proposing alternative interventions, and impact evaluation will provide evidence for decision-makers and donors on the need to develop alternative malaria control strategies, which necessitate funds and support.

Methods of evaluation should use a combination of interviews with key informants who are credible to gather more information, questionnaires, records, and documentation research. For impact evaluation, community dialog and surveys within target population could also be used [27–29].

4.4 Ethical considerations

Some ethical concerns such as handling of data and their confidentiality must be considered, as people from the community would be involved. In addition, when it comes to proposing alternative strategies, there are a number of other ethical issues related to malaria and vector research that need to be addressed such as environmental aspects and climate change, the use of products or chemicals and experimentation on vulnerable groups among others [30–32]. In some cases, humans are used as mosquito 'traps' to measure mosquito or malaria density; it will be essential to balance potential harms to a few individuals against benefits to the wider community [30].

As alternative ways of combatting malaria, the use of vaccines and genetically modified (GM) mosquitoes have been suggested. While vaccines provide some protection against severe malaria in children but not infants, the question of using placebo or other vaccine as control arm in other trials is raised. For the use GM mosquitoes, the ecological consequences are not well understood, and ethical issues relate to the balance between potential improvements in population health and possible environmental harms, since it would be difficult to control these mosquitoes once they have been released [30].

Further research on ethical issues related to malaria is needed, to inform ethics review processes linked to control interventions, and assist health workers, researchers, and policymakers in pursuing ethically sound malaria control efforts [30].

4.5 Evaluation process for new vector control products (WHO)

Before being used, any product for vector control needs to pass through a rigorous process put in place by the WHO and aiming at improving access to high-quality vector control and promoting the best use and management of vector control tools. Product with a WHO policy recommendation pass through a prequalification pathway while those without policy recommendation need to be first assessed on their public health value [33].

4.6 Use of randomized controlled trials and mathematical modeling

Financial and other constraints are likely to prevent the need to conduct necessary field trials to evaluate novel vector control tools; nevertheless, some authors proposed that new products within the same product category be evaluated through smaller scale experiments, especially where links between entomological and epidemiological indicators are well-known [34]. Other authors tested the utilization of mathematical modeling that may reduce the need for phase III studies in some instances but conclude that a better understanding is required to inform predications of impact [34].

5. Investigating novel strategies for 'limited-resources' contexts

There are new vector control tools and strategies that need an interdisciplinary approach to overcome malaria vector resistance that have been tested, from household-level vector control tools to biotechnological control of mosquitoes. Some examples include the use of attractive toxic sugar baits, eave tubes, nano-synthesized pesticides loaded with microbial and plant-borne compounds, biocontrol agents with little non-target effect, new adult repellents, oviposition deterrents, even acoustic larvicides. Their concrete application remains limited since most countries rely on IRS and LLINs [35]. In low-resources contexts, some authors have observed that simple changes in the built environment or housing could have great benefit. Further research is needed, and the combination of several strategies would have a better impact [35, 36].

In the future, other areas could be explored such as the development of targeted sugar baits, transgenic fungi that will be disseminated from bait stations, and even the potential role of volatile odor compounds, bioinsecticides and technologies for improving the incorporation of insecticides and repellents into clothing and other materials [34–36].

6. Conclusions

Despite a certain number of studies on malaria vector resistance, there is still a need for research on insecticide resistance, given the fact that vector control using these chemical products remains one of the most important strategies towards malaria elimination. This literature review provides elements to help us understanding the status of the resistance towards the four main classes of insecticides and some of its mechanisms, but also to perceive the gap in addressing this kind of research, especially in countries with limited resources.

Novel strategies could involve the use of alternative chemicals, such as non-pyrethroid ones, and/or some methods like auto dissemination with novaluron that could be useful to manage Anopheles populations, with regards to the need for a method that is cost efficient, sustainable, and requires minimal human intervention. However, there is a need to perform more experiences in the field to ensure the reproducibility of such study.

We are confident that further projects and research would be implemented and would contribute to better address insecticide resistance by proposing alternative ways of controlling malaria and its vectors.

Conflict of interest

We declare no competing interests.

Author details

Benjamin Jr Fouda Abougou
Walden University Alumni, Yaoundé, Cameroon

*Address all correspondence to: foudabenjamin@yahoo.fr

References

[1] World malaria report 2020: 20 years of global progress and challenges. Geneva: World Health Organization; 2020. Licence: CC BY-NC-SA 3.0 IGO

[2] National Strategic Plan (NSP) (2018). Retrieved from https://www.pmi.gov/docs/default-source/default-document-library/malaria-operational-plans/fy-2018/fy-2018-cameroon-malaria-operational-plan.pdf?sfvrsn=5#:~:text=The%20goal%20of%20the%20NSP,from%202000%20levels%20by%202018

[3] Karunamoorthi K, Sabesan S. Insecticide Resistance in Insect Vectors of Disease with Special Reference to Mosquitoes: A Potential Threat to Global Public Health, Health Scope. 2013; 2(1):4-18. doi: 10.17795/jhealthscope-9840.

[4] World Health Organization (WHO) (2020b). Malaria. Insecticide resistance. Retrieved from https://www.who.int/malaria/areas/vector_control/insecticide_resistance/en/

[5] Venter, N., Oliver, S.V., Muleba, M. et al. Benchmarking insecticide resistance intensity bioassays for anopheles malaria vector species against resistance phenotypes of known epidemiological significance. Parasites Vectors 10, 198 (2017). https://doi.org/10.1186/s13071-017-2134-4

[6] Awolola, T.S., Oduola, O.A. Strode, C., Koekemoer, L.L., Brooke, B. and Ranson, H. (2009). Evidence of multiple pyrethroid resistance mechanisms in the malaria vector *Anopheles gambiae* sensu stricto from Nigeria. Transactions of The Royal Society of Tropical Medicine and Hygiene, Volume 103, Issue 11, November 2009, Pages 1139-1145, ttps://doi.org/10.1016/j.trstmh.2008.08.021

[7] Etang, J., Fondjo, E., Chandre, F., Morlais, I., Brengues, C., Nwane, P., Chouaibou, M., Ndjemai, H., Simard, F. (2006). First report of knockdown mutations in the malaria vector *Anopheles gambiae* from Cameroon. The American Journal of Tropical Medicine and Hygiene, Volume 74, Issue 5, 1 May 2006, p. 795 – 797; DOI: https://doi.org/10.4269/ajtmh.2006.74.795

[8] Walden University. (2014). 2014 social change impact report. Retrieved from http://www.waldenu.edu/about/social-change/impact-report-2014

[9] Ministry of Public Health, 2002 & 2013, paper version

[10] Antonio-Nkondjio, C., Ndo, C., Njiokou, F. et al. Review of malaria situation in Cameroon: Technical viewpoint on challenges and prospects for disease elimination. Parasites Vectors 12, 501 (2019). https://doi.org/10.1186/s13071-019-3753-8

[11] President's Malaria Initiative Cameroon (PMI) (2018). Retrieved from https://www.pmi.gov/docs/default-source/default-document-library/malaria-operational-plans/fy-2018/fy-2018-cameroon-malaria-operational-plan.pdf?sfvrsn=5

[12] Catteruccia, F. (2007). Malaria vector control in the third millennium: Progress and perspectives of molecular approaches. Pest Management Science Pest Manag Sci 63:634-640 (2007) ; DOI: 10.1002/ps.1324

[13] Institut National de la Statistique. 2015. Enquête par grappes à indicateurs multiples (MICS5), 2014, Rapport Final. Yaoundé, Cameroun, Institut National de la Statistique.

[14] Kleinschmidt, I., Bradley, J., Knox, T.B., Mnzava, A.P., Kafy, H.T., Mbogo, C.....Donnelly, M.J. (2018). Implications

of insecticide resistance for malaria vector control with long-lasting insecticidal nets: a WHO-coordinated, prospective, international, observational cohort study. Lancet Infect Dis 2018; 18: 640-49. http://dx.doi.org/10.1016/S1473-3099(18)30172-5

[15] Ranson, H., N'Guessan, R., Lines, J., Moiroux, N., Nkuni, Z. and Corbel, V. (2010). Pyrethroid resistance inAfrican anopheline mosquitoes: What are the implications for malaria control? Trends in Parasitology 1-8 1 doi:10.1016/j.pt.2010.08.004

[16] Hemingway J, Beaty BJ, Rowland M, Scott TW, Sharp BL. The innovative vector control consortium: Improved control of mosquito-borne diseases. Trends Parasitol. 2006 Jul;22(7):308-312. doi: 10.1016/j.pt.2006.05.003. Epub 2006 May 18. PMID: 16713358.

[17] Antonio-Nkondjio, C., Sonhafouo-Chiana, N., Ngadjeu, C.S. et al. Review of the evolution of insecticide resistance in main malaria vectors in Cameroon from 1990 to 2017. Parasites Vectors 10, 472 (2017). https://doi.org/10.1186/s13071-017-2417-9

[18] Riveron, J.M., Watsenga, F., Irving, H., Irish, S.R., and Wondji, C.S. (2017). High plasmodium infection rate and reduced bed net efficacy in multiple insecticide-resistant malaria vectors in Kinshasa, Democratic Republic of Congo. The Journal of Infectious Diseases; 217:320-328

[19] Jacob M Riveron, Silvie Huijben, Williams Tchapga, Magellan Tchouakui, Murielle J Wondji, Micareme Tchoupo, Helen Irving, Nelson Cuamba, Mara Maquina, Krijn Paaijmans, Charles S Wondji, Escalation of Pyrethroid Resistance in the Malaria Vector Anopheles funestus Induces a Loss of Efficacy of Piperonyl Butoxide–Based Insecticide-Treated Nets in Mozambique, The Journal of Infectious Diseases, Volume 220, Issue 3, 1 August 2019, Pages 467-475, https://doi.org/10.1093/infdis/jiz139

[20] Swale DR, Li Z, Kraft JZ, Healy K, Liu M, David CM, et al. (2018) Development of an autodissemination strategy for the deployment of novel control agents targeting the common malaria mosquito, Anopheles quadrimaculatus say (Diptera: Culicidae). PLoS Negl trop dis 12(4): e0006259. Ttps://doi.org/10.1371/journal. Pntd.0006259

[21] Mandeng SE, Awono-Ambene HP, Bigoga JD, Ekoko WE, Binyang J, et al. (2019) Spatial and temporal development of deltamethrin resistance in malaria vectors of the Anopheles gambiae complex from North Cameroon. PLOS ONE 14(2): e0212024. https://doi.org/10.1371/journal.pone.0212024

[22] Kisinza, W.N., Nkya, T.E., Kabula, B. et al. Multiple insecticide resistance in Anopheles gambiae from Tanzania: A major concern for malaria vector control. Malar J 16, 439 (2017). https://doi.org/10.1186/s12936-017-2087-2

[23] Malima, R., Emidi, B., Messenger, L.A. et al. Experimental hut evaluation of a novel long-lasting non-pyrethroid durable wall lining for control of pyrethroid-resistant Anopheles gambiae and Anopheles funestus in Tanzania. Malar J 16, 82 (2017). https://doi.org/10.1186/s12936-017-1710-6

[24] Schell, S. F., Luke, D. A., Schooley, M. W., Elliott, M. B., Herbers, S. H., Mueller, N. B., & Bunger, A. C. (2013). Public health program capacity for sustainability: A new framework. Implementation Science, 8(1), 1-9.

[25] Haughey, D. (2014). SMART goals. Retrieved from http://www.projectsmart.co.uk/smart-goals.php

[26] University of Minnesota (2020). Why Program Evaluation? Retrieved

from https://cyfar.org/why-program-evaluation

[27] Centers for Disease Control and Prevention, Division of STD Prevention [CDC] (n.d.). Types of evaluation. Retrieved September 12, 2019, from https://www.cdc.gov/std/Program/pupestd/Types%20of%20 Evaluation.pdf

[28] Hallfors, D., Cho, H., Mbai, I., Milimo, B., & Itindi, J. (2012). Process and outcome evaluation of a community intervention for orphan adolescents in Western Kenya. Journal of Community Health, 37(5), 1101-1109.

[29] Joosen, M., Frings-Dresen, M., & Sluiter, J. (2011). Process and outcome evaluation of vocational rehabilitation interventions in patients with prolonged fatigue complaints. International Journal of Behavioral Medicine, 18(2), 160-171.

[30] Jamrozik, E., de la Fuente-Núñez, V., Reis, A., Ringwald, P. and Selgelid, M.J. (2015). Ethical Aspects of Malaria Control and Research; Malar Journal (2015) 14:518; DOI 10.1186/s12936-015-1042-3

[31] Ndebele, P., Musesengwa R. (2012). View point: Ethical dilemmas in malaria vector research in Africa: Making the difficult choice between mosquito, science and humans. Malawi Medical Journal; 24 (3):65-68 September 2012

[32] World Health Organization (WHO) (2017). Ethical issues associated with vector-borne diseases. Report of a WHO scoping meeting Geneva, 23-24 February 2017. Retrieved from https://apps.who.int/iris/bitstream/handle/10665/259687/WHO-HTM-NTD-VEM-2017.07-eng.pdf

[33] World Health Organization (WHO) (2017). The evaluation process for vector control products. Retrieved from https://apps.who.int/iris/bitstream/handle/10665/255644/WHO-HTM-GMP-2017.13-eng.pdf;sequence=1

[34] Jones RT, Ant TH, Cameron MM, Logan JG. 2021 Novel control strategies for mosquito-borne diseases. Phil. Trans. R. Soc. B 376: 20190802. https://doi.org/10.1098/rstb.2019.0802

[35] John C. Beier, André B.B. Wilke and Giovanni Benelli (July 18th 2018). Newer approaches for malaria vector control and challenges of outdoor transmission, Towards Malaria Elimination - A Leap Forward, Sylvie Manguin and Vas Dev, IntechOpen, DOI: 10.5772/intechopen.75513. Available from: https://www.intechopen.com/books/towards-malaria-elimination-a-leap-forward/newer-approaches-for-malaria-vector-control-and-challenges-of-outdoor-transmission

[36] Vincent Corbel and Raphael N'Guessan (July 24th 2013). Distribution, Mechanisms, Impact and Management of Insecticide Resistance in Malaria Vectors: A Pragmatic Review, Anopheles mosquitoes - New insights into malaria vectors, Sylvie Manguin, IntechOpen, DOI: 10.5772/56117. Available from: https://www.intechopen.com/books/anopheles-mosquitoes-new-insights-into-malaria-vectors/distribution-mechanisms-impact-and-management-of-insecticide-resistance-in-malaria-vectors-a-pragmat

Chapter 2

Plasmodium Species and Drug Resistance

Sintayehu Tsegaye Tseha

Abstract

Malaria is a leading public health problem in tropical and subtropical countries of the world. In 2019, there were an estimated 229 million malaria cases and 409, 000 deaths due malaria in the world. The objective of this chapter is to discuss about the different Plasmodium parasites that cause human malaria. In addition, the chapter discusses about antimalarial drugs resistance. Human malaria is caused by five *Plasmodium* species, namely *P. falciparum*, *P. malariae*, *P. vivax*, *P. ovale* and *P. knowlesi*. In addition to these parasites, malaria in humans may also arise from zoonotic malaria parasites, which includes *P. inui* and *P. cynomolgi*. The plasmodium life cycle involves vertebrate host and a mosquito vector. The malaria parasites differ in their epidemiology, virulence and drug resistance pattern. *P. falciparum is* the deadliest malaria parasite that causes human malaria. *P. falciparum* accounted for nearly all malarial deaths in 2018. One of the major challenges to control malaria is the emergence and spread of antimalarial drug-resistant Plasmodium parasites. The *P. vivax* and *P. falciparum* have already developed resistance against convectional antimalarial drugs such as chloroquine, sulfadoxine-pyrimethamine, and atovaquone. Chloroquine-resistance is connected with mutations in pfcr. Resistance to Sulfadoxine and pyrimethamine is associated with multiple mutations in pfdhps and pfdhfr genes. In response to the evolution of drug resistance *Plasmodium* parasites, artemisinin-based combination therapies (ACTs) have been used for the treatment of uncomplicated falciparum malaria since the beginning of 21th century. However, artemisinin resistant *P. falciparum* strains have been recently observed in different parts of the world, which indicates the possibility of the spread of artemisinin resistance to all over the world. Therefore, novel antimalarial drugs have to be searched so as to replace the ACTs if Plasmodium parasites develop resistance to ACTs in the future.

Keywords: Malaria, Plasmodium species, antimalarial drug resistance

1. Introduction

Malaria is a leading public health problem in tropical and subtropical countries of the world. The disease is caused by Plasmodium parasites that are transmitted by the bites of infected female Anopheles mosquitoes. In 2019, there were an estimated 229 million malaria cases and 409, 000 deaths due the disease in the world. Children aged under 5 years are the most vulnerable group, which accounted for 67% of all malaria deaths occurred in 2019. Nearly 94% of all malaria cases in 2019 occurred in Africa [1].

IntechOpen

In addition to its health burden, malaria has also placed a heavy economic burden in Africa. Since 2000, the average annual cost of case management alone has been estimated nearly USD 300 million in Africa [2]. One of the main challenges of controlling malaria is the evolution of drug resistant strains of Plasmodium species against available antimalarial drugs [3–5]. In this chapter, antimalarial drugs resistance has been discussed. Furthermore, the life cycle, clinical features and chemotherapy of the different species of human malaria parasites have been discussed.

2. Plasmodium species causing human malaria

2.1 Diversity of human malaria parasites

Malaria is caused by protozoan parasites that belongs to the genus Plasmodium. There are over 200 plasmodium species that have been proven to cause malaria. But human malaria is caused by only by five Plasmodium species, namely: - *Plasmodium falciparum (P. falciparum); Plasmodium vivax* (*P. vivax); Plasmodium malariae* (*P. malariae*), *Plasmodium ovale* (*P. ovale)* and *Plasmodium knowlesi* (*P. knowlesi*) [6]. While the first four plasmodium species (*P. falciparum, P. vivax, P. malariae* and *P. ovale)* naturally cause malaria only in humans, *P. knowlesi* causes zoonotic malaria in South East Asia, that is naturally maintained in macaque monkeys. The malaria parasites differ in their epidemiology, virulance and drug resistance pattern. Of the five human malaria parasites, *P. vivax and P. falciparum* pose the greatest threat. *P. falciparum* is the most dangerous malaria parasite that is responsible for high morbidity and mortality [7, 8]. *P. falciparum* is the most prevalent human malaria parasite in Africa, that accounted for 99.7% of the estimated malaria cases in 2018 [9].

Plasmodium parasites belong to the order *Haemosporidia* [10]. The different Plasmodium species have different host range. For example, the host range of *P. relictum* is so broad, that can infect more than 100 different species of birds, that belong to different orders and families [11]. Whereas, the host range of *P. falciparum* is so narrow that only infects humans [12]. In contrast to mammalian malaria parasites, that are only transmitted by are mosquitoes of the genus *Anopheles*, *Plasmodium* species that infect birds are transmitted by a wide variety of mosquitoes including *Culex* and *Aedes* [13].

2.2 The life cycle of malaria parasites

The life cycle of human malaria parasites is generally the same [14]. The plasmodium life cycle involves two hosts (has two parts). In the first part, the parasite infects a vertebrate host such as human being and in the second part, the plasmodium parasite infects the mosquito vector.

The Plasmodium life cycle starts when sporozoites enter the blood of the vertebrate host following a bite by the mosquito vector [15]. Then, the sporozoites rapidly move to the liver and invade hepatocytes where they multiply asexually by a process called schizogony (exo-erythrocytic schizogony) and produce merozoites [16, 17]. The merozoites are released back into the blood and infect erythrocytes [18]. In only *P. ovale and P. vivax* infection, some of the merozoites in the liver may differentiate into a dormant stage (hypnozoite), which may recure again (cause relapse by invading blood stream) after some time in the future unless treated with primaquine. In the infected erythrocyte, each merozoite multiplies by schizogony (erythrocytic schizogony) to produce between 8 and 64 new merozoites, depending on the species of the plasmodium parasite [19]. The newly produced merozoites are released back to the blood, and continues its intraerythrocytic propagation cycle every 72 (*P. malariae*) hours; every 24 hours (*P. knowlesi*), and every 48 hours (*P. falciparum, P. ovale, P. vivax*). Some of the merozoites differentiate into male and female gametocytes for sexual reproduction [20, 21].

The second part of the plasmodium life cycle starts when the insect vector bites infected vertebrate host (such as infected person) and the insect ingests the blood containing gametocytes. The gametocyte completes its development in the lumen of the mosquito midgut and the male and the female gametes fuse to produce a zygote [22], which is the only stage with diploid chromosome (genome) [23].

Following fertilization, the zygote undergoes meiosis and differentiates into ookinete (motile form) that has a haploid genome [24]. Then ookinete penetrates the wall of the midgut of the mosquito and forms an oocyst [25]. In the oocyst, mitosis take place repeatedly, and numerous sporozoites are produced by sporogony [26, 27]. When the oocyst matures, it ruptures and releases sporozoites into the haemolymph. Then, the sporozoites migrate to the salivary glands, where they mature and acquire the capacity to infect vertebrate host cells [28]. This cycle (second part of the plasmodium parasite life cycle (from gametocytes to sporozoites) takes about 10–18 days.

2.3 *Plasmodium falciparum*

P. falciparum is the deadliest Plasmodium species that causes human malaria [29]. According to the World Health Organization (WHO), *P. falciparum* accounted for nearly all malarial deaths (99.7%) in 2018, which caused an estimated 405,000 deaths [9]. With the exception of Europe, *P. falciparum* is found in all continents of the world. Before 1970s, *P. falciparum* malaria was common in Europe. But interventions which includes appropriate case management, insecticide spraying, and environmental engineering since the early 20th century resulted in complete eradication in the 1970s [30]. Unlike other malaria endemic countries in which non-falciparum malaria predominates, over 75% of malaria cases were due to *P. falciparum* in Sub-Saharan Africa [31], where 94% of malaria deaths occur [9].

The average incubation period of *P. falciparum* malaria is 11 days (ranging from 9 to 30 days) [32], which is the shortest among Plasmodium species. The sign and symptoms of uncomplicated malaria include fever, headache, nausea, vomiting, and diarrhea. If left untreated, *P. falciparum* malaria usually develops to sever malaria, which may bring about death. Children with severe malaria frequently develop severe anemia and or respiratory distress [33]. Multi-organ failure is common in adults with sever malaria. Acute respiratory distress occurs in 5–25% of adults and up to 29% of pregnant women [34].

The WHO recommends Artemisinin-based combination therapies (ACTs) as first-line treatment for uncomplicated *P. falciparum* malaria. The ACTs that are recommended by the WHO for the treatment of uncomplicated *P. falciparum* malaria include Artemether/lumefantrine, dihydroartemisinin/piperaquine, artesunate/amodiaquine, artesunate/mefloquine, and artesunate/sulfadoxine-pyrimethamine [35]. The choice of ACT that be used in different parts of the world is different, that depends on the level of resistance to the constituents in the ACT. In a condition when first line therapy fails, the following alternative antimalarial drugs can be used as second-line treatment: - artesunate plus tetracycline or doxycycline or clindamycin, and quinine plus tetracycline or doxycycline or clindamycin which is given for seven days.

The recommended first-line treatment of uncomplicated *P. falciparum* malaria in pregnant women during the first trimester is quinine plus clindamycin for seven days [35]. The second line therapy for the treatment of uncomplicated *P. falciparum* malaria in pregnant women is artesunate plus clindamycin for 7 days. Atovaquone/proguanil, or artemether/lumefantrine or quinine plus doxycycline or clindamycin are recommended for treatment of malaria in travelers returning to non-malaria endemic countries [35]. The recommended treatment for sever *P. falciparum* malaria in adults is intravenous (IV) or intramuscular (IM) artesunate. Quinine is also recommended as an alternative treatment of sever *P. falciparum* malaria if parenteral artesunate is not available [35]. Whereas, artesunate (IV or IM), quinine (IV or IM), and artemether IM are recommended for treatment of sever *P. falciparum* malaria in children, especially in malaria-endemic areas of Africa [35].

2.4 *Plasmodium vivax*

P. vivax is the second important malaria parasite after *P. falciparum*, that causes significant morbidity. The parasite can cause severe disease and even death that is usually associated with splenomegaly [36, 37]. One of the important features that distinguishes *P. vivax* from *P. falicparum* is the occurrence of dormant stage in the liver (hypnozoites) that can be reactivated later in life.

The burden of *P. vivax* malaria differ from one region of the world to the other, which is mainly seen in central Asia (82%), the Americas (6%), Southeast Asia (9%), some parts of Africa (3%) [38, 39]. *P. vivax* has wider distribution than *P. falciparum*, which is associated with the dormant stage of *P. vivax* and the ability of *P. vivax* to survive and reproduce in the mosquito vector at lower temperatures and higher altitudes. In Africa, *P. vivax* is limited to parts of horn of Africa and Madagascar, unlike the other parts of Africa that is not affected by *P. vivax* infection due to the deficiency of Duffy antigen (which serves as receptor for the parasite) in the population [40]. It has been suggested that *P. vivax* originated in Africa. This is based on the fact that gorillas and wild chimpanzees in central Africa are naturally infected with plasmodium parasite that are closely related to the *P. vivax* that causes human malaria [41].

Usually, *P. vivax* causes mild disease, that causes fever, cough, abdominal pain and diarrhea. However, the parasite may cause serious conditions like respiratory distress. In pregnant women, *P. vivax* infection brings about low birth weight. In rare cases, complications might arise from *P. vivax* infection, which includes acute kidney failure, neurological abnormalities, hypoglycemia and low blood pressures, jaundice and coagulation defects [42]. Chloroquine is the drug of choice for the treatment of malaria that is caused by *P. vivax* [43]. However, in areas where the parasite has developed resistance for Chloroquine, such as Papua New Guinea, Korea, and India where chloroquine resistance has grown up to 20% resistance [44], chloroquine has been replaced by other drugs.

2.5 Plasmodium *ovale*

P. ovale is one of the five human malaria parasites. Unlike *P. falciparum* and *P. vivax, P. ovale* accounts very small proportion (5%) of the disease [45]. The species *P. ovale* is consisted of two subspecies, *P. ovale curtisi* and *P. ovale wallikeri* [46]. *P. ovale* is mainly found in Islands in western pacific and Sub-Saharan Africa [45, 47]. But the parasite also exists in Thailand [48], Vietnam [49] Guinea [50], Bangladesh [51], Cambodia [52] India, [53] and Myanmar [54]. The incubation period of *P. ovale* ranges from 12 to 20 days. The parasite causes very mild disease and it is less dangerous than *P. falciparum.* Like *P. vivax, P. ovale* has a dormant stage in the liver (hypnozoites) that can be reactivated later in life [45]. Chloroquine is the drug of choice for the treatment of malaria that is caused by *P. ovale* [55].

2.6 Plasmodium malariae

P. malariae is one of the five human malaria parasites. It causes mild disease, which is therefore called benign malaria. *P. malariae* is found in the Amazon Basin of South America, sub-Saharan Africa, much of southeast Asia, Indonesia, and on many of the islands of the western Pacific [56]. The parasite causes a chronic infection that may sometimes last for a lifetime. Some of the major defining features of *P. malariae* include its longer (72-hour developmental cycle) (quartan periodicity) (compared with the 48-hour cycle of *P. vivax* and *P. falciparum)* and lower parasitemia compared to those in patients infected with *P. falciparum* or *P. vivax* [57, 58]. The signs and symptoms of *P. malariae* malaria include fever, chills and nausea and edema and the nephrotic syndrome has been documented with some *P. malariae* infections [57]. Like that of *P. vivax* and *P. ovale*, Chloroquine is also highly effective against *P. malariae* malaria [55].

2.7 Plasmodium knowlesi

P. knowlesi is the only human malaria parasite that can naturally cause malaria in humans and other non-human primates (NHP) such as macaque monkeys [59, 60]. *P. knowlesi* is closely related to *P. vivax* and other Plasmodium species that infect non-human primates [61].

The parasite exists in South East Asia [62]. *P. knowlesi* rarely reported from areas outside South East Asia because its vector (the mosquitoes it infects: *Anopheles hacker* and *Anopheles latens*) are restricted to South East Asia [63, 64]. *P. knowlesi* has three subspecies which includes *P. knowlesi edesoni, P. knowlesi sintoni*, and *P. knowlesi arimai* [65, 66].

In humans, the parasite can cause both sever and uncomplicated malaria [67]. Uncomplicated *P. knowlesi* malaria is manifested by fever, chills, headaches, joint pain, malaise, abdominal pain, diarrhea, and loss of appetite [67]. In contrast to the other human malarias, *P. knowlesi* malaria has daily or quotidian malaria (a fever that that spike every 24 hours) [67, 68]. Like that of *P. vivax*, *P. malariae* and *P. ovale*, Chloroquine is also highly effective against *P. knowlesi* malaria [55].

2.8 Zoonotic malaria parasites

In addition to *P. knowlesi*, other Plasmodium species have also reported to cause zoonotic malaria [69, 70]. Macaques has been reported to be reservoir of six Plasmodium species, namely *P. knowlesi, P. inui, P. cynomolgi, P. coatneyi, P. fieldi* and *P. simiovale* in Sarawak in Malaysian Borneo [71]. From these six Plasmodium species, *P. cynomolgi* has been shown to naturally cause human infection [72], and *P. inui* can cause infection in experimental condition [73], suggesting that these species might became the next Plasmodium species that may affect human health in the future.

Zoonotic malaria has also been reported from other parts of the world. Zoonotic malaria that are caused by *P. simium* [74] and *P. brasilianum* [75], that naturally infect platyrrhine monkeys have been reported in South America. *P. simium* and *P. brasilianum* are closely related with *P. vivax* and *P. malariae*, respectively [76].

3. Antimalarial drugs resistance

There are five groups of antimalarial drugs that are currently used for treatment of human malaria, that are classified on basis of their structure and action [77, 78].

The five classes include: - (1). antifolates (pyrimethamine, proguanil, sulfadoxine), (2). 4-aminoquinolines (like chloroquine, amodiaquine, hydroxychloroquine, and aryl amino alcohols (such as quinine, mefloquine) (3). Endoperoxides (like artemisinin and its derivatives), (4) naphthoquinones (like atovaquone), and (5). 8-aminoquinolines (primaquine, tafenoquine). 4- aminoquinolines, anitifolates, naphthoquinones and aryl amino alcohols cause inhibition by detoxification of haem, pyrimidine biosynthesis and mitochondrial cytochrome b involved in oxidoreduction, respectively. Whereas endoperoxides, such as artemisinin, act on multiple cellular processes involving reactive oxygen species in Plasmodium cells [78].

One of the major challenges to control malaria is the emergence and spread of antimalarial drug-resistant plasmodium parasites [3–5]. The most important plasmodium parasites (*P. vivax* and *P. falciparum*) have already developed resistance against convectional antimalarial drugs such as chloroquine, sulfadoxine-pyrimethamine, atovaquone [79–85]. In response to the evolution of drug resistance strains of *P. falciparum* malaria, since the mid-2000s, artemisinin-based combination therapies (ACTs) constitute the standard of care for uncomplicated falciparum malaria and are increasingly also taken into consideration for the treatment of non-falciparum malaria (*P. ovale, P. vivax, P. knowlesi* and *P.* malariae) [35].

The artemisinin and its derivatives in ACTs confer rapid and potent effectiveness, whereas their partner drugs are longer-lived antimalarial (such as lumefantrine, mefloquine, piperaquine (PPQ), amodiaquine or sulfadoxine-pyrimethamine). The reason for use of ACTs is the fact that the artemisinin and its derivatives rapidly eliminate the majority of the parasites within days by mechanisms that are distinct from those of the partner drug, which eliminates residual parasites over weeks, so that parasites that may develop resistance to the artemisinin drug would still be eliminated by the partner drug [86].

There is also widespread resistance of *P. vivax* to chloroquine and sulfadoxine-pyrimethamine [84, 85, 87, 88]. Since the early 1990s chloroquine-resistant *P. vivax* (CRPV) has been reported from different parts of the world, mostly from Papua New Guinea, the Solomon Islands and Indonesia, Burma (Myanmar), India, Vietnam, Turkey, and Central and South America [83]. In Africa, chloroquine resistance started in late 1970s, and treatment failure became alarmingly high until the introduction of ACT in 2005 [89, 90]. Now, the recommended drugs for the treatment of CRPV malaria by the U.S. Centers for Disease Control and Prevention (CDC) succeeded by primaquine include; quinine sulfate plus either doxycycline or tetracycline; atovaquone-proguanil; and mefloquine [91]. ACTs has been demonstrated to be effective for both chloroquine-resistant and chloroquine-sensitive strains of *P. vivax* malaria. Therefore, ACTs can be now used to treat malaria caused by P vivax [92–94]. So far, there are no reports of *P. vivax* resistance to artemisinins. The main drawback of using ACTs for the treatment of *P vivax* malaria with ACTs is that the dormant liver-stage (hypnozoites) are not targeted by the ACTs, and, therefore, primaquine is necessarily required in combination with ACTs to prevent relapse.

Chloroquine targets the polymerization of free haem (the toxic substance for the parasite) within the food vacuole of the parasite. The drug disrupts haemozoin formation so that the parasite dies by the effect of the poisonous haem. The mechanism of chloroquine resistance is drug efflux via the *P. falciparum* chloroquine-resistance transporter (encoded by pfcrt) located at the food vacuole. Chloroquine-resistance was connected with mutations in pfcrt [95–97].

Sulfadoxine and pyrimethamine inhibit two enzymes of *P. falciparum* that involve in the folate pathway, that are dihydropteroate synthase (PfDhps) and dihydrofolate reductase (PfDhfr), respectively. Resistance to these antimalarials arises from multiple mutations in pfdhps and pfdhfr genes [98–101]. In Ethiopia, *P. falciparum* resistance to Sulfadoxine-pyrimethamine (SP) had led to replacement of SP with ACT, which is composed of consisted of artemether and lumefantrine (Coartem) in 2004 [102]. However, artemisinin resistance in *P. falciparum* has emerged in different parts of the world, especially in Southeast Asia and Africa [103–106], which indicates the possibility of the spread of artemisinin resistance to all over the world.

4. Conclusions

Malaria remains the major public health problem in tropical and subtropical countries of the world. Human malaria is caused by five Plasmodium species, namely *P. falciparum*, *P. malariae*, *P. vivax*, *P. ovale* and *P. knowlesi*. In addition to these parasites, malaria in humans can sometimes arise from zoonotic malaria parasites, which includes *P. inui, P. cynomolgi, P. coatneyi, P. fieldi, P. simiovale, P. simium* and *P. brasilianum.* The plasmodium life cycle involves two hosts (has two parts). In the first part, the parasite infects a vertebrate host such as human being and in the second part, the plasmodium parasites infect the mosquito vector. The malaria parasites differ in their epidemiology, virulence and drug resistance pattern. *P. falciparum is* the deadliest Plasmodium species that causes human malaria. *P. falciparum* accounted for nearly all malarial deaths (99.7%) in 2018. One of the major challenges to control malaria is the emergence and spread of antimalarial drug-resistant plasmodium parasites. The most important Plasmodium parasites (*P. vivax* and *P. falciparum*) have already developed resistance against convectional antimalarial drugs such as chloroquine, sulfadoxine-pyrimethamine, atovaquone. In response to the evolution of drug resistance Plasmodium parasites, ACTs have been used as first line therapy for treatment of uncomplicated falciparum malaria since the beginning of 21th century. However, artemisinin resistant *P. falciparum* strains have been recently observed in different parts of the world, which indicates the possibility of the spread of artemisinin resistance to all over the world. Therefore, novel antimalarial drugs have to be searched so as to replace the ACTs if Plasmodium parasites develop resistance to ACTs in the future.

Acknowledgements

I would like to thank IntechOpen for giving me the opportunity to write a book chapter on malaria, which is the very important parasitic disease in SSA Africa.

Conflict of interest

The author declares no conflict of interest.

Author details

Sintayehu Tsegaye Tseha[1,2]

1 PhD Candidate at the Department of Microbial, Cellular and Molecular Biology, Addis Ababa University, Addis Ababa, Ethiopia

2 Lecturer of Biomedical Sciences at the Department of Biology, Arba Minch University, Ethiopia

*Address all correspondence to: sintayehu.tsegaye@amu.edu.et; sintayehutsegaye783@gmail.com

References

[1] WHO (2020). Malaria. Key facts. https://www.who.int/news-room/fact-sheets/detail/malaria. Accessed 4 April, 2021

[2] WHO (2015). World Malaria Report 2015. Available from: http://www.who.int/malaria/media/world-malaria-report-2015

[3] Mita T, Tanabe K, Kita K. Spread and evolution of *Plasmodium falciparum* drug resistance. Parasitol Int. 2009;**58**:201-209.

[4] Ashley EA, Dhorda M, Fairhurst RM, Amaratunga C, Lim P, Suon S, et al. Spread of artemisinin resistance in Plasmodium falciparum malaria. N Engl J Med. 2014;371:411-423

[5] Wellems TE, Plowe CV. Chloroquine-resistant malaria. J Infect Dis. 2001;184: 770-776

[6] WHO (2010). Malaria. http://www.who.int/media- centre/factsheets/fs094/en/index.html.

[7] Wongsrichanalai C, Pickard A, Wernsdorfer W, Mesh- nick S. Epidemiology of drug-resistant malaria. Lancet Infectious Diseases 2002; **2**:209-218.

[8] Kiwanuka GN. Genetic diversity in *Plasmodium falciparum* merozoite surface protein 1 and 2 coding genes and its implications in malaria epidemiology: a review of published studies from 1997-2007. Journal of Vector Borne Diseases. 2009; **46**:1-12.

[9] WHO (2019). The "World malaria report 2019" at a glance. https://www.who.int/news-room/featurestories/detail/worldmalariareport2019019#:~:text=The%2011%20million%20pregnant%20women,due%20to%20malaria%20in%20pregnancy. Accessed November 2/2020.

[10] Galen SC, Borner J, Martinsen ES, Schaer J, Austin CC, West CJ, et al. The polyphyly of Plasmodium : comprehensive phylogenetic analyses of the malaria parasites (order Haemosporida) reveal widespread taxonomic conflict. R Soc Open Sci. 2018;5: https://doi.org/10.1098/rsos.171780.

[11] Valkiūnas G, Ilgūnas M, Bukauskaitė D, Fragner K, Weissenböck H, Atkinson CT, et al. Characterization of Plasmodium relictum, a cosmopolitan agent of avian malaria. Malar J. 2018;**17**:184

[12] Liu W, Li Y, Learn GH, Rudicell RS, Robertson JD, Keele BF, et al. Origin of the human malaria parasite Plasmodium falciparum in gorillas. Nature. 2010; **467**:420-425

[13] Perkins SL. Malaria's many mates: past, present, and future of the systematics of the order haemosporida. J Parasitol. 2014;**100**:11-25

[14] Votýpka J, Modrý D, Oborník M, Šlapeta J, Lukeš J. Apicomplexa. In: Archibald J, et al., editors. Handbook of the Protists. Cham: Springer International Publishing; 2016. p. 1-58. https://doi.org/10.1007/978-3-319-32669-6_20-1.

[15] Perkins SL. Malaria's many mates: past, present, and future of the systematics of the order haemosporida. J Parasitol. 2014;**100**:11-25.

[16] Frischknecht F, Matuschewski K. Plasmodium sporozoite biology. Cold Spring Harb Perspect Med. 2017;7:a025478

[17] Amino R, Thiberge S, Martin B, Celli S, Shorte S, Frischknecht F, et al. Quantitative imaging of Plasmodium transmission from mosquito to mammal. Nat Med. 2006;12:220-224

[18] Prudêncio M, Rodriguez A, Mota MM. The silent path to thousands of merozoites: the Plasmodium liver stage. Nat Rev Microbiol. 2006;4: 849-856

[19] Sturm A, Amino R, van de Sand C, Regen T, Retzlaff S, Rennenberg A, et al. Manipulation of host hepatocytes by the malaria parasite for delivery into liver sinusoids. Science. 2006;313:1287-1290

[20] Gerald N, Mahajan B, Kumar S. Mitosis in the human malaria parasite *Plasmodium falciparum*. Eukaryot Cell. 2011;**10**:474-482

[21] Josling GA, Llinás M. Sexual development in Plasmodium parasites: knowing when it's time to commit. Nat Rev Microbiol. 2015;**13**:573-587

[22] Bancells C, Llorà-Batlle O, Poran A, Nötzel C, Rovira-Graells N, Elemento O, et al. Revisiting the initial steps of sexual development in the malaria parasite Plasmodium falciparum. Nat Microbiol. 2019;**4**:144-154

[23] Bennink S, Kiesow MJ, Pradel G. The development of malaria parasites in the mosquito midgut. Cell Microbiol. 2016;**18**:905-918

[24] Sinden RE, Hartley RH. Identification of the meiotic division of malarial parasites. J Protozool. 1985;**32**:742-744

[25] Siciliano G, Costa G, Suárez-Cortés P, Valleriani A, Alano P, Levashina EA. Critical steps of Plasmodium falciparum ookinete maturation. Front Microbiol. 2020;11: 269.

[26] Araki T, Kawai S, Kakuta S, Kobayashi H, Umeki Y, Saito-Nakano Y, et al. Three-dimensional electron microscopy analysis reveals endopolygeny-like nuclear architecture segregation in Plasmodium oocyst development. Parasitol Int. 2020;76:102034

[27] Vaughan JA. Population dynamics of Plasmodium sporogony. Trends Parasitol. 2007;23:63-70

[28] Smith RC, Jacobs-Lorena M. Plasmodium–mosquito interactions. A tale of roadblocks and detours. Adv Insect Physiol. 2010;39(C):119-149.

[29] Rich S. M, Leendertz F. H, Xu G, Lebreton M, Djoko C. F, Aminake M. N, Takang E. E et al The origin of malignant malaria. Proceedings of the National Academy of Sciences. 2009; 106 (35): 14902-14907.

[30] Piperak E.T, Daikos G.L. (2016). Malaria in Europe: emerging threat or minor nuisance Clinical Microbiology and Infection. 2016; **22** (6): 487– 493.

[31] World Malaria Report 2008 (http://whqlibdoc.who.int/publications/2008/9789241563697_eng. pdf) (PDF). World Health Organisation. 2008. p. 10

[32] Andrej T, Matjaz J, IgorM, Rajesh MP. Clinical review: Severe malaria. Critical Care. 2003; 7 (4): 315-323.

[33] WHO. Malaria. Key facts. https://www.who.int/news-room/fact-sheets/detail/malaria

[34] Bruce-Chwatt L.J. Falciparum nomenclature. Parasitology Today.1987; **3** (8): 252

[35] Guidelines for the treatment of malaria, second edition. WHO. 2010. https://www.who.int/malaria/publication s/atoz/9789241547925/en/index.html.

[36] Kevin B. Neglect of Plasmodium vivax malaria. Trends in Parasitology. 2007; **23** (11): 533-539.

[37] Nicholas MA, Nicholas MD. Poespoprodjo, Jeanne R.; Price, Ric N. Plasmodium vivax. Advances in Parasitology. 2012; **80**:51-201

[38] CDC. Biology: Malaria Parasites. Malaria. CDC. 2008.

[39] Lindsay Sw, Hutchinson Ra. Malaria and deaths in the English marshes – Authors' reply. The Lancet. 2006; **368**: 1152.

[40] Langhi D, Bordin J. Duffy blood group and malaria. Hematology. 2013; **11**:389-398

[41] Weimin L, Yingying L, Katharina S. Gerald H, Lindsey J, Jordan et al. African origin of the malaria parasite Plasmodium vivax". Nature Communications. 2014; **5** (1): 3346.

[42] Control of Communicable Diseases Manual. https://ccdm.aphapublications.org/doi/book/10.2105/CCDM.2745

[43] *World Health organization. 2015.* Guidelines for the treatment of malaria

[44] Hyong K, Joon-Sup Y; Sil L, Suk K, Jae-Won P, Gyo J, et al. Chloroquine-resistant Plasmodium vivax in the Republic of Korea. The American Journal of Tropical Medicine and Hygiene. 2009; **80** (2): 215-217.

[45] Collins WE, Jeffery GM. Plasmodium ovale: parasite and disease. Clinical Microbiology Reviews. 2005; **18** (3): 570-581.

[46] Sutherland CJ, Tanomsing N, Nolder D, Oguike M, Jennison C, Pukrittayakamee S, et al. Two nonrecombining sympatric forms of the human malaria parasite Plasmodium ovale occur globally. The Journal of Infectious Diseases. 2010; **201** (10): 1544-50

[47] Faye FB, Konaté L, Rogier C, Trape JF (1998). Plasmodium ovale in a highly malaria endemic area of Senegal. Transactions of the Royal Society of Tropical Medicine and Hygiene. 2008; **92** (5): 522-525.

[48] Cadigan FC, Desowitz RS. Two cases of Plasmodium ovale malaria from central Thailand. Transactions of the Royal Society of Tropical Medicine and Hygiene. 1969; **63** (5): 681-682

[49] Gleason NN, Fisher GU, Blumhardt R, Roth AE, Gaffney GW. Plasmodium ovale malaria acquired in Viet-Nam. Bulletin of the World Health Organization. 1970; **42** (3): 399-403.

[50] Baird JK, Hoffman SL. Primaquine therapy for malaria. Clinical Infectious Diseases. 2004; **39** (9): 1336-1345.

[51] Fuehrer HP, Starzengruber P, Swoboda P, Khan WA, Matt J, Ley B, et al. Indigenous Plasmodium ovale malaria in Bangladesh. The American Journal of Tropical Medicine and Hygiene. 2010; **83** (1): 75-78.

[52] Incardona S, Chy S, Chiv L, Nhem S, Sem R, Hewitt S, et al. Large sequence heterogeneity of the small subunit ribosomal RNA gene of Plasmodium ovale in Cambodia. The American Journal of Tropical Medicine and Hygiene. 2005; **72** (6): 719-724.

[53] Snounou G, Viriyakosol S, Jarra W, Thaithong S, Brown KN. Identification of the four human malaria parasite species in field samples by the polymerase chain reaction and detection of a high prevalence of mixed infections. Molecular and Biochemical Parasitology. 1993; **58** (2): 283-292.

[54] Nana L, Daniel MP, Zhaoqing Y, Qi F, Guofa Z, Guoping A. Risk factors associated with slide positivity among febrile patients in a conflict zone of north-eastern Myanmar along the China-Myanmar border. Malaria Journal. 2013; **12** (1): 361.

[55] Griffith KS, Lewis LS, Mali S, Parise M. Treatment of malaria in the United States: a systematic review. Jama. 2007; **297**:2264-2277

[56] Westling J, Yowell CA, Majer P, Erickson JW, Dame JB, Dunn BM. Plasmodium falciparum, P. vivax, and P. malariae: a comparison of the active site properties of plasmepsins cloned and expressed from three different species of the malaria parasite. Experimental Parasitology. 1997; **87** (3): 185-193.

[57] Collins WE, Jeffery GM. Plasmodium malariae: parasite and disease. Clinical Microbiology Reviews. 2007; **20** (4): 579-592

[58] Bruce MC, Macheso A, Galinski MR, Barnwell JW (May 2007). Characterization and application of multiple genetic markers for Plasmodium malariae. Parasitology. 2007; **134**: 637-650.

[59] Chin W, Contacos PG, Coatney GR, Kimball HR. A naturally acquired quotidian-type malaria in man transferable to monkeys. Science. 1965;**149**: 865

[60] Fong YL, Cadigan FC, Robert CG. A presumptive case of naturally occurring Plasmodium knowlesi malaria in man in Malaysia. Trans R Soc Trop Med Hyg. 1971;**65**:839-840.

[61] Lee KS, Divis PC, Zakaria SK, Matusop A, Julin RA, Conway DJ, et al. Plasmodium knowlesi: Reservoir Hosts and Tracking the Emergence in Humans and Macaques. PLOS Pathog. 2011; **7** (4): e1002015.

[62] Garrido-Cardenas JA, Gonzalez-Ceron L, Manzano-Agugliaro F, Mesa-Valle C. Plasmodium genomics: an approach for learning about and ending human malaria. Parasitology Research. Springer. 2019; **118** (1): 1-27.

[63] Collins WE. Plasmodium knowlesi: A Malaria Parasite of Monkeys and Humans. Annual Review of Entomology. 2012; **57**: 107-121.

[64] Millar SB, Cox-Singh J. Human infections with Plasmodium knowlesi-zoonotic malaria. Clinical Microbiology and Infection. 2015; 21 (7): 640-648

[65] Butcher GA, Mitchell GH. The role of Plasmodium knowlesi in the history of malaria research. Parasitology. Cambridge University Press. 2016; 145 (1): 6-17.

[66] Garnham PC. A new sub-species of Plasmodium knowlesi in the long-tailed macaque. J Trop Med Hyg. 1963; **66**: 156-158.

[67] Singh B, Daneshvar C. Human Infections and Detection of Plasmodium knowlesi. Clinical Microbiology Reviews. 2013; **26** (2): 165-184.

[68] Chin W, Contacos PG, Coatney RG, Kimbal HR. A naturally acquired quotidian-type malaria in man transferable to monkeys. Science. 1965; **149** (3686): 865.

[69] Faust C, Dobson AP. Primate malarias: diversity, distribution and insights for zoonotic Plasmodium. One Heal. 2015; **1**:66-75.

[70] Ramasamy R. Zoonotic malaria - global overview and research and policy needs. Front Public Heal. 2014;**2**:1-7.

[71] Raja TN, Hu TH, Zainudin R, Lee KS, Perkins SL, Singh B. Malaria parasites of long- tailed macaques in Sarawak, Malaysian Borneo: a novel species and demographic and evolutionary histories. BMC Evol Biol. 2018;**18**:49

[72] Ta TH, Hisam S, Lanza M, Jiram AI, Ismail N, Rubio JM. First case of a naturally acquired human infection with Plasmodium cynomolgi. Malar J. 2014;**13**:68

[73] Coatney GR, Chin W, Contacos PG, King HK. Plasmodium inui, a quartan-type malaria parasite of old world

monkeys transmissible to man. J Parasitol. 1966;**52**:660

[74] Brasil P, Zalis MG, de Pina-Costa A, Siqueira AM, Júnior CB, Silva S, et al. Outbreak of human malaria caused by Plasmodium simium in the Atlantic Forest in Rio de Janeiro: a molecular epidemiological investigation. Lancet Glob Heal. 2017;**5**:e1038–e1046.

[75] Lalremruata A, Magris M, Vivas-Martínez S, Koehler M, Esen M, Kempaiah P, et al. Natural infection of Plasmodium brasilianum in humans: man and monkey share quartan malaria parasites in the Venezuelan Amazon. EBioMedicine. 2015;**2**:1186-1192

[76] Tazi L, Ayala FJ. Unresolved direction of host transfer of Plasmodium vivax v.P. simium and P. malariae v. P. brasilianum. Infect Genet Evol. 2011;**11**:209– 221

[77] Ross LS, Fidock DA. Elucidating mechanisms of drug-resistant Plasmodium falciparum. Cell Host Microbe. 2019; **26**:35-47

[78] Bray PG, Hawley SR, Ward SA. 4-Aminoquinoline resistance of Plasmodium falciparum: insights from the study of amodiaquine uptake. Mol. Pharmacol. 1996; **50** (6): 1551-1558

[79] Shah NK, Dhillon G, Dash A, Arora U, Meshnick S, Valecha N, et al. Antimalarial drug resistance of Plasmodium falciparum in India: changes over time and space. Lancet. Infect. Dis. 2011; **11**: 57-64.

[80] Tumwebaze P, Tukwasibwe S, Taylor A, Conrad M, Ruhamyankaka E, Asua V. Changing antimalarial drug resistance patterns identified by surveillance at three sites in Uganda. J. Infect. Dis. 2017; **215:** 631-635.

[81] Costa G, Amaral L, Fontes C, Carvalho L, Brito C, de Sousa Tet al. Assessment of copy number variation in genes related to drug resistance in Plasmodium vivax and Plasmodium falciparum isolates from the Brazilian Amazon and a systematic review of the literature. Malar. J. 2017; **16**: 152.

[82] Peterson DS, Walliker D, Wellems TE. Evidence that a point mutation in dihydrofolate reductase-thymidylate synthase confers resistance to pyrimethamine in falciparum malaria. Proc. Natl Acad. Sci. USA. 1988; **85**; 9114-9118.

[83] Price RN, Douglas NM, Anstey NM. New developments in Plasmodium vivax malaria: severe disease and the rise of chloroquine resistance. Curr Opin Infect Dis 2009; **22**:430-435

[84] Witkowski B, Amaratunga C, Khim N, Sreng S, Chim P, Kim S et al. Novel phenotypic assays for the detection of artemisinin-resistant Plasmodium falciparum malaria in Cambodia: in-vitro and ex-vivo drug-response studies. Lancet. Infect. Dis. 2013; **13**: 1043-1049.

[85] Paloque L, Ramadani AP, Mercereau-Puijalon O, Augereau JM, Benoit-Vical F. Plasmodium falciparum: multifaceted resistance to artemisinins. Malar. 2016; **15:** 149.

[86] Taguchi K, Yamamoto M. The KEAP1-NRF2 System in Cancer. Front. Oncol. 2017; **7**:

[87] Meshnick SR, Taylor TE, Kamchonwongpaisan S. Artemisinin and the antimalarial endoperoxides: from herbal remedy to targeted chemotherapy. Microbiol. Rev. 1996; **60**, 301-315.

[88] Fairhurst RM, Dondorp AM Artemisinin-Resistant Plasmodium falciparum Malaria. Microbiol. Spectr. 2016; **4**: 3.

[89] Mohamed AO, Eltaib EH, Ahmed OA, Elamin SB, Malik EM. The

efficacies of artesunate–sulfadoxine–pyrimethamine and artemether–lumefantrine in the treatment of uncomplicated, Plasmodium falciparum malaria, in an area of low transmission in central Sudan. Ann Trop Med Parasitol. 2006; **100**:5-10.

[90] Adeel AA. Drug-resistant malaria in Sudan: a review of evidence and scenarios for the future. Sudan J Paediatr. 2012;**12**:8

[91] Arnold J, Hockwald R, Clayman C, Dern R, Beutler E, Flanagan C. Potentiation of the curative action of primaquine in vivax malaria by quinine and chloroquine. J Lab Clin Med 1955; **46**:301-306

[92] 92, Hwang J, Alemayehu BH, Reithinger R, Tekleyohannes S, Teshi T, Birhanu S, et al. In vivo efficacy of artemether/lumefantrine and chloroquine against Plasmodium vivax: a randomized open label trial in central Ethiopia. PLoS One. 2013;**8**:e63433.

[93] Yohannes AM, Teklehaimanot A, Bergqvist Y, Ringwald P. Confirmed vivax resistance to chloroquine and effectiveness of artemether-lumefantrine for the treatment of vivax malaria in Ethiopia. Am J Trop Med Hyg. 2011; **84**:137-140

[94] Krudsood S, Tangpukdee N, Muangnoicharoen S, Thanachartwet V, Luplertlop N, Srivilairit S, et al. Clinical efficacy of chloroquine versus artemetherlumefantrine for Plasmodium vivax treatment in Thailand. Korean J Parasitol 2007;**45**:111-114.

[95] Cooper RA, Ferdig M, Su X, Ursos L, Mu J, Nomura T, et al. Alternative mutations at position 76 of the vacuolar transmembrane protein PfCRT are associated with chloroquine resistance and unique stereospecific quinine and quinidine responses in Plasmodium falciparum. Mol. Pharmacol. 2002; **61**: 35-42.

[96] Cooper RA, Lane K, Deng B, Mu J, Patel J, Wellems T, et al. Mutations in transmembrane domains 1,4 and 9 of the Plasmodium falciparum chloroquine resistance transporter alter susceptibility to chloroquine, quinine and quinidine. Mol. Microbiol. 2007; **63**: 270-282.

[97] Petersen I, Gabryszewski S, Johnston G, Dhingra S, Ecker A, Lewis R, et al. Balancing drug resistance and growth rates via compensatory mutations in the Plasmodium falciparum chloroquine resistance transporter. Mol. Microbiol. 2015; **97**: 381-395

[98] Shah NK, Dhillon G, Dash A, Arora U, Meshnick S, Valecha N et al. Antimalarial drug resistance of Plasmodium falciparum in India: changes over time and space. Lancet. Infect. Dis. 2011; **11**: 57-64.

[99] Tumwebaze P, Tukwasibwe S, Taylor A, Conrad M, Ruhamyankaka E, Asua V, et al. Changing antimalarial drug resistance patterns identified by surveillance at three sites in Uganda. J. Infect. Dis. 2017; **215**, 631-635.

[100] Costa GL, Amaral L, Fontes C, Carvalho L, Brito C, Sousa T, et al. Assessment of copy number variation in genes related to drug resistance in Plasmodium vivax and Plasmodium falciparum isolates from the Brazilian Amazon and a systematic review of the literature. Malar. J. 2017; **16**

[101] Gregson A, Plowe CV. Mechanisms of resistance of malaria parasites to antifolates. Pharmacol. Rev. 2005; **57**: 117-145.

[102] Gebreyohannes E, Bhagavathula A, Seid M, Tegegn H. Anti-malarial treatment outcomes in Ethiopia: a systematic review and meta-analysis. Malaria journal. 2017; **16.** https://malariajournal.biomedcentral.com/articles/10.1186/s12936-017-1922-9

[103] EMEP. Ethiopia malaria elimination strategic plan: 2021-2025. august 2020, Addis Ababa. http://www.moh.gov.et/ejcc/sites/default/files/2020/Ethiopia%20Malaria%20Elimination%20Strategic%20Plan%202021-2025-Agust%2031.pdf

[104] Baykika-Kibwika P, Lamorde M, Mayanja-Kizza H, Merry C, Colebunders B, Van Geertruyden JP (2011). Update on the efficacy, effectiveness and safety of artemether-lumefantrine combination therapy for treatment of uncomplicated malaria. Ther. Clin. Risk Manag. 2011; 6:11-20

[105] Kamau E, Campino S, Amenga-Etego L, Drury E, Ishengoma D, Johnson K, et al. (2015). K13 propeller polymorphisms in Plasmodium falciparum parasites from sub-Saharan Africa. J Infect Dis. 2015; **211**:1352-1355.

[106] Taylor SM, Parobek CM, DeConti DK, Kayentao K, Coulibaly SO, Greenwood BM, et al. Absence of putative artemisinin resistance mutations among Plasmodium falciparum in sub-Saharan Africa: a molecular epidemiologic study. J Infect Dis. 2015; **211**:680-688.

Chapter 3

Recent Advances in Antimalarial Drug Discovery: Challenges and Opportunities

Imrat, Ajeet Kumar Verma and Pooja Rani Mina

Abstract

Malaria is a global health problem that needs attention from drug discovery scientists to investigate novel compounds with high drug efficacy, safety and low cost to encounter the malaria parasites that are resistant to existing drug molecules. Antimalarial drug development follows several approaches, ranging from modifications of existing agents to the design of novel agents that act against novel targets. Most of market and clinical drugs act on blood schizonticide are in current therapy for malaria reduction. This chapter will intend to highlight the currently available drugs including various novel agents. In addition, emphasis has been given on the prospective pharmacophores that are likely to emerge as effective clinical candidates in the treatment of malaria. Besides all aspects, some alternative approaches will also be highlight.

Keywords: Antimalarial, drug resistance, current drug, Plasmodium, chemotherapeutic target

1. Introduction

Malaria is a prevalent infectious disease, affecting about 150 million people globally and responsible for around 4, 45,000 deaths annually [1]. Geographically, it is prevalent in 106 countries of the tropical and semitropical world. Africa accounts for 80% of total malaria cases and 90% global death. Malaria is caused by the apicomplexan protozoa *Plasmodium* genus which is transmitted from one to another through bitting by female *Anopheles mosquito* [2]. Five species are known to cause malaria fever in human *i.e. P. vivax*, *P. falciparum*, *P.ovale, P. malariae* and *P. knowelsi* [3, 4].

Among all plasmodium species, *P. vivax* is prevalent in central and South America, Asia [5]. *P. ovale* infections are rare and occur only in Africa i.e. <0.5% [6] *P. malariae* is present at the globe irregularly. *P. falciparum* is most fatal, because it produces large progeny in a short time and has the ability to cause cerebral malaria which is a severe complication and leads to death of the patient. Malaria has been a long-term health issue in world. In earlier 1960s to 1980s incidence of malaria prevalence have been highest, but now, there are several effort and projects handle by the international government to reverse malaria burden. Chemotherapy against the malaria parasite had been a vital component. However, resistance to existing

IntechOpen

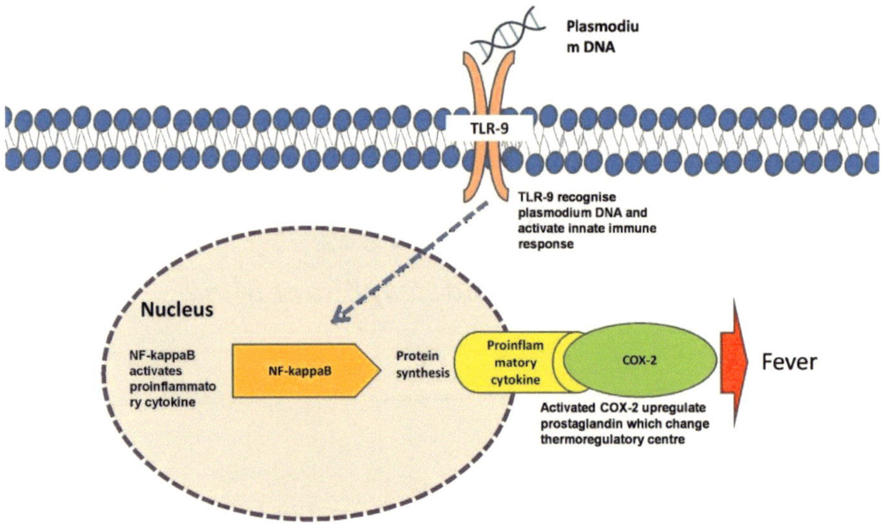

Figure 1.
Schematic representation of malaria pathogenesis in the host cell.

medicines is always a risk. Consequently, all treatments must be combinations of two or more active ingredients such that no compound is exposed as a monotherapy to high levels of parasites for a significant period of time wherever possible [7]. Artemisinin-based and nonartemisinin based combination with partner drug has been approved. This chapter will provides an overview of malaria, focusing on progress in drug discovery efforts, clinical development and the future highlight of malaria eradication agenda.

1.1 Malaria pathogenesis

Symptoms of malaria arose from hemozoin that released after rupture of infected RBCs. Hemozoin cause inflammation and take part in the immunogenic action in the blood which activates pro-inflammatory and anti-inflammatory cytokines [8]. Some studies have shown that IL-1B, IL-6, IL-8, and TNF-alpha increased in late-onset severe disease [9, 10]. Pathogenic phase of malaria is outcome of secreted cytokines tumor necrosis factor (TNF-α), interferon-γ (INF-γ), IL-6, IL-8, from macrophage and endothelial, and elevated level of as superoxide and nitric oxide (NO) [11]. These increased factor play role in dys-erythropoietic anemia, TNF-α may contribute to cerebral malaria through up-regulation of intracellular adhesion molecule-1 (ICAM-1) in cerebral blood vessel endothelium [12]. Pro-inflammatory cytokine induce cytokinemia and fever through interacting intracellularly with Toll-like receptor-9 (**Figure 1**), which lead to release of proinflammatory cytokines that can induce COX-2 up regulating prostaglandins [13, 14].

2. Diagnosis

Diagnosis of malaria infection in a patient is of critical importance since symptoms of complicated malaria may develop suddenly, causing the death of the patient. Clinical diagnosis based on the patient's symptoms and on physical findings at examination

- Microscopic diagnosis parasite can be identified by examining under the microscope a drop of the patient's blood, spread out as a "blood smear" on a microscope slide stained with Giemsa stain [15].

- A rapid diagnostic test based on antigen detection, this type of immunologic test most often uses an antigen-coated dipstick which gives results in 2–15 minutes. These "Rapid Diagnostic Tests" (RDTs) offer less time taking and more accurate results over microscopy [16, 17].

- Diagnosis of nuclei of the parasite through PCR (polymerase chain reaction) which is a quicker method [18].

- In serum-based diagnosis, malaria parasite responding antibodies generated in the human body can be detected indirectly by immunofluorescence (IFA) or enzyme-linked immunosorbent assay (ELISA). Serology can detect past exposure but unable to detect current infection [19].

3. Life cycle

Asexual Phase (Human) stage completed in humans after the invading of sporozoite to the liver which further infected other RBCs after parasitemia establishment. **Sexual Phase (Mosquito)** completed in the gut of mosquito [20]. When parasite bite infected humans, gametocytes occur in female and male form reach in their salivary gland and enter into the gut of the mosquito. The male and female gametes are fused in the gut of the mosquito to form zygotes [21]. After fertilization of gametes, ookinetes form which penetrates the gut epithelial cells and finally converts into an oocyst. The oocyst multiplies by asexual replication and produces sporozoites. Rupture of the mature oocyst releases the sporozoites into the hemocoel (body cavity) of the mosquito, from where they travel to the mosquito salivary glands [22]. When an infected mosquito has a blood meal, it injects saliva containing the parasite (sporozoites) into the human bloodstream, causing malaria infection in the new human host. Now the sporozoites travel through the circulatory system to the liver and invade hepatocytes, where the sporozoites multiply and grow through asexual replication known as exoerythrocytic schizogony. Each sporozoite develops into a schizont containing thousands of merozoites, which are released into the bloodstream. In the case of *P. vivax* and *P. ovale,* they live in a latent form in the liver-cell which can be dormant up to months or years. These hypnozoites relapse when a new primary infection reaches to liver cells [23]. The erythrocytic life cycle begins when free merozoites invade through erythrocytes. The erythrocytic cycle is responsible for all clinical manifestations of the disease. Merozoites invade erythrocytes by multiple receptor-ligands interactions within a few seconds. The early trophozoite is often called 'ring form' because of its morphology. Ring stage is developed into the trophozoite stage by metabolizing host cytoplasm and degradation of hemoglobin into globin and amino acids. The trophozoite is developed to schizont by multiple rounds of nuclear division without cytokinesis and produces 8–32 daughter merozoites [24, 25]. Mature merozoites came outside the red blood cell and released merozoites invade new RBCs and this cycle repeats. This blood stage cycle is responsible for the pathology related to malaria. Asexual stage converted into sexual stages i.e. male, female gametocyte [26, 27]. Which helps in the transmission of the infection to others through the female Anopheles mosquitoes, wherein they continue the sexual phase of the parasite's life cycle.

4. Treatment of malaria

This classification of candidate drugs is strictly based on the stage in which they exhibit their potency within the parasite life cycle. In this classification, drugs are divided into five major categories (**Table 1**) [28].

- **Blood schizontocides**: These drugs act on the blood stages of parasites and therefore prevent spreading out of malaria. The common members of this class include artemisinin (ART) and its derivatives, chloroquine (CQ), quinine (QN), mefloquine (MQ), halofantrine (HF), pyrimethamine and sulfadoxine.

- **Tissue schizontocides for causal prophylaxis**: These drugs act on the hypnozoites (liver forms of Plasmodium) occurring prior to the erythrocytic stage. These drugs are very important since they could prevent the onset and development of clinical infection at the early stage of the disease, e.g. Primaquine (PQ) and pyrimethamine.

- **Tissue schizonticides for relapse prevention**: These drugs act on the sporozoites of *P.vivax* and *P.ovale* in host liver cells, which is responsible for the relapse of malaria symptoms and regeneration of the disease e.g. primaquine.

- **Gametocytocidal**: These drugs target the gametocyte of the parasite in the blood and also prevent the transmission parasitic stages to the mosquito. CQ and QN have gametocytocidal activity against *P. vivax* and *P. malariae* but not against *P. falciparum*, but ART has activity against *P. falciparum*. Primaquine found to suppress *P. vivax* as well as *P. falciparum*.

5. Drug resistance in *P. falciparum*

Drug resistance is the reduction in the effectiveness of a medication such as an antimicrobial or an antineoplastic in curing a disease or condition [29]. The term is used in the context of pathogen that acquired survival potential in presence of drug. When an organism is resistant to more than one drug, it is said to be multidrug resistant.

P. falciparum resistance to chloroquine and sulphadoxine–pyrimethamine first developed on the in Southeast Asia and South America in the late 1950s and 1960s, respectively. The spread of resistant parasite strains elsewhere, including Africa, have been well documented retrospectively with molecular markers of the resistance to each drug. Chloroquine has been replaced by the combination of sulphadoxine and pyrimethamine (SP) in 1973. SP is widely used antimalarial worldwide and also used as the first line of treatment for malaria alone or in combination with other antimalarial drugs. SP resistance also became a big challenge to malaria control programs. For tackling this problem, SP was replaced by mefloquine but resistance to this new drug developed very rapidly. Mefloquine resistance was first observed in the late 1980s again in the same endemic area near the Thai-Cambodian border which spread out to Southeast Asia, South America and some pockets in Africa [30]. Resistance to SP was first described from the Thai-Cambodian border [31]. After chloroquine and sulphadoxine–pyrimethamine failures, Thailand introduced mefloquine in place of SP. For tackling this problem, Thailand imposed strict controls on its use but mefloquine resistance was first observed in the late 1980s and early 1990s again in the same endemic area near the Thai-Cambodian border. The increasing morbidity

Drug class	Drug	Target of action	Mode of Action	Clinical use
4-Aminoquanoline	Chloroquine	Blood-stage schizonticides	Direct heme binding, Inhibit heme Fe(II) FPIX Polymerase	Treatment and chemoprophylaxis of sensitive parasites
Cinchona alkaloid	Quinine	Erythrocyte schizonticides	Same as CQ	Treatment of CQ-resistant *P. falciparum*
Quinoline-methanol	Mefloquine	Blood-stage schizonticides	Formation of a toxic substance, Swelling of the food vacuole	Chemoprophylaxis and treatment of *P. falciparum*
8-Aminoquanoline	Primaquine	Tissue-stage schizonticides & gametocytocidales	Generation of toxic metabolites, Oxygen radicals in Plasmodial mitochondria	Radical cure and terminal prophylaxis of *P. vivax & P. ovale*
Amino alcohol	Halofantrine/ Pyronaridine	Erythrocyticschizonticides	Inhibit heme polymerase, inhibit vacuolar degradation	Treatment of CQ-resistant *P. falciparum*
Naphthoquinone	Atovaquone	Blood-stage schizonticides	Inhibit mitochondrial electron transport	Treatment and chemoprophyla xis of *P. falciparum*, in combination with Proguanil
Diaminopyrimidine/ Sulfonamide	Pyrimetham ine/ Sulfadoxine	Blood-stage schizonticides	Inhibitor of dhfr-ts/dhps, thereby, inhibit parasitic DNA	A headache. SJS, Skin rash Treatment of CQ-resistant *P. falciparum* (in combination as SP)
Biguanide	Proguanil	Erythrocyticschizonticides	Inhibit dhfr and stops pyrimidine biosynthesis	Chemoprophyla xis (with CQ)
Tetracyclines	Tetracycline/ Doxycyclin e	Blood-stage schizonticides	Inhibit mitochondrial protein synthesis, block nucleic acid synthesis	Treatment and chemoprophyla xis of *P. falciparum*
Sesquiterpene lactone	Artemisinin and its derivatives	Erythrocyticschizonticides & gametocytocidales	Formation of iron catalyzed free radical, alkylation of heme, membrane damage by free radical	Treatment of multidrug-resistant *P. falciparum*

Table 1.
Common antimalarial drugs and their mechanism of action.

rate was reversed with the introduction of artemisinin. The introduction of the artemisinin saved millions of lives around the world [32]. Artemisinin leads to a high rate of recrudescence (reinfection of parasites) other drugs are required to clear the body of all parasites and prevent recurrence hence several more potent derivatives were synthesized *viz*., artesunate, arte-ether, arte-mether and dihydroartemisinin [33]. In 1995, Thailand replaced mefloquine with artesunate–mefloquine. The same combination was the first-line therapy in Cambodia from 2000 to 2012.

5.1 Resistance to artemisinin-based combination therapies

To linger off artemisinin resistance, treatment for malaria is given as artemisinin based combination therapy (ACTs) in place of artemisinin alone or its derivative to treat uncomplicated malaria. ACT must include 1 artemisinin or its derivative another is other antimalarial drug or compound as prescribed by WHO 2001. ACTs are more efficient medicine today that is available, as it has great potential; it replaced antifolates and quinoline drug class which was used as the first-line treatment for *P. falciparum.*

Presently, artemisinin resistance is only prevalent in to the Cambodia, Thailand, Lao people's Democratic Republic [34], Viet Nam, Myanmar, and the Myanmar-China-India border area. In 2006, the declined efficacy of ASMQ (artesunate/mefloquine) was suspected for the first time on the Cambodia-Thailand border [35]. Thereafter, ASMQ clinical failures were reported on the Thailand-Myanmar border in correlation with delayed parasite clearance time [36]. Reason for resistance toward artemisinin derivatives because it promotes selection for partner-drug resistance mainly due to mismatches in the pharmacokinetics of the two drugs, causing frequent treatment failure of ACTs [37], amplification of pfmdr1 gene copy numbers. Clinical failures after dihydroartemisinin-piperaquine (DHA/PPQ) treatment have been reported, first in Cambodia in 2013 [38] and later in Vietnam in 2017 [39, 40] five and twelve years, respectively, after DHA/PPQ treatment introduction. DHA/PPQ resistance was confirmed by several reports and correlated with pfk13polymorphism, plasmepsin 2–3 gene amplification and single copies of the pfmdr1 gene [41]. Clinical failure rates greater than 10% have now been reported for the 5 ACTs in Cambodia, for 2 ACTs in Thailand and Lao PDR and for 1 ACT in Viet Nam, Myanmar, and in the Chinese and Indian border regions with Myanmar. It has been demonstrated that plasmepsin 2–3 gene amplification in DHA/PPQ resistant parasites is associated with pfmdr1 gene single copies, so these resistant parasites are sensitive to mefloquine [42]. In contrast, ASMQ-resistant parasites with pfmdr1 gene amplification are sensitive to piperaquine [37]. Based on the amplification of pfmdr1 gene copy numbers of ACT-resistant parasites, the alternating use of ASMQ and DHA/PPQ is under consideration.

5.2 Potential chemotherapeutic target

Developing resistance toward antimalarial drug has tinted requirement of new compound with antimalarial activity. To overcome this problem new validated drug target needed with detailed study of biochemical and metabolic processes of the parasite [43]. One way is to search for new drug(s) which inhibit parasite growth and cure malaria, secondly to find ways to reverse drug resistance mechanism. Research over the years have identified a number of potential drug targets mainly proteins in the parasite that can be utilized as drug targets.

6. Drug development research in during 2010–2019

There is continuous efforts has been given after resistance toward existing drug chloroquine, mefloquine, piperaquine, sulphadoxine-pyrimethamine, artemisinin derivatives, in Southeast Asia. Resistance to the partner drug, not artemisinin, is the primary driver for failure of ACT. Hence along with combination therapy of artemisinin second alternative drug is needed. Medicine of malaria venture is a non governmental organization which support collaborations with a library of antimalarial leads drug discovery (www.mmv.org.in). Clinically used antimalarial combination dose described in (**Table 2**).

A study of literature peformed to find out the new leads and their clinical stage along with survey on www.mmv.org, www.mpmp.huji, and ClinicalTrials.gov website (https://www.clinicaltrials.gov/). Major new drugs focus the blood schizonticide stage of uncomplicated *P. falciparum*. These potential inhibitor of plasmodium cycle must be single dose with minimum exposure and minimized toxicity in pregnant women and children with quite affordability to common people of minimum income.

There are at least 13 agents in clinical development (**Table 3**). Krintafel (tafenoquine) developed by Glaxosmith in collaboration with MMV has the potential to clear hypnozoites is approved for a single dose by regulatory authorities as a treatment for *Plasmodium vivax* relapse prevention. This represents an advance over standard 14-day primaquine regimens; however, the risk of acute haemolytic anemia in patients with glucose-6-phosphate dehydrogenase deficiency remains. Cipargamin (KAE609), developed by Novartis in collaboration with MMV. Cipargamin targets a cell membrane channel in the parasite, which is the new molecular target for malaria in more than 20 years. 75 mg for over 8 days require killing parasite in blood, and also having malaria transmission blocking. Intravenous formulation for severe malaria is also planned for 2020. One of the leading pipeline combinations are artefenomel (OZ439)–ferroquine and lumefantrine-KAF156, both in Phase 2b. Artefenomel is nonartemisinin based drug which has been designed by joint sanofi and mmv effort for children and to allow for once-daily. The combination is currently in a phase IIb trial, which is completed in the 2018. A novel trioxane 97/78, contains 1,2,4-trioxane nucleus similar to artemisinin developed by Central Drug Research Institute (CDRI), India, has shown promising antimalarial activity and is currently in clinical trials phase I. This 97/78 target, plasmodial phospholipid metabolism responsible for their pharmacological activity. Firstly 97/63 was synthesized but, due to its poor bioavailability, it was resynthesized as a hemisuccinate derivative and coded as 97/78. Upon administration of 97/78 it gets converted into its active *in vivo* metabolite 97/63. The concentrations of 97/63 and 97/78 can be measured by validated LC–MS/MS method [44].

7. Conclusion

In last ten years of discovery and development of new anti-malarial medicines showed an explosion in new molecules in the malaria pipeline. These current leads are result of a dramatic increase in the number and diversity of new molecules presently in pre-clinical and early clinical development. MMV itself and along with collaboration make this discovery possible. When malaria remains a challenge because of drug failure resist toward current line therapies time to time in parallele a successful drug discovery programmes also been run that provide satisfactory results with no reason to worry. The malaria drug development pipeline, at

Combinations	Dosing schedule and summary	Trade name/associated organization	Year of Launching
Artemether-lumefantrine	• Dosing twice/day for three days • Qualified WHO prequalification in Feb 2009 • Approved from the US-FDA • Several generic version of this have been produced.	(Coartem®/Novartis, MMV)	2008
Artesunate-amodiaquine	• Dosing once/day for three days. • Approved in 31 countries including 25 in Africa • Prequalified in 2008 by WHO.	(Carsucam®; (Sanofi/DNDi/MMV)	2008
Artesunate-Mefloquine	• It given once/day over three days. • Prequalified by WHO in September 2012 • Registered in India.	(Cephalon/DNDi/ Cipla/MMV)	2008
Dihydroartemisinin-piperaquine	• It given once/day for three days. Approved by EMA in 2011. • Prequalified by WHO • Included in the malaria treatment guidelines of WHO in 2011.	(Eurartesim®/Artekin®/sigma-Tau/MMV/Pfizer)	2010
Artesunate-Pyronaridine	• It given once/day for three days • Approved by the KFDA in 2011 and by the EMA in 2012. • Prequalified by WHO.	(Pyramax®/ShingPoong/MMV)	2011

Table 2.
Antimalarial combination along with prescribed dose.

Company	Supporter of fund		project	Clinical Phase
AbbVie	MMV	DSM265, MMV390048, DSM421	PK studies, formulation evaluation, PD and metabolite sample analysis, pathology peer review, technical consulting	I, II, preclinical
Eisai	Fiocruz	E6446	TLR9 antagonist for cerebral Malaria	Preclinical
	St. Jude, MMV, GHIT -	SJ733	Inhibitor of Plasmodium ATP4	Phase I
GlaxoSmithKline	MMV	Tafenoquine	(radical cure of *P. vivax*)	Approved
Novartis	Company	Coartem 80/480	developing a new formulation with 75% reduced pill burden for patients with body weight 35 kg+	Phase IV
	Wellcome, MMV, BPRC, Swiss TPH	Imidazolopiperazines (KAF156):	developing an NCE for patients with artemisinin-resistant strains of malaria	Phase II
		Spiroindolone (KAE609):	developing an NCE for patients with artemisinin-resistant strains of malaria	Phase II
	MMV	Coartem®	Dispersible: developing a new formulation for younger children	Phase IV
Sanofi	MMV	Oz 439/Ferroquine		Phase IIb
		Ferroquine (SSR97193)		Phase II
		MMV533		Phase-I
Takeda	MMV, GHIT	DSM265		Phase II

Company	Supporter of fund		project	Clinical Phase
		DSM421 Preclinical (plans to go into Phase I in 2017)		-pta kro
Zydus Cadila (AstraZeneca)		MMV253		Phase-I
CDRI		CDRI97/78		Phase-II

Table 3.
Antimalarial pipeline drugs.

present, is in a state where we still have leads in final stage to be released at market level. Currently Tafenoquine is permit to use for *P.vivax* malaria. With the current scenario of drug development against malaria we are able to control the situation and in next year we will be on the path of control malaria eradication. In many countries encouraging progress toward malaria elimination achieved e.g. Sri Lanka, China. With new clinically approved agents (arterolane, cipargamin, KAF156) on the horizon show potential to replace failing artemisinin combination therapies as part of novel combinations. Malaria drug discovery studies are in the successive direction where we can stay with malaria free country till of 2030 aim of malaria controlled region.

Author details

Imrat[1], Ajeet Kumar Verma[2] and Pooja Rani Mina[3]*

1 Institute of Bioresources and Sustainable Development (IBSD), Takyelpat Institutional Area, Imphal, Manipur, India

2 Ohio State University, Columbus, Ohio, United States

3 Central Institute of Medical and Aromatic Plant, Lucknow, Uttar Pradesh, India

*Address all correspondence to: pmeena28@gmail.com

References

[1] W.H. Organization, World malaria report 2020: 20 years of global progress and challenges, (2020)

[2] S.E. Afifi, M. Spencer, P.B. Hudson, N.W. Tavil, Biting prevalence and malaria transmission patterns in the Anopheles punctulatus complex (Diptera: Culicidae) in Papua New Guinea, Australian Journal of Experimental Biology and Medical Science 58(1) (1980) 1-17.

[3] D.P. Mason, F.E. McKenzie, Blood-stage dynamics and clinical implications of mixed Plasmodium vivax-Plasmodium falciparum infections, The American journal of tropical medicine and hygiene 61(3) (1999) 367-374.

[4] A.A. Escalante, E. Barrio, F.J. Ayala, Evolutionary origin of human and primate malarias: evidence from the circumsporozoite protein gene, Molecular biology and evolution 12(4) (1995) 616-626.

[5] E.D. MANGONI, C. Severini, M. Menegon, R. Romi, G. Ruggiero, G. Majori, Case report: An unusual late relapse of Plasmodium vivax malaria, The American journal of tropical medicine and hygiene 68(2) (2003) 159-160.

[6] S.C. Murphy, J.G. Breman, Gaps in the childhood malaria burden in Africa: cerebral malaria, neurological sequelae, anemia, respiratory distress, hypoglycemia, and complications of pregnancy, The American journal of tropical medicine and hygiene 64 (1_suppl) (2001) 57-67.

[7] R. Rueangweerayut, A.P. Phyo, C. Uthaisin, Y. Poravuth, T.Q. Binh, H. Tinto, L.K. Pénali, N. Valecha, N.T. Tien, S. Abdulla, Pyronaridine–artesunate versus mefloquine plus artesunate for malaria, New England Journal of Medicine 366(14) (2012) 1298-1309.

[8] A. Wroczyńska, W. Nahorski, A. Bąkowska, H. Pietkiewicz, Cytokines and clinical manifestations of malaria in adults with severe and uncomplicated disease, International maritime health 56(1-4) (2005) 103-114.

[9] G. Trinchieri, Proinflammatory and immunoregulatory functions of interleukin-12, International reviews of immunology 16(3-4) (1998) 365-396.

[10] H.C. van der Heyde, J. Nolan, V. Combes, I. Gramaglia, G.E. Grau, A unified hypothesis for the genesis of cerebral malaria: sequestration, inflammation and hemostasis leading to microcirculatory dysfunction, TRENDS in Parasitology 22(11) (2006) 503-508.

[11] F.C. Fang, Perspectives series: host/pathogen interactions. Mechanisms of nitric oxide-related antimicrobial activity, The Journal of clinical investigation 99(12) (1997) 2818-2825.

[12] H. Brown, T. Hien, N. Day, N. Mai, L. Chuong, T. Chau, P. Loc, N. Phu, D. Bethell, J. Farrar, Evidence of blood-brain barrier dysfunction in human cerebral malaria, Neuropathology and applied neurobiology 25(4) (1999) 331-340.

[13] R.T. Gazzinelli, C. Ropert, M.A. Campos, Role of the Toll/interleukin-1 receptor signaling pathway in host resistance and pathogenesis during infection with protozoan parasites, Immunological reviews 201(1) (2004) 9-25.

[14] R.R. Schumann, Malarial fever: Hemozoin is involved but Toll-free, Proceedings of the National Academy of Sciences 104(6) (2007) 1743-1744.

[15] R. Christophers, Microscopic diagnosis of malaria, British medical journal 1(4697) (1951) 75.

[16] A. Moody, Rapid diagnostic tests for malaria parasites, Clinical microbiology reviews 15(1) (2002) 66-78.

[17] D. Bell, R.W. Peeling, Evaluation of rapid diagnostic tests: malaria, Nature Reviews Microbiology 4(9) (2006) S34-S38.

[18] L. Andrews, R.F. Andersen, D. Webster, S. Dunachie, R.M. Walther, P. Bejon, A. Hunt-Cooke, G. Bergson, F. Sanderson, A.V. Hill, Quantitative real-time polymerase chain reaction for malaria diagnosis and its use in malaria vaccine clinical trials, The American journal of tropical medicine and hygiene 73(1) (2005) 191-198.

[19] C. Joos, L. Marrama, H.E. Polson, S. Corre, A.-M. Diatta, B. Diouf, J.-F. Trape, A. Tall, S. Longacre, R. Perraut, Clinical protection from falciparum malaria correlates with neutrophil respiratory bursts induced by merozoites opsonized with human serum antibodies, PLoS One 5(3) (2010).

[20] S. James, P. TATE, New knowledge of the life-cycle of malaria parasites, Nature 139(3517) (1937) 545-545.

[21] R. Sinden, G. Butcher, O. Billker, S. Fleck, Regulation of infectivity of Plasmodium to the mosquito vector, Advances in parasitology, Elsevier1996, pp. 53-117.

[22] A. Ghosh, L. Moreira, M. Jacobs-Lorena, Plasmodium–mosquito interactions, phage display libraries and transgenic mosquitoes impaired for malaria transmission, Insect biochemistry and molecular biology 32(10) (2002) 1325-1331.

[23] N.J. White, Determinants of relapse periodicity in Plasmodium vivax malaria, Malaria Journal 10(1) (2011) 297.

[24] L. Bannister, J. Hopkins, R. Fowler, S. Krishna, G. Mitchell, A brief illustrated guide to the ultrastructure of Plasmodium falciparum asexual blood stages, Parasitology today 16(10) (2000) 427-433.

[25] M. Prudêncio, A. Rodriguez, M.M. Mota, The silent path to thousands of merozoites: the Plasmodium liver stage, Nature Reviews Microbiology 4(11) (2006) 849-856.

[26] L.A. Baton, L.C. Ranford-Cartwright, Spreading the seeds of million-murdering death: metamorphoses of malaria in the mosquito, TRENDS in Parasitology 21(12) (2005) 573-580.

[27] P. Alano, R. Carter, Sexual differentiation in malaria parasites, Annual review of microbiology 44(1) (1990) 429-449.

[28] J.N. Alumasa, New insights on the structure-function principles and design of quinoline antimalarial drugs, Georgetown University, 2010.

[29] J.H. Goldie, A.J. Coldman, The genetic origin of drug resistance in neoplasms: implications for systemic therapy, Cancer research 44(9) (1984) 3643-3653.

[30] U. Farooq, R. Mahajan, Drug resistance in malaria, Journal of vector borne diseases 41(3/4) (2004) 45.

[31] M.T. Alam, S. Vinayak, K. Congpuong, C. Wongsrichanalai, W. Satimai, L. Slutsker, A.A. Escalante, J.W. Barnwell, V. Udhayakumar, Tracking origins and spread of sulfadoxine-resistant Plasmodium falciparum dhps alleles in Thailand, Antimicrobial agents and chemotherapy 55(1) (2011) 155-164.

[32] L.H. Miller, X. Su, Artemisinin: discovery from the Chinese herbal garden, Cell 146(6) (2011) 855-858.

[33] G.A. Balint, Artemisinin and its derivatives: an important new class of

antimalarial agents, Pharmacology & therapeutics 90(2-3) (2001) 261-265.

[34] M. Manske, O. Miotto, S. Campino, S. Auburn, J. Almagro-Garcia, G. Maslen, J. O'Brien, A. Djimde, O. Doumbo, I. Zongo, Analysis of Plasmodium falciparum diversity in natural infections by deep sequencing, Nature 487(7407) (2012) 375-379.

[35] C. Wongsrichanalai, S.R. Meshnick, Declining artesunate-mefloquine efficacy against falciparum malaria on the Cambodia–Thailand border, Emerging infectious diseases 14(5) (2008) 716.

[36] K. Na-Bangchang, P. Muhamad, R. Ruaengweerayut, W. Chaijaroenkul, J. Karbwang, Identification of resistance of Plasmodium falciparum to artesunate-mefloquine combination in an area along the Thai-Myanmar border: integration of clinico-parasitological response, systemic drug exposure, and in vitro parasite sensitivity, Malaria Journal 12(1) (2013) 1-14.

[37] M. Ouji, J.-M. Augereau, L. Paloque, F. Benoit-Vical, *Plasmodium falciparum* resistance to artemisinin-based combination therapies: A sword of Damocles in the path toward malaria elimination, Parasite 25 (2018).

[38] F. Gobbi, D. Buonfrate, M. Menegon, G. Lunardi, A. Angheben, C. Severini, S. Gori, Z. Bisoffi, Failure of dihydroartemisinin-piperaquine treatment of uncomplicated Plasmodium falciparum malaria in a traveller coming from Ethiopia, Malaria Journal 15(1) (2016) 1-4.

[39] B.Q. Phuc, C. Rasmussen, T.T. Duong, L.T. Dong, M.A. Loi, D. Ménard, J. Tarning, D. Bustos, P. Ringwald, G.L. Galappaththy, Treatment failure of dihydroartemisinin/piperaquine for Plasmodium falciparum malaria, Vietnam, Emerging infectious diseases 23(4) (2017) 715.

[40] N.V. Thanh, N. Thuy-Nhien, N.T.K. Tuyen, N.T. Tong, N.T. Nha-Ca, H.H. Quang, J. Farrar, G. Thwaites, N.J. White, M. Wolbers, Rapid decline in the susceptibility of Plasmodium falciparum to dihydroartemisinin–piperaquine in the south of Vietnam, Malaria Journal 16(1) (2017) 1-10.

[41] A.P. Phyo, P. Jittamala, F.H. Nosten, S. Pukrittayakamee, M. Imwong, N.J. White, S. Duparc, F. Macintyre, M. Baker, J.J. Möhrle, Antimalarial activity of artefenomel (OZ439), a novel synthetic antimalarial endoperoxide, in patients with Plasmodium falciparum and Plasmodium vivax malaria: an open-label phase 2 trial, The Lancet Infectious Diseases 16(1) (2016) 61-69.

[42] B. Witkowski, V. Duru, N. Khim, L.S. Ross, B. Saintpierre, J. Beghain, S. Chy, S. Kim, S. Ke, N. Kloeung, A surrogate marker of piperaquine-resistant Plasmodium falciparum malaria: a phenotype–genotype association study, The Lancet Infectious Diseases 17(2) (2017) 174-183.

[43] P.L. Olliaro, Y. Yuthavong, An overview of chemotherapeutic targets for antimalarial drug discovery, Pharmacology & therapeutics 81(2) (1999) 91-110.

[44] M. Wahajuddin, S.P. Singh, I. Taneja, K.S.R. Raju, J.R. Gayen, H.H. Siddiqui, S.K. Singh, Development and validation of an LC-MS/MS method for simultaneous determination of piperaquine and 97-63, the active metabolite of CDRI 97-78, in rat plasma and its application in interaction study, Drug testing and analysis 8(2) (2016) 221-227.

Chapter 4

Adaptive Drug Resistance in Malaria Parasite: A Threat to Malaria Elimination Agenda?

Moses Okpeku

Abstract

Malaria is a global disease of importance, especially in the sub-Saharan African region, where malaria accounts for great losses economically and to life. Fight to eliminate this disease has resulted in reduced disease burden in many places where the diseases is endemic. Elimination strategies in most places is focus on the use of treated nets and drug application. Exposure of malaria parasites to anti-malaria drugs have led to the evolution of drug resistance in both parasites and host. Development of drug resistance vary but, studies on adaptive drug resistance has implications and consequences. Our knowledge of this consequences are limited but important for the pursuit of an uninterrupted malaria elimination agenda. This chapter draws our attention to this risks and recommends interventions.

Keywords: adaptive resistance, drug-resistance, malaria, plasmodium, parasite

1. Introduction

1.1 Malaria - a global infectious disease

Malaria is a global deadly communicable disease [1], caused by plasmodium species, an apicomplexan microbe transmitted by the mosquito vector. Five major plasmodia parasites (*P falciparum, P vivax, P ovale, P malariae* and *P knowlesi*) have been implicated in malaria infections [2]. Of these, *Plasmodium falciparum* (*P. falciparum*) and *Plasmodium vivax (P. vivax)* are more widely distributed [3]. In sub-Saharan Africa, *P. falciparum* is the cause of most malaria cases while *P. vivax* is reported to cause most of the malaria cases in Asia; *P. falciparum* cause more fatal disease [4].

In 2019 alone, about 229 million positive malaria infections were reported globally, mortality from was estimated at about 409,000, with children under 5 years accounting for about 67% of death [5]. The disease is common among in poor communities [6], especially rural communities of the underdeveloped/ developing countries of the world. Economic, social and health importance of this disease in terms of loss of life (particularly; young children), reduction in productivity of affected adult population, and negative social and health implication of the disease makes it one of the high ranking microbial, infectious disease in the world.

1.2 Malaria elimination agenda

Among the diseases which have great public health impact, malaria is a significant public health concern [7–9]. The fight to eliminate malaria is an aged long battle globally. Elimination programmes were launched after the Second World War [6], with chloroquine as the major frontline anti-malaria drug [10] and Dichlorodiphenyltrichloroethane DDT used for vector control [11]. Malaria eliminations efforts in Africa began with the World Health Organisation (WHO) roll back malaria initiatives started in 1998 [1]; these efforts focused on entomology control (to reduce transmitting vectors) using indoor insecticides, and treated mosquito nets introduced for protection and prevention [6].

The success of these elimination programmes is why over one hundred countries have been awarded malaria free status [12] and thirty-four others accorded elimination status [13], and most malaria endemic countries working very hard towards the attainment of elimination status. Today the disease burden continues to decrease across the world [14] relative to the era, before the launch of the global elimination programmes.

Success stories leading to this elimination stage in malaria control had been heavily dependent on traditional entomology surveillance and drug use. However, the plasmodium is a ubiquitous parasites that has evolved, complex systems of survival [15]. Among these survival strategies is the development of drug resistance to nearly all know malaria drugs. Resistance to chloroquine (the major frontline medicine for the treatment of malaria) was reported and widespread [13] long before the roll-back-malaria initiatives. Better understanding of the biology of the parasites and the life cycle led to the development of a range of other anti-malaria drugs some of which are still actively being used, but resistance to almost all know malaria drugs have been reported [16–19].

Drug resistance vary, and is transferable from pathogen to host [20]. Of the different types of drug resistance, adaptive drug resistance is usually not permanent, but is capable of producing strains of parasites not targeted by known drugs. This chapter aims at reviewing the different types of drug resistance with focus on adaptive drug resistance in plasmodium and the implication to malaria elimination programme.

2. Brief history of anti-malaria drug resistance

The fight against drug resistance in pathogenic microbes is global. The life of these microbes are so inter-twined with human wellness that if overlooked could be very costly in terms of treatment cost and loss of life. As efforts are being up-scaled towards malaria elimination, the issue of drug resistance continues to surface as a major challenge to cope with. This is because the malaria parasite continues to evolve and regularly develop mechanisms for surviving the toxic effect of drugs. These mechanisms result with fixed mutations in the genetic architecture that confers fitness and resistance to withstand or evade targeting drugs, thereby hindering or completely preventing binding between drug compounds and their target.

The history of evolution of drug resistance in plasmodium dates back to the 1930s when chloroquine (CQ) resistance in *P. falciparum* arose independently in Columbia and Thailand [21], and rapidly spread throughout the world. Research efforts to truncate this spread led to the development of different variants of malaria drugs to replace CQ. However, the plasmodium in it's unique way continue to adapt and evolve new mutations for survival and resistance to drugs which are harmful to it [22]. Advances in molecular technology has made it possible to

Mutation sites associated with drug resistance in plasmodium	References
Mutation resulting in polymorphism at the position 76 (K76T) in the transmembrane protein, known as *Plasmodium falciparum* chloroquine resistance transporter (PfCRT).	[23, 24]
The N86Y and Y184F amino-terminal mutations falciparum multidrug resistance transporter 1 (PfMDR1) has been implicated commonly in CQ and other anti-malaria drug resistance in Asian and African parasites.	[17, 25, 26]
Mutation of dihydrofolate reductase (DHFR) associated with *Plasmodium falciparum* sulfadoxine-pyrimethamine resistance.	[27]
Mutation of dihydropteroate synthetase (DHPS) enzymes implicated in *Plasmodium falciparum* sulfadoxine-pyrimethamine resistance.	[27]
mutations in *pvmdr1*, *pvcrt-o*, *pvdhfr*, and *pvdhps* genes in temperate-zone of *P. vivax* *associated with malaria drug resistance*	[28, 29]

Table 1.
Common mutations associated with P. falciparum *malaria drug resistance.*

uncover different mutations in the plasmodium parasites associated with drug resistance (**Table 1**). Evolution of these mutations are dynamic and difficult could be difficult to track and eliminate, especially when novel parasite results, against which known anti-malaria drugs is ineffective.

3. Drug resistance types: how much do we know in plasmodium?

Drug resistance types include Intrinsic, acquired and adaptive resistance. Intrinsic drug resistance is a natural phenomenon, and an innate ability in pathogen for resisting drug or harmful substance without prior record of susceptibility [30, 31], pathogens do not necessarily develop mutation for this to occur [32]. Acquired drug resistance builds up in human host, and makes them unresponsive to a drug that should normally eliminate known pathogenic parasite from the host system [33], these are both stable forms of drug resistance. Adaptive resistance [34, 35] develops in a pathogen in response to stimuli [36].

While "intrinsic and acquired resistance are stable and can be transmitted vertically to subsequent generations "[32] adaptive resistance is temporal, unstable, and is often lost ([17]; [37]). [38] observed that "unstable adaptation contains modulation of gene expression, which results in phenotypic changes due to changes in environmental markers that are sensed by the microorganisms" but it is not certain how long this resistance is, or could be sustained [39]. Adaptive resistance is acquired through mutation and binding genetic plasticity that enables transfer of genes [20] from parasites to host. These different mode of drug resistance have been extensively studied and reported for bacteria [36, 40–42], but not much is seen in literature regarding adaptive resistance in plasmodium.

4. Adaptive drug resistance has implications and consequences

Development of drug resistance interferes with disease control, increase the cost of treatment and management of control programs and if not quickly address could thwart control programmes. The evolution of drug resistance in malaria parasites have been a focus of many research but there is a dearth of information regarding adaptive resistance in malaria parasite and the consequence in their human hosts. It is quite understandable since adaptive resistance only confers a temporal resistance and is reversible. Although temporal and reversible, The possibility of mutation and evolution of a unique strain of parasite is possible, on which known drugs would be ineffective. However, the period between active activation of adaptive resistance in plasmodium, the product of activation (whether lethal or not, or novel and insensitive to known drugs or not), the consequence in gene transfer to host and a host of other factors are unknown.

5. Discovering and tackling adaptive drug resistance in plasmodium: recommendations

Evolution of resistance to drugs is a survival mechanism influenced by many factors that produce mutation in the parasites. Common among causes of resistance is exposure to non-lethal doses of anti-malaria drugs [15]. Malaria parasites have unique ability to evolving mechanisms for evading the immune response in humans [43] and they are actively evolving resistance to anti-plasmodia drugs [44]. But there is a dearth of information are to the effect of plasmodia resistance to drug, especially adaptive resistance, which though is temporal, could influence the development of novel plasmodium stains not targeted by currently available anti-malaria drug. This development is a threat to malaria elimination agenda and should not be encouraged.

A host of resistance gene markers in plasmodium for drug resistance is an active field of malaria research [16, 18, 19, 45, 46], and still counting, but not much is written about the role or influence of adaptive resistance on these markers this is a conspicuous research gap in malaria biology and genetics requiring urgent attention. Selective sweep resulting in sudden change in an advantageous gene under strong positive selection [47] has been reported as product of evolution of resistance to drug. It is possible to scanning the genome for signature of selective sweeps, to identify genes undergoing adaptive evolution [48]. Similar studies revealed the mutations in presently known markers used in the study of malaria drug resistance [49–52], but none is focused on adaptive resistance. This kind of studies leverage of the NEXT GENERATION sequencing technology which is very limited and still very expensive in developing countries, especially in countries with no direct funding of research by government, where malaria is endemic.

6. Pertinent questions and suggestions for the way forward

Is adaptive resistance in malaria parasites a challenge? Does it have a significant influence on combating and elimination of malaria particularly in malaria endemic regions in Africa? Understanding the effects of adaptive malaria drug resistance, in plasmodium, the vector and the human host will greatly contribute to malaria elimination agenda and reposition the malaria elimination programmes across the world with focus on sub-Saharan Africa as the hub. In addition, different populations respond differently to the same drugs. These differential responses are influenced by genetic variability in different ethnic groups within a population, which in turn can be associated with variation in resistance to given drugs. Identification of genes and gene pathways involved in adaptive resistance is also vital for developing markers for prediction and diagnosis and should be pursued.

Kim and Schneider [48] observed that, "by examining selective sweeps in many endemic areas with different demographic and epidemiologic characteristics" it would be possible to identify factors associated with adaptive resistance to malaria drugs and track epidemiological variables [53–56] for transmission and development of treatment regimes, accurate drug prescription and be able to determine costs of resistance. Understanding the implication and consequences of adaptive resistance alongside other forms of drug resistances will play significant role in policy formulation and implementation for disease control, give vivid picture of how to manage malaria control and modelling of disease transmission.

Author details

Moses Okpeku
Discipline of Genetics, School of Life Sciences, University of Kwa-Zulu Natal, South Africa

*Address all correspondence to: okpekum@ukzn.ac.za

References

[1] World Health Organization 2015. Global Malaria Programme. Eliminating malaria. Geneva: World Health Organization. World Health. 2015;243.

[2] Talapko, J., Škrlec, I., Alebić, T., Jukić, M. and Včev, A. 2019. Malaria: The past and the present. Microorganisms, 7(6), 179. MDPI AG. http://dx.doi.org/10.3390/microorganisms7060179

[3] White, M.T., Karl, S., Koepfli, C. Longley, R.J., Hofmann, N.E., Wampflier, R., Felger, I., Smith, T., Nguitragool, W., Sattabongkot, J., Robinson, L. Ghani, A. and Mueller I. 2018. Plasmodium vivax and plasmodium falciparum infection dynamics: re-infections, recrudescences and relapses. Malar J 17 (170). https://doi.org/10.1186/s12936-018-2318-1

[4] de Jong, S.E., van Unen, V., Manurung, M.D. et al. Systems analysis and controlled malaria infection in Europeans and Africans elucidate naturally acquired immunity. Nat Immunol 22, 654-665 (2021). https://doi.org/10.1038/s41590-021-00911-7

[5] World Health Organization 2020. World Malaria Report. https://www.who.int/malaria/publications/world-repot-malaria-report-2019/en/. Accessed 10 September, 2020.

[6] Maharaj, R., Kissoon, S., Lakan V. and Kheswa, N. 2019. Rolling back malaria in Africa – Challenges and opportunities to winning the elimination battle. South African Medical Journal 2019;109(11b):53-56. DOI:10.7196/SAMJ.2019.v109i11b.14250

[7] Dewald, J.R., Fuller, D.O., Müller, G.C. et al. A novel method for mapping village-scale outdoor resting microhabitats of the primary African malaria vector, Anopheles gambiae . Malar J 15, 489 (2016). https://doi.org/10.1186/s12936-016-1534-9

[8] Gwitira, I., Murwira, A., Mberikunashe, J. et al. Spatial overlaps in the distribution of HIV/AIDS and malaria in Zimbabwe. BMC Infect Dis 18, 598 (2018). https://doi.org/10.1186/s12879-018-3513-y

[9] Shi, S. M., Shi, T. Q., Chen, S. B., Cui, Y. B., Kassegne, K., Okpeku, M., Chen, J. H., & Shen, H. M. (2021). Genome-Wide Scans for Ghanaian Plasmodium falciparum Genes Under Selection From Local and Chinese Host Populations. Frontiers in cellular and infection microbiology, 11, 630797. https://doi.org/10.3389/fcimb.2021.630797

[10] Sweeney, A.W. 2000. Wartime research on malaria chemotherapy. Parassitologia 42:33-46

[11] Russell, P.F. 1951. Some epidemiological aspects of malaria control with reference to DDT. *J Natl Malar Soc.*10:257-265

[12] WHO, (2019): Global Malaria Program - Countries and territories certified malaria-free by WHO https://www.who.int/teams/global-malaria-programme/elimination/countries-and-territories-certified-malaria-free-by-who (accessed February 2021)

[13] Cotter, C., Sturrock, HJW, Hsiang, MS., Liu, J., Phillips, AA., Hwang, J., Gueye, CS., Fullman, N., Gosling, RD & Feachem, RGA. 2013. The changing epidemiology of malaria elimination: new strategies for new challenges. The Lancet, 382(9895), 900-911, https://doi.org/10.1016/S0140-6736(13)60310-4.

[14] Nkumama I.N, O'Meara W.P, Osier F.H.A. Changes in malaria epidemiology in Africa and new challenges for elimination. Trends Parasitol. 2017;33:128-140.

[15] Fernández L, Breidenstein E.B, Hancock R.E 2011. Creeping baselines

and adaptive resistance to antibiotics. Drug Resist Updat 14: 1-21.

[16] Huang B, Deng C, Yang T, et al. 2015 Polymorphisms of the artemisinin resistant marker (K13) in plasmodium falciparum parasite populations of Grande Comore Island 10 years after artemisinin combination therapy. Parasites and Vectors. 8:1-8.

[17] Idowu, A.O., Oyibo, W.A., Bhattacharyya, S. Khubbar, M. Mendie, U.E., Bumah, V.V., Black, C., Igietseme, J. and Azenabor A.A. 2019. Rare mutations in *Pfmdr1* gene of *Plasmodium falciparum* detected in clinical isolates from patients treated with anti-malarial drug in Nigeria. Malar J 18, 319. https://doi.org/10.1186/s12936-019-2947-z

[18] Kamau E, Campino S, Amenga-Etego L, et al. 2015 K13-propeller polymorphisms in plasmodium falciparum parasites from sub-saharan Africa. J infect dis.211:1352-5.

[19] Oboh MA, Ndiaye D, Antony HA, et al. 2018. Status of Artemisinin Resistance in Malaria Parasite Plasmodium Falciparum from Molecular Analyses of the Kelch13 Gene in Southwestern Nigeria. Biomed Res Int.

[20] Dhawale A and Rath A 2014. Antibiotic resistance: A threat and challenge to society. Ann Appl Biosci 1: R1-R6.

[21] Zareen S, Rehman H.U, Gul N, et al. 2016. Malaria is still a life threatening disease review. *J Entomol Zool Stud JEZS*.105:105-12.

[22] Laxminarayan R. 2004 . Act now or later? Economics of malaria resistance. Am J Trop Med Hyg. 71(2 Suppl):187-195. PMID: 15331837.

[23] Johnson, D. J., Fidock, D. A., Mungthin, M., Lakshmanan, V., Sidhu, A. B., Bray, P. G., & Ward, S. A. 2004. Evidence for a central role for PfCRT in conferring plasmodium falciparum resistance to diverse antimalarial agents. Molecular cell, *15*(6), 867-877. https://doi.org/10.1016/j.molcel.2004.09.012

[24] Lakshmanan, V., Bray, P. G., Verdier-Pinard, D., Johnson, D. J., Horrocks, P., Muhle, R. A., Alakpa, G. E., Hughes, R. H., Ward, S. A., Krogstad, D. J., Sidhu, A. B., & Fidock, D. A. 2005. A critical role for PfCRT K76T in Plasmodium falciparum verapamil-reversible chloroquine resistance. *The EMBO journal*, *24*(13), 2294-2305. https://doi.org/10.1038/sj.emboj.7600681

[25] Calçada C, Silva M, Baptista V, Thathy V, Silva-Pedrosa R, Granja D, Ferreira PE, Gil JP, Fidock DA, Veiga MI. 2020. Expansion of a specific plasmodium falciparum PfMDR1 haplotype in Southeast Asia with increased substrate transport. *mBio* 11: e02093-20. doi:10.1128/mBio.02093-20.

[26] Veiga, M. I., Dhingra, S. K., Henrich, P. P., Straimer, J., Gnädig, N., Uhlemann, A. C., Martin, R. E., Lehane, A. M., & Fidock, D. A. (2016). Globally prevalent PfMDR1 mutations modulate plasmodium falciparum susceptibility to artemisinin-based combination therapies. Nature communications, *7*, 11553. https://doi.org/10.1038/ncomms11553

[27] Ahmed, A., Bararia, D., Vinayak, S., Yameen, M., Biswas, S., Dev, V., Kumar, A., Ansari, M. A., & Sharma, Y. D. 2004. Plasmodium falciparum isolates in India exhibit a progressive increase in mutations associated with sulfadoxine-pyrimethamine resistance. Antimicrobial agents and chemotherapy, *48*(3), 879-889. doi:10.1128/aac.48.3.879-889.2004

[28] Lu, F., Wang, B., Cao, J., Sattabongkot, J., Zhou, H., Zhu, G., Kim, K., Gao, Q., & Han, E. T. 2012.

Prevalence of drug resistance-associated gene mutations in plasmodium vivax in Central China. The Korean journal of parasitology, 50(4), 379-384. https://doi.org/10.3347/kjp.2012.50.4.379

[29] Zhao, Y., Wang, L., Soe, M.T. Aung, P.L, Wei, H., Liu, Z., Ma, T., Huang, Y., Menezes, L.J., Wang, Q., Kyaw, M.P., Nyunt, M.H., Cui, L. & Cao, Y. 2020. Molecular surveillance for drug resistance markers in *Plasmodium vivax* isolates from symptomatic and asymptomatic infections at the China–Myanmar border. Malar J 19, 281. https://doi.org/10.1186/s12936-020-03354-x

[30] Cox G, Wright GD. Intrinsic antibiotic resistance: Mechanisms, origins, challenges and solutions. Int J Med Microbiol. 2013;303(6-7):287-292. doi: 10.1016/j.ijmm.2013.02.009.

[31] Impey R.E., Hawkins D. A., Sutton J.M. and Soares da Costa T.P. 2020. Overcoming intrinsic and acquired resistance mechanisms associated with the Cell Wall of gram-negative bacteria. Antibiotics 9:(623), 1 – 19. doi:10.3390/antibiotics9090623.

[32] Rizi K.S, Ghazvini K, Noghondar M.K 2018. Adaptive antibiotic resistance: Overview and perspectives. J Infect Dis Ther 6: 363. doi:10.4172/2332-0877.1000363.

[33] Kempker R.R, Kipiani M, Mirtskhulava V, Tukvadze N, Magee M.J, Blumberg H.M. 2015. Acquired drug resistance in mycobacterium tuberculosis and poor outcomes among patients with multidrug-resistant tuberculosis. Emerg Infect Dis. 21(6):992-1001. doi:10.3201/eid2106.141873.

[34] Coleman SR, Bains M, Smith ML, Spicer V, Lao Y, Taylor PK, Mookherjee N, Hancock REW. 2021. The small RNAs PA2952.1 and PrrH as regulators of virulence, motility, and iron metabolism in *Pseudomonas aeruginosa*. Appl Environ Microbiol 87: e02182-e02120. doi:10.1128/AEM.02182-20.

[35] Coleman SR, Blimkie T, Falsafi R, Hancock R.E.W. 2020. Multidrug adaptive resistance of *Pseudomonas aeruginosa* swarming cells. Antimicrob Agents Chemother 64: e01999-e01919. doi:10.1128/AAC.01999-19.

[36] Fernández, L., & Hancock, R. E. 2012. Adaptive and mutational resistance: Role of porins and efflux pumps in drug resistance. Clinical microbiology reviews, 25(4), 661-681. https://doi.org/10.1128/CMR.00043-12

[37] Baquero F 2001. Low-level antibacterial resistance: A gateway to clinical resistance. Drug Resist Updat 4: 93-105.

[38] López-Maury L, Marguerat S, Bähler J 2008. Tuning gene expression to changing environments: From rapid responses to evolutionary adaptation. Nat Rev Genet 9: 583-593.

[39] Jahn L.J, Munck C, Ellabaan M.M, Sommer M.O .2017. Adaptive laboratoryevolution of antibiotic resistance using different selection regimes lead to similar phenotypes and genotypes. Front Microbiol 8: 816.

[40] Li, X. Z., Zhang, L., & Nikaido, H. 2004. Efflux pump-mediated intrinsic drug resistance in mycobacterium smegmatis. Antimicrobial agents and chemotherapy, 48(7), 2415-2423. https://doi.org/10.1128/AAC.48.7.2415-2423.2004

[41] Motta, S.S., Cluzel, P. & Aldana, M. 2015. Adaptive resistance in bacteria requires epigenetic inheritance, genetic noise, and cost of efflux pumps. PLoS ONE 10(3): e0118464. https://doi.org/10.1371/journal.pone.0118464

[42] Olaitan, A.O., Morand, S. & Rolain, J.M. 2014 Mechanisms of polymyxin

resistance: Acquired and intrinsic resistance in bacteria. Front. Microbiol. 5:643. doi: 10.3389/fmicb.2014.00643

[43] Dinko B, Pradel G. 2016. Immune evasion by plasmodium falciparum parasites converting a host protection mechanism for the parasite's benefit. Advances in Infectious Diseases.06(02):82-95.

[44] Niba, P.T.N., Nji, A.M., Evehe, MS. et al. 2020. Drug Resistance Markers within an Evolving Efficacy of Anti-Malarial Drugs in Cameroon: A Systematic Review and Meta-Analysis 1998–Malar J 20, 32 (2021). https://doi.org/10.1186/s12936-020-03543-8.

[45] Conrad MD, Bigira V, Kapisi J, et al. 2014. Polymorphisms in K13 and falcipain-2 associated with artemisinin resistance are not prevalent in Plasmodium falciparum isolated from Ugandan children. PLoS One. 9. 1 – 10.

[46] Ouattara A, Kone A, Adams M, et al. 2015. Polymorphisms in the K13-propeller gene in artemisinin-susceptible plasmodium falciparum parasites from Bougoula-Hameau and Bandiagara, Mali. Am J Trop Med Hyg. 92:1202-1206.

[47] Maynard, Smith J. & Haigh, J. (1974). The hitch-hiking effect of a favourable gene. Genetical Research 23, 23-35.

[48] Kim, Y. & Schneider, K. A. (2013) Evolution of drug resistance in malaria parasite populations. Nature Education Knowledge 4(8):6

[49] Wootton JC, Feng X, Ferdig MT, Cooper RA, Mu J, Baruch DI, Magill AJ, Su XZ. Genetic diversity and chloroquine selective sweeps in Plasmodium falciparum. Nature. 2002 Jul 18;418(6895):320-323. doi: 10.1038/nature00813. PMID: 12124623.

[50] Nair, S., Williams, JT., Brockman, A., Paiphun, L., Mayxay, M., Newton, PN., Guthmann, J., Smithuis, FM., Hien, TT., White, NJ., Nosten, F. & Anderson, TJC. 2003. A Selective Sweep Driven by Pyrimethamine Treatment in Southeast Asian Malaria Parasites, Molecular Biology and Evolution. 20(9) 1526-1536, https://doi.org/10.1093/molbev/msg162

[51] Nash D, Nair S, Mayxay M, Newton PN, Guthmann JP, Nosten F, Anderson TJ. 2005. Selection strength and hitchhiking around two anti-malarial resistance genes. Proc Biol Sci. 272(1568):1153-61. doi: 10.1098/rspb.2004.3026. PMID: 16024377; PMCID: PMC1559806.

[52] Vinayak, Sumiti and Alam, Tauqeer and Mixson-Hayden, Tonya and McCollum, Andrea M. and Sem, Rithy and Shah, Naman K. and Lim, Pharath and Muth, Sinuon and Rogers, William O. and Fandeur, Thierry and Barnwell, John W. and Escalante, Ananias A. and Wongsrichanalai, Chansuda and Ariey, Frederick and Meshnick, Steven R. and Udhayakumar, Venkatachalam. 2010. Origin and Evolution of Sulfadoxine Resistant Plasmodium falciparum. PLOS Pathogens. 3. e1000830. Doi:10.1371/journal.ppat.1000830

[53] Belachew E.B. 2018. Immune response and evasion mechanisms of plasmodium falciparum parasites. J Immunol Res. 2018: 6529681.

[54] Escalante, A. A., Smith, D. L., & Kim, Y. (2009). The dynamics of mutations associated with anti-malarial drug resistance in Plasmodium falciparum. Trends in parasitology, 25(12), 557-563. https://doi.org/10.1016/j.pt.2009.09.008

[55] Schneider KA, Kim Y. An analytical model for genetic hitchhiking in the evolution of antimalarial drug resistance. Theor Popul Biol. 2010 Sep;78(2):93-108. doi: 10.1016/j.tpb.2010.06.005. Epub 2010 Jun 19.

PMID: 20600206; PMCID: PMC2916054.

[56] Maharaj, L., Adeleke, VT., Fatoba, AJ., Adeniyi A A., Tshilwane, SI., Adeleke, MA., Maharaj, R. & Okpeku, M. 2021. Immunoinformatics approach for multi-epitope vaccine design against P. falciparum malaria. Infection, Genetics and Evolution. 92 104875. https://doi.org/10.1016/j.meegid.2021.104875.

Chapter 5

Treatment of Malaria Infection and Drug Resistance

Bernard Kofi Turkson, Alfred Ofori Agyemang, Desmond Nkrumah, Reinhard Isaac Nketia, Michael Frimpong Baidoo and Merlin Lincoln Kwao Mensah

Abstract

Malaria is a public health challenge that requires prompt treatment for those infected to make a full recovery. Treatment of malaria infection is to be started as soon as a diagnosis is confirmed. Antimalarial medications are administered to prevent and also to treat malaria. The type of medication used and the duration of therapy is dependent on the type of malaria-causing *plasmodium species*, the severity of the symptoms, geographical area where malaria infection occurred and the medication used to prevent malaria and whether there is pregnancy. Treatment of malaria from public health perspective is to reduce transmission of the infection to others, by reducing the infectious reservoir and to prevent the emergence and spread of resistance to antimalarial medicines. Medications used in the treatment of malaria infection come from the following five groups of chemical compounds: quinolines and aryl amino alcohols, antifolate, artemisinin derivatives, hydroxynaphthoquinones and antibacterial agents. The treatment of malaria is not initiated until the diagnosis has been established through laboratory testing. Artemisinin-based Combination Therapy (ACTs) has been used for the treatment of uncomplicated malaria. ACTs are also to enhance treatment and protect against the development of drug resistance. IV artesunate is used in the treatment of severe malaria, regardless of infecting species.

Keywords: Malaria, treatment, drug resistance, ACTs, drugs and plasmodium specie

1. Introduction

Plasmodium species are protozoan parasites that cause malaria, a life-threatening infectious ailment in humans. Five different species of *Plasmodium* are known to infect man: *P. falciparum, P. malariae, P. ovale, P. vivax* and *P. knowlesi*. *Plasmodium falciparum* is the commonest malaria-causing parasite in the World Health Organization (WHO) African Region, accounting for 99.7% of estimated malaria cases in 2018, as well as in the WHO Eastern Mediterranean Region (71%), the WHO Western Pacific Region (65%), and WHO South-East Asia Region (50%).

Plasmodium falciparum causes a serious form of malaria infection. *Plasmodium falciparum* parasite is known to be responsible for the vast majority of malaria morbidity and mortality in Africa [1].

Plasmodium vivax, causes most of the malaria infections in the Americas (75%). Also, about 53% of the malaria cases found in Southeast Asiais caused by *P. vivax*.

In addition, *P. vivax* presents some challenges as compared to *Plasmodium falciparum* which includes; shortage of accurate diagnostics and its ability to remain dormant in a person's liver among others [2].

Plasmodium malariae is found worldwide and causes a mild form of malaria. It is not as harmful as that caused by *P. falciparum or P. vivax*. Clinical signs associated with P. malariae include fevers that reoccur just about three-day intervals (a quartan fever) and longer than the two-day (tertian) intervals of the other malarial parasites [3]. *Plasmodium malariae* gives rise to a chronic infection that in some cases can last for a long period. The *P. malariae* parasite has diverse variations between it and the other Plasmodium parasites, one being that maximum parasite counts are normally low as compared to those in patients infected with *P. falciparum* or *P. vivax* [4].

Plasmodium ovale causes tertian malaria in humans. It is rare compared to *P. falciparum* and *P. ovale* and substantially less dangerous than *P. falciparum. P. ovale* has recently been shown by genetic methods to consist of two subspecies, *P. ovale curtisi* and *P. ovale wallikeri* [5]. *P. ovale* can infect persons who are negative for the Duffy blood group. This is common in many residents of sub-Saharan.

Africa. This accounts for the significant prevalence of *P. ovale* in most of Africa rather than *P. vivax* [6].

Plasmodium knowlesi causes malaria in humans and other primates. The natural warm-blooded hosts of *P. knowlesi* are various monkeys and humans can be infected by *P. knowlesi*. It closely resembles *Plasmodium vivax* as well as other *Plasmodium* species that infect primates other than humans. Individuals with *P. knowlesi* infection can develop uncomplicated or severe malaria comparable to that brought about by *Plasmodium falciparum*. Diagnosis of *P. knowlesi* infection is burdensome as *P. knowlesi* very closely looks like other species that infect humans [7].

2. Treatment of malaria and drug resistance

Malaria is an entirely preventable and treatable ailment. The choice of therapy is dependent mainly on the infecting species, the severity of infection, age of the patient, and susceptibility of parasites to antimalarial therapies, the cost and availability of medicines. The aim of malaria treatment is to ensure rapid and total elimination of the *Plasmodium* parasites from the patient's blood to help prevent the progression of uncomplicated malaria to complicated illness that leads to malaria-related anemia and death. From a public health perspective, treatment is meant to reduce transmission of the infection to others, by reducing the infectious reservoir and preventing the emergence and spread of resistance to antimalarial medicines [8, 9].

Drugs used in the treatment of malaria infection come from the following five groups of chemical compounds: quinolines and aryl amino alcohols, antifolate, artemisinin derivatives, the hydroxynaphthoquinones and antibacterial agents [10].

i. **Quinolines** include 4-aminoquinolines (chloroquine, amodiaquine and piperaquine), 8-aminoquinolines (e.g., primaquine and pamaquine) belong to the quinolines. **Chloroquine** (**Figure 1**), a 4-aminoquinoline manifests its antimalarial activity mostly on the mature trophozoites stage of the parasite by causing inhibition of the hemozoin (Hz) formation from hemoglobin digestion. Free heme causes lysis of membrane and parasite death. The side-effects of chloroquine include pruritus, skin-rashes, cephalgia, gastrointestinal disturbances and rarely bone marrow suppression, alopecia and convulsions [11]. Chloroquine was withdrawn from use because of a

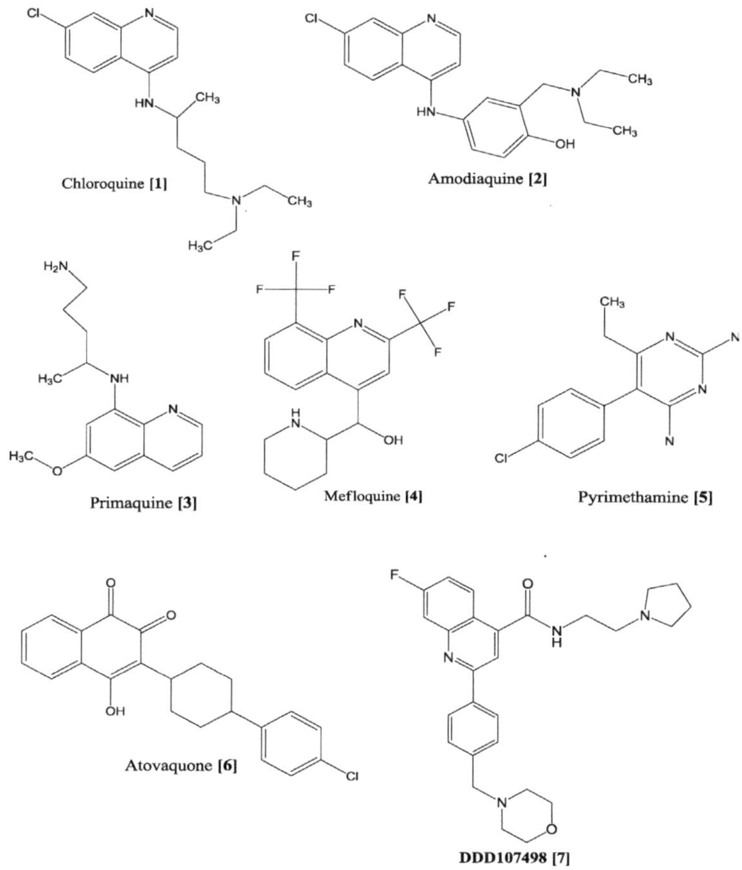

Figure 1.
Chemical structures of some synthetic compounds used as antimalarial.

decline in effectiveness resulting from resistant strains of the plasmodium parasite and fatal side effects [12]. *Plasmodium* parasite resistance against chloroquine and treatment failure is associated with multiple mutations in *Plasmodium falciparum* chloroquine-resistant transporter (PfCRT), a protein that probably functions as a transporter in the parasite's digestive vacuole membrane which results in reduced intracellular drug concentrations [13]. Chloroquine is currently on the Model List of Essential Medicines (MLEM) for the treatment of *P. vivax* infection in regions where resistance has not developed [14]. **Amodiaquine [2]**, also a Mannich base 4-aminoquinoline and its mechanism of action involve the suppression of the breakdown of hemoglobin. The drug also suppresses the glutathione-dependent destruction of ferriprotoporphyrin IX in the malaria parasite, leading to the accumulation of this peptide, which is unsafe to the survival of the parasite. Amodiaquine is therapeutically potent as compared to chloroquine in treating chloroquine-resistant *Plasmodium falciparum* malaria infections. These two drugs were widely used in the past for both prophylaxis and treatment of malaria. However, amodiaquine has serious adverse effects of hepatitis and agranulocytosis associated with its long-term use and therefore not generally recommended in malaria treatment [15]. Resistance to amodiaquine by plasmodium parasite has been associated with single nucleotide polymorphism (SNP) alleles *pfcrt* 76 T, *pfmdr1* 86Y, 184Y and 1246Y (c). Also, PfCRT, has been found to contribute to resistance to amodiaquine [16].

Primaquine [3] is a member of the 8-aminoquinoline range of antimalarials that includes tafenoquine and pamaquine. Primaquine is mainly used in the treatment of *P. vivax* or *P. ovale* malaria, specifically to get rid of the inactive liver forms of these parasites (hypnozoites). To achieve this, a 14-day course of primaquine is required [17]. The usual adverse effects associated with the administration of primaquine include nausea, vomiting, and stomach cramps. The most dangerous adverse effect of primaquine is haemolysis in patients who are deficient in Glucose-6-phosphate dehydrogenase (G6PD) enzyme, Africans or Caucasians of Mediterranean descent. Primaquine is the only antimalarial currently recommended as a therapy in *P vivax* malaria [18]. Resistance to primaquine is known to occur due to CYP-4502D6 mutation, which affects its metabolism and activation [19].

Piperaquine is a bisquinoline compound which was first synthesized in the 1960s and was widely used in China and Southeast Asia (Indochina) as a preventive agent for treatment purposes for over 20 years. Due to resistant strains of *P. falciparum* and the introduction of artemisinin-based antimalarial products, the usage of piperaquine declined [20]. Currently, piperaquine is used in combination with dihydroartemisinin to treat malaria [21]. Piperaquine resistance has been reported and the genetic markers plasmepsin 2 (*pfpm2*), exonuclease (*pfexo*) and chloroquine resistance transporter (*pfcrt*) genes are implicated for the resistance [22].

Mefloquine [4] is a quinoline methanol compound that resembles quinine and it is active against the asexual stages of malaria; however, its precise mode of action is not known. Mefloquine is therapeutically potent as a preventive agent against malaria and is extensively used in therapy against chloroquine-resistant *P. falciparum* malaria infection. Mefloquine is effective against all five strains of malaria parasites known to affect humans [23]. Frequent treatment using mefloquine is associated with asymptomatic, transient serum enzyme elevations in up to 18 per cent of patients. Adverse reactions such as skin-rash and autoantibody formation are also rare. Reported side effects of mefloquine include nausea, vomiting, abdominal pains, dizziness, neurotoxic effects and chronic neuropsychiatric adverse effects [24, 25]. Mefloquine is currently not widely used due to the perception of central nervous system toxicity [23]. Resistance to mefloquine result from increased amplification in *pfmdr1* in falciparum malaria [26].

ii. **Arylaminoalcohols.** Quinine, quinidine, mefloquine, lumefantrine and halofantrine, belong to the arylamino alcohols. **Quinine** is a drug obtained from the stem bark of the cinchona tree and was the first therapy used for malaria [27]. The most common adverse effects of quinine involve a group of symptoms called cinchonism; headache, vasodilation and sweating, nausea, tinnitus, hearing impairment, vertigo or dizziness, blurred vision, and interference in color perception. Quinine is a common cause of drug-induced disorders, including thrombocytopenia and thrombotic microangiopathy [28]. Quinine can also have severe adverse effects involving multiple organ systems, among which are immune system effects and fever, hypotension, haemolytic anemia, acute kidney injury, liver toxicity, and blindness. Quinine excites the secretion of insulin and may lead to hyperglycaemia which is a risk in pregnancy [29]. The mode of action of quinine is not clear but it is believed to interfere with the parasite's ability to breakdown hemoglobin leading to the inhibition of self-generated formation of beta-haematin (haemozoin or malaria pigment) which is a poisonous product of the breakdown of hemoglobin by the parasite [10]. Quinine is currently not used as front-line therapy for malaria due to the high-quality evidence of the efficacy superiority of artesunate over quinine in adults and children with severe malaria [21]. There is currently inadequate data on resistance to quinine in malaria therapy [30, 31].

iii. **Antifolate**. The principal antifolates are pyrimethamine **[5]** (PYR), proguanil (PG; broken-down *in vivo* to the active form cycloguanil [CG]) and Dapsone. The sulfa drugs, the most significant of the antifolate are the outstanding, sulfadoxine (SDX), and the sulfone, dapsone. Antifolates were initially made available in the late 1960, and established to be of long-term use, particularly, as a low-cost substitute to combat the CQ-resistant parasites that were distributed across Africa from the late 1970s onwards [32]. Currently, antifolate are not widely used as a preventative therapy because of high levels of resistance [33]. Resistance to *antifolate* drugs is linked to point mutations in the dihydrofolate reductase domain of the dihydrofolate-thymidylate synthetase (DHFR-TS) gene and dihydropteroate synthase region of the pyrophosphokinase-dihydropteroate synthetase (PPK-DHPS) gene of the *malaria* parasite [34].

iv. **Hydroxy naphthoquinones** have been widely investigated over the past 50 years for their anti-malarial effect [35]. Atovaquone **[6]** is a hydroxyl naphthoquinone that is used in combination with proguanil for prophylaxis and therapy of uncomplicated malaria [36]. Atovaquone has outstanding anti-malarial property but demonstrates poor pharmaceutical activities, such as poor bioavailability and high plasma protein binding. The mechanism of action of atovaquone is through the prevention of the electron transport system at the level of cytochrome BC1 complex. Atovaquone also ensures the breakdown of the parasite mitochondrial membrane potential. Atovaquone is used as a fixed-dose combination with proguanil for the treatment of uncomplicated malaria. No serious or life-threatening adverse effects have been reported. Hydroxy naphthoquinones are taken one dose per day and for 7 consecutive days [6, 37]. Resistance to naphthoquinones has been attributed to a single-point mutation in the cytochrome b (*Pfcytb*) gene [38].

v. **Artemisinin** and its derivatives (Artesunate, Artemether, and Dihydroartemisinin) represent a new category of antimalarials. Fixed-dose formulations (combining two different active ingredients co-formulated in one tablet, Artesunate-Amodiaquine and Artemether-Lumefantrine are ideally favored and recommended over co-blistered, co-packaged or loose tablet combinations since it enhances adherence to treatment and cuts down the possible use of the individual components of co-blistered drugs as monotherapy [39]. The WHO advocates for the use of artemisinin-based combination therapies (ACTs) for the treatment of uncomplicated malaria caused by the *P. falciparum* parasite. ACTs are the most therapeutically potent antimalarial medicines available today [40]. The current trend in the treatment of uncomplicated malaria caused by *P. falciparum* is the use of ACTs with one of the following artemisinin-based combination therapies:

- Artesunate+Amodiaquine (AS-AQ)
- Artemether+Lumefantrine (A-L)

- Dihydroartemisinin+Piperaquine (DHAP).
- Artesunate+Mefloquine
- Artesunate+ Sulfadoxine+Pyrimethamine [32].

Artemisinin-based Combination Therapy (ACTs) has been used since the year 2004 for the treatment of uncomplicated malaria. This initiative was important because the malaria parasite became resistant to Chloroquine and other monotherapies. Artemisinin is administered in combination with a second, long-acting antimalarial to enhance treatment and protect against the development of drug resistance [33]. Quite recently the malaria parasite has developed resistance to artemisinin. Reasons for artemisinin resistance include uncontrolled use of artemisinin-based combination therapy (ACT), mobile populations and migrants, artemisinin monotherapy, the use of subtherapeutic levels of artemisinin, substandard and counterfeit drugs, high treatment cost, and co-use of artemisinin derivates as prophylactic agents [41].

2.1 New product under development

DDD107498 is a compound with the chemical name 6-Fluoro-2-[4-(4-morpholinylmethyl) phenyl]-N-[2-(1-pyrrolidinyl) ethyl]-4-quinolinecarboxamide. It is a novel chemical compound developed based on a 2, 6-disubstituted quinoline-4-carboxamide scaffold against the blood stage of the multi-drug-sensitive *Plasmodium falciparum* 3D7 strain. The compound has a powerful and wide spectrum of antimalarial activity against varied life-cycle phases of the *Plasmodium* parasite, with better pharmacokinetic activities and a satisfactory safety profile. DDD107498 has sub-micromolar efficacy against parasites. The compound has shown marked activity against 3D7 strain parasites. DDD107498 averted the development of trophozoites and schizonts. It is also effective against several drug-resistant strains. It is more effective as compared to artesunate in (*ex vivo)* assays against a range of clinical isolates of both *P. falciparum* and *P. vivax* and is not toxic to human cells [42–44]. DDD107498 which is now called M5717 entered the first stages of human clinical trials in 2017 (**Figure 1**).

3. Guidelines for the treatment of malaria

Ideally, treatment of malaria should not be initiated until the diagnosis has been established by laboratory testing. Therefore, without prior laboratory testing to confirm the presence of the parasite, treatment, should only be reserved for extreme circumstances, such as strong clinical suspicion of severe disease in a setting where there are no prompt laboratory services to confirm a diagnosis. The following factors should act as a guide in the treatment of malaria:

- the Plasmodium species causing the infection;
- the clinical condition of the patient;
- the anticipated drug responsiveness of the infecting parasite as determined by the geographic location where the infection was acquired; and
- the previous utilization of antimalarials, including those taken for malaria chemoprophylaxis [45].

Treatment of malaria is dependents on the species responsible for the malaria, as well as on the seriousness of the disease. The World Health Organization's protocols for the treatment of malaria provides recommendations on topics such as:

- Treatment of uncomplicated malaria caused by *P. falciparum*
- Treatment of uncomplicated malaria caused by *P. vivax*
- Treatment of severe malaria
- Mass drug administration

4. Modes of treatment

Treatment of malaria involves two principal concepts which are suppressive and radical treatments.

4.1 Suppressive treatment

The symptoms of malaria are relieved by suppressing the erythrocytic stage of the parasitic development in the suppressive treatment. This involves the administration of appropriate blood schizonticidal agents. In all cases of non-falciparum malaria (*P. vivax*, *P. ovale*, P. malariae and *P. knowlesi*), it consists of the administration of chloroquine. Also, presumptive treatment for malaria involves administration of blood schizonticidal medicines, such as chloroquine, to suspected cases of malaria, followed by full treatment after confirmation. This plan of action has been abandoned in recent years [45].

4.2 Radical treatment

Radical treatment involves the administration of primaquine to all confirmed cases of malaria [45].

5. Treatment of uncomplicated malaria caused by *P. falciparum*

Uncomplicated malaria is defined as a patient having symptoms of malaria and a positive parasitological test (microscopy or RDT) but with no clinical manifestation of severe malaria. The clinical goals of treating uncomplicated malaria are to seek to the total elimination of all parasites from the body as rapidly as possible followed by preventing progression to severe disease. The public health goals of treatment are to prevent onward transmission of the infection to others, prevent the emergence and spread of resistance to antimalarial medicines [46].

The WHO recommends that children and adults with uncomplicated *P. falciparum* malaria (except pregnant women in their first trimester) are to be treated with one of the following recommended ACTs:

- Artemether + Lumefantrine
- Artesunate + Amodiaquine
- Artesunate + Mefloquine

- Dihydroartemisinin + Piperaquine
- Artesunate + Sulfadoxine–Pyrimethamine (SP).

The duration of ACT treatment regimens should provide 3 days' treatment with an artemisinin-derivative [46].

Pregnant women with uncomplicated *P. falciparum* malaria during the first trimester are to be treated for 7 days with quinine + clindamycin. Also, infants weighing less than 5 kg are to be treated with an ACT at the same mg/kg body weight target dose as for children weighing 5 kg. In addition, people with HIV/AIDS and having uncomplicated *P. falciparum* malaria, should avoid artesunate + SP if they are also receiving co-trimoxazole, also, they are to avoid artesunate + amodiaquine if they are also receiving efavirenz or zidovudine [46].

6. Treatment of uncomplicated malaria caused by *P. vivax*

The utilization of artemether-lumefantrine, atovaquone-proguanil, or quinine sulfate with doxycycline or tetracycline (or clindamycin for pregnant women and children <8 years old), are recommended treatment for uncomplicated malaria caused by *P. vivax*. Also, mefloquine can be used if no other options are available. In addition, primaquine phosphate can be used in combination with any of the medication options for treatment of the acute phase of infection [46].

7. Treatment of severe malaria

Patients with clinical manifestations and features of severe malaria; coma, hemoglobin of less than 7 g/dL, acute kidney injury, acute respiratory distress syndrome, shock, acidosis, jaundice should be treated promptly and aggressively with parenteral antimalarial therapy regardless of the species of malaria noted. All patients with severe malaria, regardless of infecting species, should be treated with intravenous (IV) artesunate [47].

The objective of management of severe malaria infection is to prevent deaths from the direct effect of the disease or its complications through the use of appropriate emergency supportive measures, diagnostics and the recommended anti-malaria medications. The goals of management of severe/complicated malaria are to provide:

- Urgent treatment of life-threatening problems.
- Anti-malarial treatment which is specific for severe/complicated malaria.
- Appropriate supportive care throughout illness [47].

8. Mass drug administration

Mass drug administration (MDA) is defined as the provision of a therapeutic dose of an effective anti-malarial medication to the entire target population, irrespective of infection status or symptoms. The MDA is a strategy recommended by the WHO for the elimination of *Plasmodium falciparum* malaria in areas approaching interruption of transmission, as well as where multidrug resistance is present, given the prerequisites of good access to case management, effective vector control and surveillance, and limited potential for reintroduction [48].

9. Conclusion

The treatment of malaria infection involves the utilization of various medicines and combinations however, the choice of medication is dependent on several factors, including the specific species of parasite identified, the severity of symptoms, and determination of drug resistance based on the geographic area. The anti-malarial used are administered in pill form or as an intravenous depending on the above factors. The most commonly utilized antimalarial medications are artemisinin, its derivatives and combinations. Artemisinin's are more effective acting anti-malarial agents killing young parasites. It has also been used successfully for the treatment of severe malaria. In cases of parasite resistance to drugs, combination therapies are used. In addition, malaria parasites, such as *P. vivax* and *P. ovale*, have liver stages where the parasite can live in the body for an extended period and reactivate at a later date causing a relapse of the infection. In situations like this, a second medication to prevent a relapse in the future is administered.

Acknowledgements

Thanks goes to the editor and management members of IntechOpen for the opportunity.

Conflicts of Interest

The authors declare that they have no conflicts of interest.

Abbreviations

ACT	Artemisinin-based Combination Therapy
CG	Cycloguanill
CQ	Chloroquine
CYP	Cytochrome
DHFR-TS	Dihydrofolate-Thymidylate Synthetase
G6PD	Glucose-6-phosphate dehydrogenase
MLEM	Model List of Essential Medicines
PfCRT	*Plasmodium falciparum* chloroquine resistant transporter
PG	Proguanil
PPK-DHPS	Pyrophosphokinase-Dihydropteroate Synthetase
PYR	Pyrimethamine
RDT	Rapid Diagnostic Test
SDX	Sulfadoxine
SNP	Single Nucleotide Polymorphism
WHO	World Health Organization

Author details

Bernard Kofi Turkson[1*], Alfred Ofori Agyemang[2], Desmond Nkrumah[3], Reinhard Isaac Nketia[3], Michael Frimpong Baidoo[2] and Merlin Lincoln Kwao Mensah[1]

1 Department of Herbal Medicine, Faculty of Pharmacy and Pharmaceutical Sciences, Kwame Nkrumah University of Science and Technology, Kumasi, Ghana

2 Institute of Traditional and Alternative Medicine, University of Health and Allied Sciences, Ho, Ghana

3 Department of Pharmacognosy, Faculty of Pharmacy and Pharmaceutical Sciences, Kwame Nkrumah University of Science and Technology, Kumasi, Ghana

*Address all correspondence to: bentsi2000@yahoo.com

References

[1] WHO. Meeting report of the WHO Evidence Review Group on mass drug administration for malaria: 11-13, Geneva, Switzerland. Geneva: World Health Organization; 2018. p. 2019.

[2] Worldwide Antimalarial Resistance Network. Malaria Drug Resistance. 2020. https://www.wwarn.org/about-us/malaria-drug-resistance. Accessed March 09, 2021.

[3] Mohapatra PK, Prakash A, Bhattacharyya DR, Goswami BK, Ahmed A, Sarmah B, Mahanta J. Detection and molecular confirmation of a focus of *Plasmodium malariae* in Arunachal Pradesh, India. The Indian Journal of Medical Research. 2008. 128 (1): 52-6.

[4] Collins WE, Jeffery GM. *"Plasmodium malariae: parasite and disease"*. Clinical Microbiology Reviews. 2007. **20** (4): 579-592. *doi:10.1128/CMR.00027-07*.

[5] Sutherland CJ, Tanomsing N, Nolder D, Oguike M, Jennison C, Pukrittayakamee S."Two nonrecombining sympatric forms of the human malaria parasite Plasmodium ovale occur globally". The Journal of Infectious Diseases. 2010. 201 (10): 1544-1550. doi:10.1086/652240.

[6] https://www.cdc.gov/malaria/about/biology/index.html.

[7] Garrido-Cardenas JA, Gonzalez-Ceron L, Manzano-Agugliaro F, Mesa-Valle C (January 2019). "Plasmodium genomics: an approach for learning about and ending human malaria". Parasitology Research. Springer. 2019. **118** (1): 1-27. *doi:10.1007/s00436-018-6127-9*.

[8] Ishengoma DR, Rwegoshora RT, Mdira KY, Kamugisha ML, Anga EO, Bygbjerg IC, Ronn AM, Magesa SM. Health Laboratories in the Tanga Region of Tanzania: The Quality of Diagnostic Services for Malaria and other Communicable Diseases. Ann Trop Med Parasitol. 2009. 103: 441-453. DOI: 10.1179/136485909X451726.

[9] WHO. Treating malaria. 2013. https://www.who.int/activities/treating-malaria. Accessed March 09, 2021.

[10] Salfi M.H, Beg T, Harrath A.H, Altayalan F.S.H and Al Quraishy S. Antimalarial Drugs: Mode of Action and Status of Resistance. African journal of Pharmacy and Pharmacology. 2013. Vol. 7. No. 5. Pp. 148-156. DOI: 10.5897/AJPPX12.015.

[11] Tripathi KD. Essentials of Medical Pharmacology. 6th Edition. Jaypee Brothers Medical Publishers (P) Ltd. 2006. Pp. 780-796.

[12] Fröberg, G., Jörnhagen, L., Morris, U. *et al.* Decreased prevalence of *Plasmodium falciparum* resistance markers to amodiaquine despite its wide scale use as ACT partner drug in Zanzibar. Malar J **11,** 321 (2012). https://doi.org/10.1186/1475-2875-11-321.

[13] Thomas E. Wellems, Christopher V. Plowe. Chloroquine-Resistant Malaria. The Journal of Infectious Diseases. 2001. Vol. 184. No. 6. Pp. 770-776. doi.org/10.1086/322858.

[14] Martin RE, Marchetti RV, Cowan AL. Chloroquine Transport via the Malaria Parasite's Chloroquine Resistance Transporter. Science. 2009. Vol. 325. No. 5948. Pp. 1680-1682. DOI: 10.1126/science.1175667.

[15] Parhizgar AR and Tahghighi A. Introducing New Antimalarial Analogues of Chloroquine and Amodiaquine: A Narrative Review. Iranian Journal of Medical Sciences. 2017. Vol. 42. No. 2. Pp. 115-128.

[16] Ecker A, Lehane AM, Clain J, Fidock DA. PfCRT and its role in antimalarial drug resistance. Trends Parasitol. 2012;28:504-514.

[17] Baird JK, Rieckmann KH. "Can Primaquine Therapy for Vivax Malaria be Improved?" Trends Parasitol. 2003. 19 (3): 115-120). DOI: 10.1016/s1471-4922(03)00005-9.

[18] Recht Judith, Elizabeth A. Ashley and Nicholas J. White. Use of Primaquine and Glucose-6-Phosphate Dehydrogenase Deficiency Testing: Divergent Policies and Practices in Malaria Endemic Countries. PLoS Negl Trop Dis. 2018. 12(4): e0006230. DOI: 10.1371/journal.pntd.0006230.

[19] Christopher Dijanic, Jillian Nickerson, Sunita Shakya, Amanda Dijanic, Marilyn Fabbri, "Relapsing Malaria: A Case Report of Primaquine Resistance", Case Reports in Infectious Diseases. 2018. https://doi.org/10.1155/2018/9720823.

[20] Davis TM, Hung TY, Sim IK, Karunajeewa HA, Ilett KF. "Piperaquine: A Resurgent Antimalarial Drug". Drugs. 2005. Vol. 65. No. 1. Pp. 75-87. DOI: 10.2165/00003495-200565010-00004.

[21] WHO. Guidelines for the Treatment of Malaria. 3rd Ed. World Health Organization. 2015. Pp. 33-34.

[22] Boonyalai, N., Vesely, B.A., Thamnurak, C. *et al.* Piperaquine resistant Cambodian *Plasmodium falciparum* clinical isolates: in vitro genotypic and phenotypic characterization. Malar J **19,** 269 (2020). https://doi.org/10.1186/s12936-020-03339-w.

[23] WHO. Available at https://www.who.int/malaria/areas/treatment/overview/en/. World Health Organization. 2018. Accessed January 11, 2021.

[24] Ritchie E. Cameron, J. Block, and R. Lee Nevin. "Psychiatric side effects of mefloquine: applications to forensic psychiatry," Journal of the American Academy of Psychiatry and the Law. 2013. Vol. 41. No. 2. Pp. 224-235.

[25] Nevin RL. Idiosyncratic Quinoline Central Nervous System Toxicity: Historical insights into the Chronic Neurological Sequelae of Mefloquine. Int J Parasitol Drugs Drug Resist. 2014. 4: 118-125. DOI: 10.1016/j.ijpddr.2014.03.002.

[26] Price, R. N., Uhlemann, A. C., Brockman, A., McGready, R., Ashley, E., Phaipun, L., Patel, R., Laing, K., Looareesuwan, S., White, N. J., Nosten, F., & Krishna, S. (2004). Mefloquine resistance in Plasmodium falciparum and increased pfmdr1 gene copy number. Lancet (London, England), *364*(9432), 438-447. https://doi.org/10.1016/S0140-6736(04)16767-6.

[27] Nevin RL, Croft AM. Psychiatric effects of malaria and anti-malarial drugs: historical and modern perspectives. Malar J. 2016. Vol. 5. Pp. 332.

[28] Achan, J., Talisuna, A. O., Erhart, A., Yeka, A., Tibenderana, J. K., Baliraine. Quinine, an Old Anti-Malarial Drug in a Modern World: Role in the Treatment of Malaria. Malar J. 2011. Issue10. Pp. 144. DOI: 10.1186/1475-2875-10-144.

[29] Reese Jessica A, Daniel W Bougie, Brian R Curtis, Deirdra R Terrell, Sara K Vesely, Richard H Aster, James N George. Drug-induced thrombotic Microangiopathy: Experience of the Oklahoma Registry and the BloodCenter of Wisconsin. Am J Hematol. 2015. Vol. 90. No.5. 406-410. DOI: 10.1002/ajh.23960.

[30] Kremsner, P. G., Winkler, S., Wildhng, E., Prada, J., Bienzle, U., Graninger, W. Quinine plus

Clindamycin improves Chemotherapy of Severe Malaria in Children. Antimicrob Agents Chemother. 2012. Vol. 39. No. 7. Pp. 1603-1605. DOI: 10.1128/aac.39.7.1603.

[31] Tinto H, Rwagacondo C, Karema C, Mupfasoni D, Vandoren W, Rusanganwa E, Erhart A, Van Overmeir C, Van Marck E, D'Alessandro U: In-vitro susceptibility of Plasmodium falciparum to monodes ethylamodiaquine, dihydroartemisinin and quinine in an area of high chloroquine resistance in Rwanda. Trans R Soc Trop Med Hyg. 2006, 100 (6): 509-514. 10.1016/j.trstmh.2005.09.018.

[32] Toure AO, Kone LP, Jambou R, Konan TD, Demba S, Beugre GE, Kone M: [In vitro susceptibility of P. falciparum isolates from Abidjan (Cote d'Ivoire) to quinine, artesunate and chloroquine]. Sante. 2008, 18 (1): 43-47.

[33] Hyde JE. Drug-resistant Malaria – An Insight. FEBS J. 2007. 274(18), 4688-4698.

[34] Lumb V, Das MK, Singh N, Dev V, Khan W, Sharma YD. Multiple origins of *Plasmodium falciparum* dihydropteroate synthetase mutant alleles associated with sulfadoxine resistance in India. Antimicrob Agents Chemother. 2011. Vol. 55. Pp. 2813-2817.

[35] Triglia T, Cowman AF: Primary structure and expression of the dihydropteroate synthetase gene of Plasmodium falciparum. Proc Natl Acad Sci U S A. 1994, 91: 7149-7153. 10.1073/pnas.91.15.7149.

[36] Srivastava IK, Rottenberg H, Vaidya AB. Atovaquone, a Broad Spectrum Antiparasitic Drug, Collapses Mitochondrial Potential in a Malarial Parasite. J Biol Chem. 1997. Issue 272. Pp. 3961-3966. DOI: 10.1074/jbc.272.7.3961.

[37] Baggish AL, Hill DR. Antiparasitic Agent Atovaquone. Antimicrob Agents Chemother. 2002. 46:1163-1173. DOI: 10.1128/aac.46.5.1163-1173.2002.

[38] Dressman JB and Reppas C. In Vitro-in vivo Correlations for Lipophilic, Poorly Water-soluble Drugs. Eur J Pharm Sci. 2000. 11 Suppl 2: S73-S80. DOI: 10.1016/s0928-0987(00)00181-0.

[39] Fivelman QL, Butcher GA, Adagu IS, Warhurst DC, Pasvol G. Malarone treatment failure and in vitro confirmation of resistance of *Plasmodium falciparum* isolate from Lagos, Nigeria. Malar J. 2002; 1:1.

[40] WHO. Fact sheet N°387 March 2014. World Health Organization.

[41] Ministry of Health (MOH). Guidelines for case management of malaria in Ghana. Ministry of Health edition 3rd. 2014.

[42] Cosima Chrubasik, Raymond L Jacobson. The development of artemisinin resistance in malaria: reasons and solutions. Phytother Res. 2010. Vol. 24. No. 7. Pp. 1104-6. doi: 10.1002/ptr.3133.

[43] Baragana B, Irene Hallyburton, Marcus C. S. Lee, Neil R. Norcross1, Raffaella Grimaldi, Thomas D. Otto. A Novel Multiple-Stage Antimalarial Agent that Inhibits Protein Synthesis. Nature. Macmillan Publishers Limited. 2015. Vol. 22. No. 7556. Pp. 315-331. DOI.org/10.1038/nature14451.

[44] www.glixxlabs.com. Accessed May 2, 2019.

[45] Medicines for Malaria Venture (MMV) (2018). forps://www.mmv.org/node/12787/overlay. Accessed December 12, 2019.

[46] https://www.cdc.gov/malaria/diagnosis_treatment/clinicians1.html.

[47] www.malariasite.com/
treatment-of-malaria.

[48] WHO. Meeting report of the WHO Evidence Review Group on mass drug administration for malaria: 11-13, Geneva, Switzerland. Geneva: World Health Organization; 2018.

Section 2

Molecular Markers of Drug Resistance and Stable Resistance Phenotype

Chapter 6

P. falciparum and Its Molecular Markers of Resistance to Antimalarial Drugs

Peter Hodoameda

Abstract

The use of molecular markers of resistance to monitor the emergence, and the spread of parasite resistance to antimalarial drugs is a very effective way of monitoring antimalarial drug resistance. The identification and validation of molecular markers have boosted our confidence in using these tools to monitor resistance. For example, *P. falciparum* chloroquine resistance transporter (PfCRT), *P. falciparum* multidrug resistance protein 1 (PfMDR1), *P. falciparum* multidrug *kelch 13* (*pfk13*), have been identified as molecular markers of resistance to chloroquine, lumefantrine, and artemisinin respectively. The mechanism of resistance to antimalarial drugs is mostly by; (1) undergoing mutations in the parasite genome, leading to expelling the drug from the digestive vacuole, or (2) loss of binding affinity between the drug and its target. Increased copy number in the *pfmdr1* gene also leads to resistance to antimalarial drugs. The major cause of the widespread chloroquine and sulfadoxine-pyrimethamine resistance globally is the spread of parasites resistant to these drugs from Southeast Asia to Africa, the Pacific, and South America. Only a few mutations in the parasite genome lead to resistance to chloroquine and sulfadoxine-pyrimethamine arising from indigenous parasites in Africa, Pacific, and South America.

Keywords: Plasmodium falciparum, molecular marker of resistance, antimalarial drugs, Polymerase chain reaction, DNA sequencing

1. Introduction

The monitoring and identification of drug-resistant *P. falciparum* strains is paramount to the fight against malaria. The traditional identification of resistant parasite strains is by *in vivo* and/or *in vivo* drug susceptibility assays. Although these methods are effective in identifying resistant strains, they are faced with an array of challenges. The most profound challenge being faced by both *in vivo* and *in vitro* techniques is the cost and time associated with them. Since malaria is mostly endemic in poor countries, it is imperative to identify cost-friendly methods for the surveillance and identification of resistant parasites.

One method that shows a lot of promise in the identification of resistant parasite strains is the use of polymerase chain reaction and sequencing techniques to identify the molecular markers of resistance that are associated with resistance to a particular antimalarial drug (s). The ever-improving knowledge in malaria parasite genomics has made it possible to identify mutations that are associated with resistance to antimalarial drugs. Identification of these markers in resistant strains and the validation of these markers using genome editing techniques such as Crispr-Cas9 have been possible, making us confident that, a parasite will be resistant to an antimalarial drug when the molecular marker of resistance-associated to it is identified in the parasite, without the performance of *in vitro* drug susceptibility assay. The use of molecular markers of resistance in identifying parasite-resistant strains has not just made it possible to identify resistant parasite strains, but also to predict how fast a resistant strain is emerging and how fast it is spreading. From the aforementioned advantages, it is clear that the most cost-friendly, time-saving, high through-put, and robust technique to use in identifying the emergence and spread of a resistance parasite strain by PCR and sequencing techniques to identify molecular markers of resistance to antimalarial drugs.

This chapter will focus on the *Plasmodium* parasite molecular markers of resistance responsible for antimalarial drug resistance. The mechanism of resistance due to mutations or increase in copy number in the molecular markers of resistance to the different antimalarial drugs will be elaborated. The epidemiology of different molecular markers will be also addressed.

2. Molecular markers of resistance to Quinoline-based drugs

2.1 *P. falciparum* chloroquine resistance transporter (*pfcrt*)

The *P. falciparum* Chloroquine Resistance Transporter (*pfcrt*) gene is a putative transporter, has a weight of 49 kDa, is a member of the drug transporter superfamily, and localized to the parasite digestive vacuole [1, 2]. Mutations within the *pfcrt* are the primary responsible for resistance to chloroquine. This was identified after a genetic cross experiment between CQ-sensitive HB3 and CQ-resistant Dd2 clones. Genetic analysis of the CQ-resistant progeny identified mutation in a single genetic locus on chromosome 7. A quantitative trait loci (QTL) analysis mapped a mutation on the 13-exon of the *pfcrt* gene [1, 3]. Studies by [4] have confirmed that mutation in the *pfcrt* gene is associated with chloroquine resistance in a genome-wide association study. A single mutation, resulting in the change in amino acid from K76T confers resistance to CQ in both labs adapted and field isolated *P. falciparum* strains. Removal of this mutation in CQ-resistant strains (Dd2 from Southeast Asia and 7G8 from South Africa) resulted in the total loss of resistance to chloroquine in these strains [5].

The mechanism of CQ resistance after the replacement of a positively charged lysine (K) with a neutral threonine (T) results in the expulsion of deprotonated CQ out of the digestive vacuole. The expulsion is achieved through either active transport or facilitated diffusion. This results in decreasing access of the CQ to heme, which is its target [6].

There are other mutations in the *pfcrt* gene which introduce different amino acids in the wild-type amino acids CVMNK, which compensates for the altered PfCRT function due to *pfcrt* K76T mutation and may subsequently modulate drug susceptibility in the parasite. These mutations occur in the surroundings of K76T (position 72–76). These mutations that occur at positions 72–76 may be unique to a particular geographic location. For example, the CVIET mutations at positions 72–76 are mostly found in parasites from Africa and Southeast Asia, while the SVMNT mutations at position 72–76 are found in South America, the Philippines, and Papua New Guinea [7].

The use of *pfcrt* K76T mutations in epidemiology surveillance does not only apply to chloroquine resistance but also some partner drugs used in artemisinin-based combination therapy. For example, the introduction of mutant *pfcrt* into CQ-sensitive GC03 strain resulted in reduced susceptibility to both amodiaquine and its primary metabolite desethylamodiaquine (DEAQ) [8]. Studies conducted by [9] using field isolates showed the selection of *pfcrt* K76T in AQ recrudescence treatment outcome. Parasite resistance to AQ or DEAQ is not solely dependent on *pfcrt* mutation, but rather a combination of mutation(s) in both the *pfcrt* and *pfmdr1* gene [10].

The *pfcrt* K76T mutation does not only results in resistance to CQ and AQ but also results in increased susceptibility to lumefantrine [11], quinine, halofantrine, mefloquine, artemisinin and its derivatives [8, 12].

2.2 *P. falciparum* multidrug resistance protein 1

The *P. falciparum* multidrug resistance protein 1 (*pfmdr1*) is a member of the ATP-binding cassette (ABC). The *pfmdr1* is also known as the P-glycoproteins homolog 1 (Pgh-1) [6]. The PfMDR1 is localized in the membrane of the DV. The PfMDR1 is a transporter and functions by regulating drug accumulation in the parasite's DV [6].

The *pfmdr1* plays a very important role in the parasite response to different antimalarial drugs. The two mechanisms used by the *pfmdr1* gene to regulate antimalarial drug response are through increased *pfmdr1* copy number or by introducing mutations in the gene. Increased copy number of *pfmdr1* has been associated with reduced *in vitro* susceptibility to halofantrine, quinine, mefloquine, dihydroartemisinin, and artesunate [13]. Most importantly, increased *pfmdr1* copy number in clinical isolates is the cause of mefloquine monotherapy [14] or artesunate-mefloquine combination treatment failures [15]. The validation of increased *pfmdr1* copy number and its involvement in mefloquine, lumefantrine, halofantrine, quinine, and artemisinin resistance was proven in an experiment that involved the knockout of one of the two copies of drug-resistant FCB strains, resulting in the reversal of its resistance to make it susceptible to mefloquine, lumefantrine, halofantrine, quinine, and artemisinin [16].

The polymorphisms which occur in different haplotypes of *pfmdr1* result in resistance to different antimalarial drugs. These mutations alter the substrate specificity of *pfmdr1* [17]. The *pfmdr1* N86Y mutation has been associated with CQ and AQ treatment failure, although the association to CQ is weak [18]. The *pfmdr1* D1246Y have been reported to be involved in resistance to AQ/DEAQ. In East Africa, the *pfmdr1* 86Y-184Y-1246Y haplotype was selected for an AQ recrudescence treatment outcome [19]. In other studies using field isolates from Columbia observed high AQ IC_{50} for parasites with *pfmdr1* D1246Y [20]. The *pfmdr1* N86-F184-D1246 haplotype is associated with resistance to lumefantrine in Africa [21, 22] whiles the *pfmdr1* N1042D was associated with increased in vitro lumefantrine IC_{50} values in isolates from the Thai-Myanmar border [23]. The *pfmdr1* S1034C/N1042D/D1246Y mutations are associated with reduced susceptibility to quinine [24]. The *pfmdr1* and *pfcrt* alleles may interact to confer higher resistance to AQ and DEAQ [10].

2.3 *P. falciparum* multidrug resistance-associated protein (PfMRP)

The *P. falciparum* Multidrug Resistance-Associated Protein (*pfmrp*) belongs to the ABC transporter family [25]. The *pfmrp* acts as a transport regulatory protein. Mutations in the *pfmrp* have been associated with resistance to some antimalarial drugs such as quinine and chloroquine [25]. The Y191H and A437S have been shown to have a weak association to CQ-resistance in Asia and the Americas respectfully, while Y191H and A437S are associated with quinine resistance in the Americas. Recent studies have also reported the selection of *pfmrp* 856I alleles following the use of artemether-lumefantrine for the treatment of malaria [26]. The *pfmrp* 1466 K has been reported in sulfadoxine-pyrimethamine recrudescence treatment outcome [26].

The validation of the contribution of *pfmrp* to quinine and CQ resistance was reported by [27] after showing that knock out of PfMRP in CQ-resistant strain W2 rendered the parasite to be susceptible to CQ and quinine. Parasite with disrupted PfMRP also showed reduced IC_{50} values for primaquine, piperaquine, and artemisinin. The reduced IC_{50} for these drugs was modest, showing a reduced IC_{50} ranging from 38–57%. These may suggest that *pfmrp* might act as a secondary determinant in the modulation of parasite resistance to these antimalarial drugs [28].

2.4 *P. falciparum* Na+/H + exchanger 1 (*Pfnhe-1*)

The *P. falciparum* Na^+/H^+ exchanger 1 (*Pfnhe-1*) gene is a putative Na^+/H^+ exchanger found on chromosome 13 in the parasite genome. Some polymorphisms in the *pfnhe-1* are involved in resistance to some antimalarial drugs whiles other polymorphisms result in increased susceptibility to other antimalarial drugs [3]. Parasites with the D-and N-rich polymorphism (microsatellite ms4760–1) have been reported to be resistant to quinine in clinical isolates from Asia, Southeast Asia, and Central and South America [3]. Resistance to quinine by this locus is ambiguous, with some scientists reporting increased quinine IC50 values in one study [29], and decreased quinine IC_{50} values in another study [30].

The destruction of *pfnhe-1* in CQ and quinine resistant parasite strains 1BB5 and 3BA6 lead to an approximately 30% decrease in quinine mean IC_{50} values, but the knockdown of *pfnhe-1* in CQ-sensitive GC03 strain did not lead to the reduction in quinine mean IC_{50} values [31]. These results suggest that *pfnhe-1* contributes to quinine resistance in a strain-specific manner, and also other parasite genetic background factors are required for quinine resistance in parasites [28].

2.5 Plasmepsin II &III (*pfmp2* and *pfmp3*)

The plasmepsins are aspartic proteases in *P. falciparum* that are involved in the degradation of hemoglobin. They are approximately 38-kDa in weight. The *pfmp2* and *pfmp3*cleave hemoglobin in the parasite's digestive vacuole [32]. Piperaquine, an aminoquinoline drug targets the *pfmp2* and *pfmp3* to inhibit them as its mode of action. An increase in *pfmp2* and *pfmp3* copy numbers have been associated with piperaquine resistance [33].

3. Molecular markers for resistance to antifolates

The antifolates used in malaria treatment are pyrimethamine, sulfadoxine, and proguanil. The proguanil is a cycloguanil metabolite that functions by interfering with folate metabolism [34]. The mode of action of pyrimethamine and cycloguanil is by inhibiting the dihydrofolate reductase (DHFR) enzyme, whiles sulfadoxine acts by inhibiting the dihydropteroate synthase (DHPS) enzyme, all involved in the folate metabolism pathway [34]. The sulfadoxine–pyrimethamine is used in a combination therapy to treat CQ-resistant parasites mostly in pregnant women in most malaria-endemic countries in Africa [34, 35].

Mutations in the DHFR are associated with resistance to pyrimethamine and cycloguanil, while mutations in DHPS are associated with sulfadoxine [36]. The *pfdhfr* S108N, N51I, C59R, and I164L are associated with pyrimethamine resistance, while *pfdhfr* A16V/S108T confers greater resistance to cycloguanil compared to pyrimethamine [37]. The quadruple mutant (S108N/N51I/C59R/I164L combination), which is mostly found in Asia but rare in Africa confers high levels of resistance to sulfadoxine–pyrimethamine [38]. The *pfdhps* S436A/F, A437G, K540E, A581G, and A613S/T mutations have been associated with resistance to sulfadoxine, with the *pfdhps* A437G mutation observed either alone or in combination with other mutations in field isolates [39]. The amplification of GTP-cyclohydrolase I, a gene involved in the upstream biosynthesis of folate is mostly seen with the *pfdhfr* I164L mutation in *P. falciparum* clinical isolates, and this is taught to compensate for the reduced efficiency of the *pfdhfr* I164L mutation in the parasite [40].

4. Molecular markers of resistance to artemisinin

Artemisinin and its derivatives are the current in-use antimalarial drug in most malaria-endemic countries. Clinical resistance to artemisinin and its derivatives has not yet been defined, but what has been reported is delayed parasite clearance in clinical isolates from Cambodia. The emergence of delayed parasite clearance to artemisinin and its derivatives calls for concerns as it may emerge into full resistance [41]. This makes it important to identify molecular markers of resistance to artemisinin and its derivatives. A molecular marker that has been suggested to cause partial resistance to artemisinin and its derivatives is the ATP-consuming calcium-dependent *P. falciparum* SERCA ortholog, *Pfatp6*. The *Pfatp6* L263E mutation has been associated with increased artemisinin and dihydroartemisinin IC_{50} values in D10 parasite strains. Parasite clinical isolates from France with the *pfatp6* S769N mutation have been reported to have high IC_{50} values to artemether [42]. Another gene that has been associated with artemisinin and its derivatives is the *Kelch 13* gene. The *kelch 13* encodes 726 amino acids and located on chromosome 13 [43]. The kelch family of proteins has diverse functions, including organizing and interacting with other proteins. Mutations in the *Kelch 13* gene that have been associated with artemisinin resistance include Y493H, R539T, I543T, F446L, P574L, and C580Y [43, 44].

5. Molecular markers for resistance to atovaquone

Atovaquone has been in use since the 1980s when it was first developed for the treatment of malaria. Despite its high efficacy in the past, it is faced with a high level of recrudescence of approximately 30% when used as a monotherapy [45, 46]. Currently, atovaquone is used in combination with proguanil as a prophylaxis or treatment of malaria [47].

Atovaquone acts by inhibiting the electron transport in the mitochondria by interacting with the cytochrome b1 complex [48]. This makes the cytochrome b gene a molecular marker for the monitoring of atovaquone resistance (**Table 1**) [49]. The cytochrome b Y268S/C/N mutations have been associated with resistance to atovaquone. These mutations have been validated to cause resistance to atovaquone, in a study that introduces the mutation Y302C in the bacterial cytochrome b (this mutation corresponds to the Y268C in the *P. falciparum*) rendered the bacterial cytochrome bc1 less sensitive to atovaquone [50].

Antimalarial drug	Molecular markers of resistance
Quinine	*pfmdr1* N86Y, Y184F, S1034C, N1042D, D1246Y [51] *pfmrp* Y191H, A437S [25]
Halofantrine	Increased *pfmdr1* copy number [16]
Mefloquine	*pfcrt* K76T, Increased *pfmdr1*copy number, *pfmdr1* N86Y [52, 53]
Lumefantrine	*pfmdr1* N86Y, Y184F, S1034C, N1042D, D1246Y [22] Increased *pfmdr1* copy number [54]
Chloroquine	*pfcrt* K76T, K76N, K76I, and [55] *pfmdr1* N86Y [28]
Amodiaquine	*pfmdr1* N86Y, Y184F, S1034C, N1042D, D1246Y *pfcrt* K72T [9, 56]
Piperaquine	Increased *pfpm2* and *pfpm3* copy numbers [33, 57]
Proguanil	*pfdhfr* S108N, N51I, and C59R [58]
Pyrimethamine	*pfdhfr* S108N, N51I, C59R, 164 I164L, and A16V [58]
Sulfadoxine	*pfdhps* S436F/A, A437G, K540E, A581G, and A613S/T [58]
Artemisinin	*pfk13* C580Y, R539T, I543T, F446L, N458Y, P547L, R56IH, Y493H [43] *pfatp6* A623E, S769N [59]
Atovaquone	*pfcytb* Y268S/C/N [60, 61]

Table 1.
Current antimalarial drugs, and their molecular markers of resistance.

6. Molecular markers for drug resistance in *P. vivax*

The study of antimalarial drug resistance in *P. vivax* is hindered by the lack of *in vitro* culture techniques for the culturing of the parasite. This has made knowledge about the genetic basis of resistance in *P. vivax* limited. Insights about the genetic basis of antimalarial drugs in *P. vivax* have been gained by comparing it with *P. falciparum*.

Orthologs of *pfcrt* and *pfmdr1* which are *pvcrt-o* and *pvmdr1* respectively in *P. vivax* have been reported. *P. vivax* isolates with the *pvmdr1* Y976F mutation are associated with higher CQ IC_{50} values. Studies show that the *pvmdr1* Y976F mutation has reached near fixation in parasite isolates from Papua New Guinea, Indonesia [62], and Brazil [63], but CQ is still highly efficacious in these countries. These provide weak evidence for using *pvmdr1* Y976F mutation as a CQ molecular marker of resistance in *P. vivax*, hence, CQ resistance in *P. vivax* may have a different genetic basis. Increased *pvndr1* copy numbers have been recorded in *P. vivax* in regions Thailand where mefloquine is used extensively, but not in regions where mefloquine is less used [62, 64].

Mutations in *dhfr* and *dhps* in *P. vivax* have been associated with decreased susceptibility to sulfadoxine-pyrimethamine [65]. Studies by [65] have identified more than 20 alleles in the *dhfr* and *dhps* genes in *P. vivax*. An example of such a mutation is the PvDHFR S58R/S117N which are homologous to PfDHFR C59R/S108N mutations. The PvDHFR S117N has been reported to prevent binding pyrimethamine [66] just like the PfDHFR S108N [67].

7. Origins and spread of CQ resistance

The notable mutations in *pfcrt* 72–76 are associated with certain geographical locations. Other mutations outside these positions have no clear geographical association

[68]. This makes it possible to identify or predict the evolution and geographical spread of chloroquine resistance-associated with mutations in *pfcrt* codons 72–76 by genotyping for these codons and the haplotype flanking this locus by microsatellite [68].

7.1 Route 1: southeast Asia to Africa

One of the most important routes, if not the most important for the spread of CQ-resistant parasite strains is the Southeast Asia to Africa route (**Figure 1a**). The CVIET (mutations in *pfcrt* from codons 72 to 76) lineage are responsible for the spread of CQ-resistance along this route. In the late 1950s, *P. falciparum* resistance to chloroquine was first identified in the Thai-Cambodian border. The spread of CQ-resistant parasites from Southeast Asia to Africa is considered to originate from the Thai-Cambodia border. The CQ-resistant parasites spread to Thailand in 1959 [68], and in Malaysia, Vietnam, and Cambodia in 1962 [68]. By the mid-1970s, CQ-resistance had been recorded in all Southeast Asia [68]. The SVMNT haplotype, which is mostly confined to the Pacific and South America has been reported in India and Laos [69, 70]. The CVIDT haplotype has also been reported [70, 71]. It remains a mystery whether these minor haplotypes found in Southeast Asia are due to new indigenous mutations or from other areas [68].

The first CQ-resistance was seen in Kenya in 1978 [68]. In the early 1980s, the CQ-resistance parasites spread to Comoro Island [68], Madagascar [68], Uganda [72], Zambia, and Malawi [68]. By the mid-1980s, CQ-resistant parasites had spread to Angola, Namibia [68]; and the western part of Africa, Nigeria, Benin, Togo, Ghana, Senegal, and Gambia [68]. The CVIET haplotype accounts for most of the CQ resistance in Africa [73]. The SVMNT haplotype has also been reported in Tanzania (in 19% of the field isolates) [74], whiles the SVIET haplotype is mostly confined to West Papua has been recorded in the Democratic Republic of Congo [75]. It remains unknown whether these haplotypes migrated from non-African regions or evolved indigenously [76].

7.2 Route 2: pacific regions

Chloroquine resistance was reported in the Pacific regions in the year 1959–1961 in West Papua, shortly after mass distribution of CQ [68]. The halting of the mass drug administration saw a reduction in the level of CQ-resistant but reemerged 10 years later [68]. The spread of resistance to other countries in the Pacific region like Papua New Guinea in 1976, the Solomon Islands in 1980, and Vanuatu in 1980 [68]. In the early 1980s, resistance was found in Sumatra and Java in Indonesia [77]. The common haplotype in the Pacific region is the SVMNT haplotype. In West Lombok in Indonesia, the CVIET haplotype is found in 10% of the *P. falciparum* clinical isolates [78]. The CVMNT has been recorded in indigenous *P. falciparum* lineage in the Philippines [79].

7.3 Route 3: south America

Chloroquine resistance was recorded in the 1960s in Columbia and Venezuela in South America [68]. Chloroquine-resistant parasites later spread to malaria-endemic regions in Brazil, Guyana in 1969, Suriname in 1972, Ecuador in 1976, Peru in 1980, and Bolivia in 1980 [68]. Two different CQ-resistant haplotypes are recorded in South America, which are the SVMNT and CVMET haplotypes with SVMNT haplotype being the most widely spread haplotype (**Figure 1b**) [1, 73]. This suggests that the SVMNT haplotype, originally found in Venezuela is responsible for the emergence of CQ-resistant isolates in South America [73, 80]. Recently, two other haplotypes; CVIET and CVMNT have been reported in Brazil and

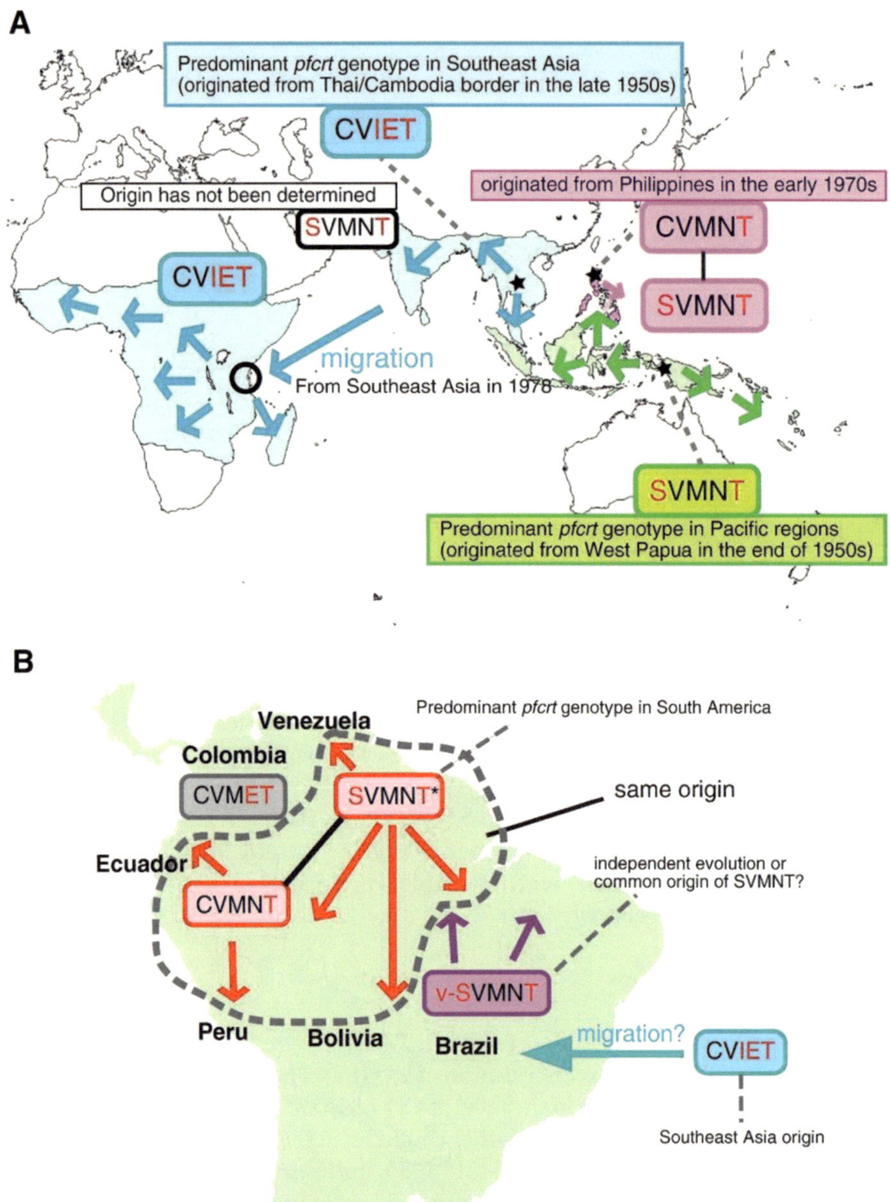

Figure 1.
Origins and geographical spread of CQ resistance. (A) Three different pfcrt *mutants; the CVIET type, SVMNT type, and CVMNT type. Migration of the CVIET type from Southeast Asia to Africa is the most notable cause of CQ resistance in Africa. Capital letters are abbreviations of amino acids at positions 72–76 in pfcrt. Red-colored letters represent mutations. (B) Four different* pfcrt *mutants; CVMET type, SVMNT type, CVMNT type, s-SVNMT type originate from South America whiles CVIET type is imported from Southeast Asia. The v-S(agt)VMNT type has different bases at position 72 from the S(tct)VMNT type originated from Venezuela. Abbreviations are the same as in (A). Adapted from [68].*

Peru respectively [81]. The CVIET haplotype might have been imported in South America from Southeast Asia or Africa [68].

7.4 Recovery of CQ resistance

The high level of CQ resistance in Malawi resulted in the ban of CQ for malaria treatment in Malawi in 1993. Just after 5 to 7 years after the CQ withdrawal, CQ sensitivity was observed [82, 83]. A decrease in the *pfcrt* K67T, which was 17% in 1998 and 2% in 2000 was observed [82]. Recovery of CQ resistance has been attributed to the expansion of wild-type *pfcrt* allele rather than a back mutation in the *pfcrt* allele [84]. This trend has also been recorded in Gabon, Vietnam [68], and China [85]. The rapid decrease in the CQ-resistance parasite population has been attributed to fitness costs incurred by the parasite as a result of the drug resistance [68].

7.5 Origins and spread of sulfadoxine-pyrimethamine resistance

Resistance to pyrimethamine was observed in the 1950s after it was used in mass drug administration and/or prophylaxis for malaria in most malaria-endemic regions [68]. Resistance to pyrimethamine led to it been used mostly as a first-line treatment option in sulfadoxine-pyrimethamine combination therapy in Thailand in the late 1960s, and most malaria-endemic countries in Southeast Asia, and South America in the 1970s and later in Africa [86].

7.6 Route 1: southeast Asia to Africa

P. falciparum resistance to SP was first reported in the 1960s at the Thai-Cambodia. Mutations in *pfdhfr* at codons 50,51,59,108, and 164 are CNRNI → CIRNI or CNRNL→CIRNL. These mutations have spread to other countries in Southeast Africa due to sulfadoxine-pyrimethamine pressure (**Figure 2A**) [87]. The *pfdhfr* quartet CIRNL mutant is dominant in Thailand [58], while the CIRNI mutant is found predominantly in Cambodia and Vietnam. The CNRNL mutant is found dominantly in Myanmar [87], while the CNRNI is found in Laos [88, 89]. Three additional genotypes, which are CNCNI, CICNI, and CICNL are also found in Southeast Asia at a very low prevalence of 5% [87]. The *pfdhfr* CIRNI mutant is predominant in many Africa countries such as South Africa, Benin, Cameroon, The Comoros, Congo, Gabon, Ghana, Guinea, Ivory Coast, Mali, Senegal, and Uganda (**Figure 2A**) [90]. This mutant is taught to have migrated to Africa from Asia [90]. It remains unknown when parasites resistant to pyrimethamine migrated to Africa, although some studies indicate the Asian origin triple mutant arrived in Kenya in 1987 [91].

7.7 Route 2: pacific region

The *pfdhfr* CNRNI double mutant is predominant in malaria-endemic regions in the Pacific. The CNRNI has been reported to have two lineages, one which is indigenous and the other from Southeast Asia [92]. Resistance to pyrimethamine was observed in the early 1960s, after its introduction in a mass drug administration [68].

7.8 Route 3: south America

Resistance to pyrimethamine was first recorded in South America in the 1950s shortly after its introduction in Venezuela [68]. *In vitro* resistance to pyrimethamine was confirmed in Brazil in the mid 1960s [93] and Columbia in 1981 [68]. Since then, sulfadoxine-pyrimethamine-resistant parasites have spread to other countries in South America [94]. Parasites with *pfdhfr* evolved indigenously in South America. Two distinct *pfdhfr* lineages resistant to pyrimethamine have been confirmed in South America. The *pfdhfr* RICNI triple mutant has been confirmed in Venezuela [95], Bolivia [96], and Brazil [97]. The *pfdhfr* RICNI triple mutant

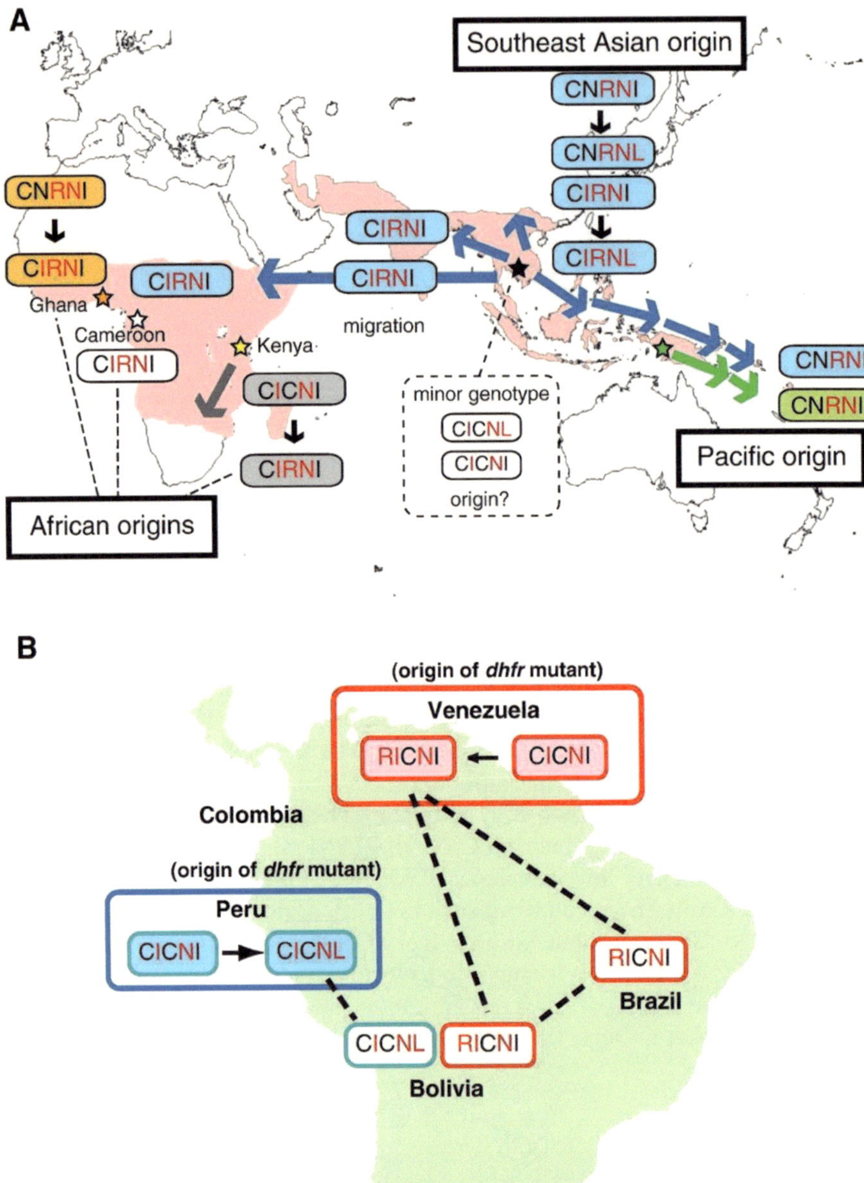

Figure 2.
Origins and spread of pyrimethamine resistance. (A) A resistant lineage having a double mutation (CNRNI), from the Thai-Cambodia border, evolved into triple (CIRNI and CNRNL) and quartet (CIRNL) types and spread to other regions in Asia and Africa. Three indigenous lineages of the dhfr triple mutant evolved in Africa. In the Pacific region, two resistant lineages having the CNRNI type have been reported: An indigenous lineage and the lineage that migrated from Southeast Asia. Capital letters are abbreviations of amino acids at positions 50, 51, 59, 108, and 164 in dhfr. Red-colored letters represent mutations. (B) Two distinct lineages of pyrimethamine resistance have been detected in South America in Venezuela and Peru. The two triple mutants (RICNI and CICNL) lineages sequentially evolved from different lineages of the CICNI type of dhfr double mutant. Abbreviations are the same as in (A). Adapted from [68].

is taught to have evolved from the CICNI double mutant. The second lineage, the CICNL triple mutant is found in Peru and Bolivia. The CICNL triple mutant has been suggested to evolve from the CICNI double mutant [96, 98].

Author details

Peter Hodoameda
West Africa Center for Cell Biology and Infectious Pathogen, University of Ghana, Accra, Ghana

*Address all correspondence to: peterhodoameda@gmail.com

References

[1] Fidock, D. A., Nomura, T., Talley, A. K., Cooper, R. A., Dzekunov, S. M., Ferdig, M. T., Ursos, L. M. B., Sidhu, A. bir S., Naude´, B., Deitsch, K. W., Su, X., Wootton, J. C., Roepe, P. D., Wellems, and T. E., Wootton, J. C., Su, X., Naudé, B., Fidock, D. A., bir Singh Sidhu, A., ... Nomura, T. (2000). Mutations in the P. falciparum digestive vacuole transmembrane protein PfCRT and evidence for their role in chloroquine resistance. Molecular Cell, *6*(4), 861-871. https://doi.org/10.1016/s1097-2765(05)00077-8

[2] Martin, R. E., & Kirk, K. (2004). The malaria parasite's chloroquine resistance transporter is a member of the drug/metabolite transporter superfamily. Molecular Biology and Evolution, *21*(10), 1938-1949. https://doi.org/10.1093/molbev/msh205

[3] Ferdig, M. T., Cooper, R. A., Mu, J., Deng, B., Joy, D. A., Su, X. Z., & Wellems, T. E. (2004). Dissecting the loci of low-level quinine resistance in malaria parasites. Molecular Microbiology, *52*(4), 985-997. https://doi.org/10.1111/j.1365-2958.2004.04035.x

[4] Mu, J., Myers, R. A., Jiang, H., Liu, S., Ricklefs, S., Waisberg, M., Chotivanich, K., Wilairatana, P., Krudsood, S., White, N. J., Udomsangpetch, R., Cui, L., Ho, M., Ou, F., Li, H., Song, J., Li, G., Wang, X., Seila, S., ... Su, X. Z. (2010). Plasmodium falciparum genome-wide scans for positive selection, recombination hot spots and resistance to antimalarial drugs. Nature Genetics, *42*(3), 268-271. https://doi.org/10.1038/ng.528

[5] Lakshmanan, V., Bray, P. G., Verdier-Pinard, D., Johnson, D. J., Horrocks, P., Muhle, R. A., Alakpa, G. E., Hughes, R. H., Ward, S. A., Krogstad, D. J., Sidhu, A. B. S., & Fidock, D. A. (2005). A critical role for PfCRT K76T in plasmodium falciparum verapamil-reversible chloroquine resistance. EMBO Journal, *24*(13), 2294-2305. https://doi.org/10.1038/sj.emboj.7600681

[6] Valderramos, S. G., & Fidock, D. A. (2006). Transporters involved in resistance to antimalarial drugs. Trends in Pharmacological Sciences, *27*(11), 594-601. https://doi.org/10.1016/j.tips.2006.09.005

[7] Bray, P. G., Martin, R. E., Tilley, L., Ward, S. A., Kirk, K., & Fidock, D. A. (2005). Defining the role of PfCRT in plasmodium falciparum chloroquine resistance. Molecular Microbiology, *56*(2), 323-333. https://doi.org/10.1111/j.1365-2958.2005.04556.x

[8] Singh Sidhu, A. B., Verdier-Pinard, D., & Fidock, D. A. (2002). Chloroquine resistance in plasmodium falciparum malaria parasites conferred by pfcrt mutations. Science, *298*(5591), 210-213. https://doi.org/10.1126/science.1074045

[9] Holmgren, G., Gil, J. P., Ferreira, P. M., Veiga, M. I., Obonyo, C. O., & Björkman, A. (2006). Amodiaquine resistant plasmodium falciparum malaria in vivo is associated with selection of pfcrt 76T and pfmdr1 86Y. Infection, Genetics and Evolution, *6*(4), 309-314. https://doi.org/10.1016/j.meegid.2005.09.001

[10] Sá, J. M., Twu, O., Hayton, K., Reyes, S., Fay, M. P., Ringwald, P., & Wellems, T. E. (2009). Geographic patterns of plasmodium falciparum drug resistance distinguished by differential responses to amodiaquine and chloroquine . Proceedings of the National Academy of Sciences, *106*(45), 18883-18889. https://doi.org/10.1073/pnas.0911317106

[11] Sisowath, C., Ferreira, P. E., Bustamante, L. Y., Dahlström, S.,

Mårtensson, A., Björkman, A., Krishna, S., & Gil, J. P. (2007). The role of pfmdr1 in plasmodium falciparum tolerance to artemether-lumefantrine in Africa. Tropical Medicine and International Health, *12*(6), 736-742. https://doi.org/10.1111/j.1365-3156.2007.01843.x

[12] Cooper, R. A. (2002). Alternative mutations at position 76 of the vacuolar transmembrane protein PfCRT are associated with chloroquine resistance and unique stereospecific quinine and quinidine responses in plasmodium falciparum. Molecular Pharmacology, *61*(1), 35-42. https://doi.org/10.1124/mol.61.1.35

[13] Wilson, C. M., Volkman, S. K., Thaithong, S., Martin, R. K., Kyle, D. E., Milhous, W. K., & Wirth, D. F. (1993). Amplification of pfmdr1 associated with mefloquine and halofantrine resistance in plasmodium falciparum from Thailand. Molecular and Biochemical Parasitology, *57*(1), 151-160. https://doi.org/10.1016/0166-6851(93)90252-S

[14] Nelson, A. L., Purfield, A., McDaniel, P., Uthaimongkol, N., Buathong, N., Sriwichai, S., Miller, R. S., Wongsrichanalai, C., & Meshnick, S. R. (2005). pfmdr1 genotyping and in vivo mefloquine resistance on the Thai-Myanmar border. American Journal of Tropical Medicine and Hygiene, *72*(5), 586-592. https://doi.org/10.4269/ajtmh.2005.72.586

[15] Alker, A. P., Lim, P., Sem, R., Shah, N. K., Yi, P., Bouth, D. M., Tsuyuoka, R., Maguire, J. D., Fandeur, T., Ariey, F., Wongsrichanalai, C., & Meshnick, S. R. (2007). PFMDR1 and in vivo resistance to artesunate-mefloquine in falciparum malaria on the Cambodian-Thai border. American Journal of Tropical Medicine and Hygiene, *76*(4), 641-647. https://doi.org/10.4269/ajtmh.2007.76.641

[16] Sidhu, A. B. S., Uhlemann, A., Valderramos, S. G., Valderramos, J., Krishna, S., & Fidock, D. A. (2006). Decreasing pfmdr1 copy number in plasmodium falciparum malaria heightens susceptibility to Mefloquine, Lumefantrine, Halofantrine, quinine, and artemisinin . The Journal of Infectious Diseases, *194*(4), 528-535. https://doi.org/10.1086/507115

[17] Volkman, S. K., Cowman, A. F., & Wirth, D. F. (1995). Functional complementation of the ste6 gene of Saccharomyces cerevisiae with the pfmdr1 gene of plasmodium falciparum. Proceedings of the National Academy of Sciences of the United States of America, *92*(19), 8921-8925. https://doi.org/10.1073/pnas.92.19.8921

[18] Picot, S., Olliaro, P., De Monbrison, F., Bienvenu, A. L., Price, R. N., & Ringwald, P. (2009). A systematic review and meta-analysis of evidence for correlation between molecular markers of parasite resistance and treatment outcome in falciparum malaria. Malaria Journal, *8*(1), 1-15. https://doi.org/10.1186/1475-2875-8-89

[19] Holmgren, G., Hamrin, J., Svärd, J., Mårtensson, A., Gil, J. P., & Björkman, A. (2007). Selection of pfmdr1 mutations after amodiaquine monotherapy and amodiaquine plus artemisinin combination therapy in East Africa. Infection, Genetics and Evolution, *7*(5), 562-569. https://doi.org/10.1016/j.meegid.2007.03.005

[20] Echeverry, D. F., Holmgren, G., Murillo, C., Higuita, J. C., Björkman, A., Gil, J. P., & Osorio, L. (2007). Short report: Polymorphisms in the pfcrt and pfmdr1 genes of plasmodium falciparum and in vitro susceptibility to amodiaquine and desethylamodiaquine. American Journal of Tropical Medicine and Hygiene, *77*(6), 1034-1038. https://doi.org/10.4269/ajtmh.2007.77.1034

[21] Dokomajilar, C., Nsobya, S. L., Greenhouse, B., Rosenthal, P. J., &

Dorsey, G. (2006). Selection of plasmodium falciparum pfmdr1 alleles following therapy with artemether-lumefantrine in an area of Uganda where malaria is highly endemic. Antimicrobial Agents and Chemotherapy, *50*(5), 1893-1895. https://doi.org/10.1128/AAC.50.5.1893-1895.2006

[22] Sisowath, C., Petersen, I., Veiga, M. I., Mårtensson, A., Premji, Z., Björkman, A., Fidock, D. A., & Gil, J. P. (2009). In vivo selection of plasmodium falciparum parasites carrying the chloroquine-susceptible pfcrt K76 allele after treatment with Artemether-Lumefantrine in Africa . Journal of Infectious Diseases, *199*(5), 750-757. https://doi.org/10.1086/596738

[23] Anderson, T. J. C., Nair, S., Qin, H., Singlam, S., Brockman, A., Paiphun, L., & Nosten, F. (2005). Are transporter genes other than the chloroquine resistance locus (pfcrt) and multidrug resistance gene (pfmdr) associated with antimalarial drug resistance? Antimicrobial Agents and Chemotherapy, *49*(6), 2180-2188. https://doi.org/10.1128/AAC.49.6.2180-2188.2005

[24] Reed, M. B., Saliba, K. J., Caruana, S. R., Kirk, K., & Cowman, A. F. (2000). Pgh1 modulates sensitivity and resistance to multiple antimalarials in plasmodium falciparum. Nature, *403*(6772), 906-909. https://doi.org/10.1038/35002615

[25] Mu, J., Ferdig, M. T., Feng, X., Joy, D. A., Duan, J., Furuya, T., Subramanian, G., Aravind, L., Cooper, R. A., Wootton, J. C., Xiong, M., & Su, X. Z. (2003). Multiple transporters associated with malaria parasite responses to chloroquine and quinine. Molecular Microbiology, *49*(4), 977-989. https://doi.org/10.1046/j.1365-2958.2003.03627.x

[26] Dahlström, S., Veiga, M. I., Mårtensson, A., Björkman, A., & Gil, J. P. (2009). Polymorphism in Pfmrp1 (plasmodium falciparum multidrug resistance protein 1) amino acid 1466 associated with resistance to sulfadoxine-pyrimethamine treatment. Antimicrobial Agents and Chemotherapy, *53*(6), 2553-2556. https://doi.org/10.1128/AAC.00091-09

[27] Raj, D. K., Mu, J., Jiang, H., Kabat, J., Singh, S., Sullivan, M., Fay, M. P., McCutchan, T. F., & Su, X. Z. (2009). Disruption of a plasmodium falciparum multidrug resistance-associated protein (PfMRP) alters its fitness and transport of antimalarial drugs and glutathione. Journal of Biological Chemistry, *284*(12), 7687-7696. https://doi.org/10.1074/jbc.M806944200

[28] Ecker, A., Lehane, A. M., Clain, J., & Fidock, D. A. (2012). *PfCRT and its role in antimalarial drug resistance Andrea*. *4*(Novenber 2012), 504-514. https://doi.org/10.1016/j.pt.2012.08.002.PfCRT

[29] Andriantsoanirina, V., Ménard, D., Rabearimanana, S., Hubert, V., Bouchier, C., Tichit, M., Le Bras, J., & Durand, R. (2010). Association of microsatellite variations of plasmodium falciparum Na+/H+ exchanger (Pfnhe-1) gene with reduced in vitro susceptibility to quinine: Lack of confirmation in clinical isolates from Africa. American Journal of Tropical Medicine and Hygiene, *82*(5), 782-787. https://doi.org/10.4269/ajtmh.2010.09-0327

[30] Henry, M., Briolant, S., Zettor, A., Pelleau, S., Baragatti, M., Baret, E., Mosnier, J., Amalvict, R., Fusai, T., Rogier, C., & Pradines, B. (2009). Plasmodium falciparum Na+/H+ exchanger 1 transporter is involved in reduced susceptibility to quinine. Antimicrobial Agents and Chemotherapy, *53*(5), 1926-1930. https://doi.org/10.1128/AAC.01243-08

[31] Nkrumah, L. J., Riegelhaupt, P. M., Moura, P., Johnson, D. J., Patel, J.,

Hayton, K., Ferdig, M. T., Wellems, T. E., Akabas, M. H., & Fidock, D. A. (2009). Probing the multifactorial basis of plasmodium falciparum quinine resistance: Evidence for a strain-specific contribution of the sodium-proton exchanger PfNHE. Molecular and Biochemical Parasitology, *165*(2), 122-131. https://doi.org/10.1016/j.molbiopara.2009.01.011

[32] Banerjee, R., Liu, J., Beatty, W., Pelosof, L., Klemba, M., & Goldberg, D. E. (2002). Four plasmepsins are active in the plasmodium falciparum food vacuole, including a protease with an active-site histidine. Proceedings of the National Academy of Sciences, *99*(2), 990-995. https://doi.org/10.1073/pnas.022630099

[33] Bopp, S., Magistrado, P., Wong, W., Schaffner, S. F., Mukherjee, A., Lim, P., Dhorda, M., Amaratunga, C., Woodrow, C. J., Ashley, E. A., White, N. J., Dondorp, A. M., Fairhurst, R. M., Ariey, F., Menard, D., Wirth, D. F., & Volkman, S. K. (2018). Plasmepsin II-III copy number accounts for bimodal piperaquine resistance among Cambodian plasmodium falciparum. Nature Communications, *9*(1). https://doi.org/10.1038/s41467-018-04104-z

[34] Wongsrichanalai, C., Pickard, A. L., Wernsdorfer, W. H., & Meshnick, S. R. (2002). *Reviews Epidemiology of drug-resistant malaria*. *2*, 209-218.

[35] Harrington, W. E., Mutabingwa, T. K., Muehlenbachs, A., Sorensen, B., Bolla, M. C., Fried, M., & Duffy, P. E. (2009). Competitive facilitation of drug-resistant plasmodium falciparum malaria parasites in pregnant women who receive preventive treatment. Proceedings of the National Academy of Sciences of the United States of America, *106*(22), 9027-9032. https://doi.org/10.1073/pnas.0901415106

[36] Peterson, D. S., Walliker, D., & Wellems, T. E. (1988). Evidence that a point mutation in dihydrofolate reductase- thymidylate synthase confers resistance to pyrimethamine in falciparum malaria (Plasmodiumfakiparum/drug resistance/folic acid antagonists/genetic linkage analysis/polymerase chain reaction). *Genetics Communicated by George H.* Hitchings, *85*(December), 9114-9118. http://www.pnas.org/content/85/23/9114.full.pdf

[37] Foote, S. J., Galatis, D., & Cowman, A. F. (1990). Amino acids in the dihydrofolate reductase-thymidylate synthase gene of plasmodium falciparum involved in cycloguanil resistance differ from those involved in pyrimethamine resistance. Proceedings of the National Academy of Sciences of the United States of America, *87*(8), 3014-3017. https://doi.org/10.1073/pnas.87.8.3014

[38] Kiara, S. M., Okombo, J., Masseno, V., Mwai, L., Ochola, I., Borrmann, S., & Nzila, A. (2009). In vitro activity of antifolate and polymorphism in dihydrofolate reductase of plasmodium falciparum isolates from the Kenyan coast: Emergence of parasites with Ile-164-Leu mutation. Antimicrobial Agents and Chemotherapy, *53*(9), 3793-3798. https://doi.org/10.1128/AAC.00308-09

[39] Price, R. N., Dorsey, G., Ashley, E. A., Barnes, K. I., Baird, J. K., D'Alessandro, U., Guerin, P. J., Laufer, M. K., Naidoo, I., Nosten, F., Olliaro, P., Plowe, C. V., Ringwald, P., Sibley, C. H., Stepniewska, K., & White, N. J. (2007). World antimalarial resistance network I: Clinical efficacy of antimalarial drugs. Malaria Journal, *6*, 1-9. https://doi.org/10.1186/1475-2875-6-119

[40] Nair, S., Miller, B., Barends, M., Jaidee, A., Patel, J., Mayxay, M., Newton, P., Nosten, F., Ferdig, M. T., & Anderson, T. J. C. (2008). Adaptive copy number evolution in malaria parasites. PLoS Genetics, *4*(10). https://doi.org/10.1371/journal.pgen.1000243

[41] Noedl, H., Se, Y., Schaecher, K., Smith, B. L., Socheat, D., & Fukuda, M. M. (2008). Evidence of artemisinin-resistant malaria in Western Cambodia. New England Journal of Medicine, *359*(24), 2619-2620. https://doi.org/10.1056/NEJMc0805011

[42] Krishna, S., Pulcini, S., Fatih, F., & Staines, H. (2010). Artemisinins and the biological basis for the PfATP6/SERCA hypothesis. Trends in Parasitology, *26*(11), 517-523. https://doi.org/10.1016/j.pt.2010.06.014

[43] Ariey, F., Witkowski, B., Amaratunga, C., Beghain, J., Langlois, A. C., Khim, N., Kim, S., Duru, V., Bouchier, C., Ma, L., Lim, P., Leang, R., Duong, S., Sreng, S., Suon, S., Chuor, C. M., Bout, D. M., Ménard, S., Rogers, W. O., ... Ménard, D. (2014). A molecular marker of artemisinin-resistant plasmodium falciparum malaria. Nature, *505*(7481), 50-55. https://doi.org/10.1038/nature12876

[44] Ashley, E. A., Dhorda, M., Fairhurst, R. M., Amaratunga, C., Lim, P., Suon, S., Sreng, S., Anderson, J. M., Mao, S., Sam, B., Sopha, C., Chuor, C. M., Nguon, C., Sovannaroth, S., Pukrittayakamee, S., Jittamala, P., Chotivanich, K., Chutasmit, K., Suchatsoonthorn, C., ... White, N. J. (2014). Spread of artemisinin resistance in plasmodium falciparum malaria. New England Journal of Medicine, *371*(5), 411-423. https://doi.org/10.1056/NEJMoa1314981

[45] Looareesuwan, S., Chulay, J. D., Canfield, C. J., Hutchinson, D. B. A., De Alencar, F., Anabwani, G., Attanath, P., Bienzle, U., Bouchaud, O., Bustos, D., Campos, P., Cerutti, C., Charoenlarp, P., Chiodini, P., Chongsuphajaisiddihi, T., Clendenes, M., Conlon, C., Coulaud, J. P., Danis, M., ... Wilairatana, P. (1999). Malarone(TM) (atovaquone and proguanil hydrochloride): A review of its clinical development for treatment of malaria. American Journal of Tropical Medicine and Hygiene, *60*(4), 533-541. https://doi.org/10.4269/ajtmh.1999.60.533

[46] Chiodini, P. L., Conlon, C. P., Hutchinson, D. B. A., Farquhar, J. A., Hall, A. P., Peto, T. E. A., Birley, H., & Warrell, D. A. (1995). Evaluation of atovaquone in the treatment of patients with uncomplicated plasmodium falciparum malaria. Journal of Antimicrobial Chemotherapy, *36*(6), 1073-1078. https://doi.org/10.1093/jac/36.6.1073

[47] Nakato, H., Vivancos, R., & Hunter, P. R. (2007). A systematic review and meta-analysis of the effectiveness and safety of atovaquone - Proguanil (Malarone) for chemoprophylaxis against malaria. Journal of Antimicrobial Chemotherapy, *60*(5), 929-936. https://doi.org/10.1093/jac/dkm337

[48] Fry, M., & Pudney, M. (1992). Site of action of the antimalarial hydroxynaphthoquinone, 2-[trans-4-(4′-chlorophenyl) cyclohexyl]-3-hydroxy-1,4-naphthoquinone (566C80). Biochemical Pharmacology, *43*(7), 1545-1553. https://doi.org/10.1016/0006-2952(92)90213-3

[49] Srivastava, I. K., Morrlsey, J. M., Darrouzet, E., Daldal, F., & Vaidya, A. B. (1999). Resistance mutations reveal the atovaquone-binding domain of cytochrome b in malaria parasites. Molecular Microbiology, *33*(4), 704-711. https://doi.org/10.1046/j.1365-2958.1999.01515.x

[50] Mather, M. W., Darrouzet, E., Valkova-Valchanova, M., Cooley, J. W., McIntosht, M. T., Daldal, F., & Vaidya, A. B. (2005). Uncovering the molecular mode of action of the antimalarial drug atovaquone using a bacterial system. Journal of Biological Chemistry, *280*(29), 27458-27465. https://doi.org/10.1074/jbc.M502319200

[51] Sidhu, A. B. S., Valderramos, S. G., & Fidock, D. A. (2005). pfmdr1

mutations contribute to quinine resistance and enhance mefloquine and artemisinin sensitivity in plasmodium falciparum. Molecular Microbiology, *57*(4), 913-926. https://doi.org/10.1111/j.1365-2958.2005.04729.x

[52] Muhamad, P., Phompradit, P., Sornjai, W., Maensathian, T., Chaijaroenkul, W., Rueangweerayut, R., & Na-Bangchang, K. (2011). Polymorphisms of molecular markers of antimalarial drug resistance and relationship with artesunate-mefloquine combination therapy in patients with uncomplicated plasmodium falciparum malaria in Thailand. American Journal of Tropical Medicine and Hygiene, *85*(3), 568-572. https://doi.org/10.4269/ajtmh.2011.11-0194

[53] Price, R. N., Uhlemann, A., Brockman, A., Mcgready, R., Ashley, E., Phaipun, L., Patel, R., Laing, K., Looareesuwan, S., White, N. J., Nosten, F., & Krishna, S. (2015). *Europe* PMC Funders Group Mefloquine resistance in Plasmodium falciparum and increased pfmdr1 gene copy number. *364*(9432), 438-447. https://doi.org/10.1016/S0140-6736(04)16767-6.Mefloquine

[54] Mungthin, M., Khositnithikul, R., Sitthichot, N., Suwandittakul, N., Wattanaveeradej, V., Ward, S. A., & Na-Bangchang, K. (2010). Association between the pfmdr1 gene and in vitro artemether and lumefantrine sensitivity in thai isolates of plasmodium falciparum. American Journal of Tropical Medicine and Hygiene, *83*(5), 1005-1009. https://doi.org/10.4269/ajtmh.2010.10-0339

[55] DJIMDÉ, A. B., DOUMBO, O. K., CORTESE, J. F., KAYENTAO, K., DOUMBO, S., DIOURTÉ, Y., DICKO, A., SU, X.-Z., OMURA, A. N., FIDOCK, D. A., WELLEMS, T. E., & PLOWE, C. V. (2001). A molecular marker for chloroquine-resistant falciparum malaria. English Journal, *344*(4), 257-263. http://www.ncbi.nlm.nih.gov/pubmed/11172152

[56] Folarin, O. A., Bustamante, C., Gbotosho, G. O., Sowunmi, A., Zalis, M. G., Oduola, A. M. J., & Happi, C. T. (2011). In vitro amodiaquine resistance and its association with mutations in pfcrt and pfmdr1 genes of plasmodium falciparum isolates from Nigeria. Acta Tropica, *120*(3), 224-230. https://doi.org/10.1016/j.actatropica.2011.08.013

[57] Witkowski, B., Duru, V., Khim, N., Ross, L. S., Saintpierre, B., Beghain, J., Chy, S., Kim, S., Ke, S., Kloeung, N., Eam, R., Khean, C., Ken, M., Loch, K., Bouillon, A., Domergue, A., Ma, L., Bouchier, C., Leang, R., ... Ménard, D. (2017). A surrogate marker of piperaquine-resistant plasmodium falciparum malaria: A phenotype–genotype association study. The Lancet Infectious Diseases, *17*(2), 174-183. https://doi.org/10.1016/S1473-3099(16)30415-7

[58] Rout, S., & Mahapatra, R. K. (2019). Plasmodium falciparum: Multidrug resistance. Chemical Biology and Drug Design, *93*(5), 737-759. https://doi.org/10.1111/cbdd.13484

[59] Pillai, D. R., Lau, R., Khairnar, K., Lepore, R., Via, A., Staines, H. M., & Krishna, S. (2012). Artemether resistance in vitro is linked to mutations in PfATP6 that also interact with mutations in PfMDR1 in travellers returning with plasmodium falciparum infections. Malaria Journal, *11*, 1-9. https://doi.org/10.1186/1475-2875-11-131

[60] Severini, C., & Menegon, M. (2015). Resistance to antimalarial drugs: An endless world war against plasmodium that we risk losing. Journal of Global Antimicrobial Resistance, *3*(2), 58-63. https://doi.org/10.1016/j.jgar.2015.02.002

[61] Olliaro, P. (2001). Mode of action and mechanisms of resistance for antimalarial drugs. Pharmacology and

Therapeutics, *89*(2), 207-219. https://doi.org/10.1016/S0163-7258(00)00115-7

[62] Suwanarusk, R., Russell, B., Chavchich, M., Chalfein, F., Kenangalem, E., Kosaisavee, V., Prasetyorini, B., Piera, K. A., Barends, M., Brockman, A., Lek-Uthai, U., Anstey, N. M., Tjitra, E., Nosten, F., Cheng, Q., & Price, R. N. (2007). Chloroquine resistant plasmodium vivax: In vitro characterisation and association with molecular polymorphisms. PLoS ONE, *2*(10), 1-9. https://doi.org/10.1371/journal.pone.0001089

[63] Gama, B. E., de Oliveira, N. K. A., de Souza, J. M., Daniel-Ribeiro, C. T., & Ferreira-da-Cruz, M. de F. (2009). Characterisation of pvmdr1 and pvdhfr genes associated with chemoresistance in Brazilian plasmodium vivax isolates. Memorias Do Instituto Oswaldo Cruz, *104*(7), 1009-1011. https://doi.org/10.1590/S0074-02762009000700012

[64] Imwong, M., Pukrittayakamee, S., Pongtavornpinyo, W., Nakeesathit, S., Nair, S., Newton, P., Nosten, F., Anderson, T. J. C., Dondorp, A., Day, N. P. J., & White, N. J. (2008). Gene amplification of the multidrug resistance 1 gene of plasmodium vivax isolates from Thailand, Laos, and Myanmar. Antimicrobial Agents and Chemotherapy, *52*(7), 2657-2659. https://doi.org/10.1128/AAC.01459-07

[65] Hawkins, V. N., Joshi, H., Rungsihirunrat, K., Na-Bangchang, K., & Sibley, C. H. (2007). Antifolates can have a role in the treatment of plasmodium vivax. Trends in Parasitology, *23*(5), 213-222. https://doi.org/10.1016/j.pt.2007.03.002

[66] Kongsaeree, P., Khongsuk, P., Leartsakulpanich, U., Chitnumsub, P., Tarnchompoo, B., Walkinshaw, M. D., & Yuthavong, Y. (2005). Crystal structure of dihydrofolate reductase from plasmodium vivax: Pyrimethamine displacement linked with mutation-induced resistance. Proceedings of the National Academy of Sciences of the United States of America, *102*(37), 13046-13051. https://doi.org/10.1073/pnas.0501747102

[67] Yuvaniyama, J., Chitnumsub, P., Kamchonwongpaisan, S., Vanichtanankul, J., Sirawaraporn, W., Taylor, P., Walkinshaw, M. D., & Yuthavong, Y. (2003). Insights into antifolate resistance from malarial DHFR-TS structures. Nature Structural Biology, *10*(5), 357-365. https://doi.org/10.1038/nsb921

[68] Mita, T., Tanabe, K., & Kita, K. (2009). Spread and evolution of plasmodium falciparum drug resistance. Parasitology International, *58*(3), 201-209. https://doi.org/10.1016/j.parint.2009.04.004

[69] Dittrich, S., Alifrangis, M., Stohrer, J. M., Thongpaseuth, V., Vanisaveth, V., Phetsouvanh, R., Phompida, S., Khalil, I. F., & Jelinek, T. (2005). Falciparum malaria in the north of Laos: The occurrence and implications of the plasmodium falciparum chloroquine resistance transporter (pfcrt) gene haplotype SVMNT. Tropical Medicine and International Health, *10*(12), 1267-1270. https://doi.org/10.1111/j.1365-3156.2005.01514.x

[70] Lim, P., Chy, S., Ariey, F., Incardona, S., Chim, P., Sem, R., Denis, M. B., Hewitt, S., Hoyer, S., Socheat, D., Merecreau-Puijalon, O., & Fandeur, T. (2003). Pfcrt polymorphism and chloroquine resistance in plasmodium falciparum strains isolated in Cambodia. Antimicrobial Agents and Chemotherapy, *47*(1), 87-94. https://doi.org/10.1128/AAC.47.1.87-94.2003

[71] Durrand, V., Berry, A., Sem, R., Glaziou, P., Beaudou, J., & Fandeur, T. (2004). Variations in the sequence and expression of the plasmodium falciparum chloroquine resistance

transporter (Pfcrt) and their relationship to chloroquine resistance in vitro. Molecular and Biochemical Parasitology, *136*(2), 273-285. https://doi.org/10.1016/j.molbiopara.2004.03.016

[72] Onori, E. (1984). The problem of plasmodium falciparum drug resistance in Africa south of the Sahara. *Bulletin of the World Health Organization*, *62*(SUPPL.), 55-62.

[73] Wootton, J. C., Feng, X., Ferdig, M. T., Cooper, R. A., Mu, J., Baruch, D. I., Magill, A. J., & Su, X. Z. (2002). Genetic diversity and chloroquine selective sweeps in plasmodium falciparum. Nature, *418*(6895), 320-323. https://doi.org/10.1038/nature00813

[74] Alifrangis, M., Dalgaard, M. B., Lusingu, J. P., Vestergaard, L. S., Staalsoe, T., Jensen, A. T. R., Enevold, A., Rønn, A. M., Khalil, I. F., Warhurst, D. C., Lemnge, M. M., Theander, T. G., & Bygbjerg, I. C. (2006). Occurrence of the southeast Asian/south American SVMNT haplotype of the chloroquine-resistance transporter gene in plasmodium falciparum in Tanzania. Journal of Infectious Diseases, *193*(12), 1738-1741. https://doi.org/10.1086/504269

[75] Severini, C., Menegon, M., Sannella, A. R., Paglia, M. G., Narciso, P., Matteelli, A., Gulletta, M., Caramello, P., Canta, F., Xayavong, M. V., Moura, I. N. S., Pieniazek, N. J., Taramelli, D., & Majori, G. (2006). Prevalence of pfcrt point mutations and level of chloroquine resistance in plasmodium falciparum isolates from Africa. Infection, Genetics and Evolution, *6*(4), 262-268. https://doi.org/10.1016/j.meegid.2005.07.002

[76] Zakeri, S., Afsharpad, M., Kazemzadeh, T., Mehdizadeh, K., Shabani, A., & Djadid, N. D. (2008). Association of pfcrt but not pfmdr1 alleles with chloroquine resistance in Iranian isolates of plasmodium falciparum. American Journal of Tropical Medicine and Hygiene, *78*(4), 633-640. https://doi.org/10.4269/ajtmh.2008.78.633

[77] Smrkovski, L. L., Hoffman, S. L., Purnomo, Hussein, R. P., Masbar, S., & Kurniawan, L. (1983). Chloroquine resistant plasmodium falciparum on the island of Flores, Indonesia. Transactions of the Royal Society of Tropical Medicine and Hygiene, *77*(4), 459-462. https://doi.org/10.1016/0035-9203(83)90112-8

[78] Mehlotra, R. K., Mattera, G., Bockarie, M. J., Maguire, J. D., Baird, J. K., Sharma, Y. D., Alifrangis, M., Dorsey, G., Rosenthal, P. J., Fryauff, D. J., Kazura, J. W., Stoneking, M., & Zimmerman, P. A. (2008). Discordant patterns of genetic variation at two chloroquine resistance loci in worldwide populations of the malaria parasite plasmodium falciparum. Antimicrobial Agents and Chemotherapy, *52*(6), 2212-2222. https://doi.org/10.1128/AAC.00089-08

[79] Chen, N., Wilson, D. W., Pasay, C., Bell, D., Martin, L. B., Kyle, D., & Cheng, Q. (2005). Origin and dissemination of chloroquine-resistant plasmodium falciparum with mutant pfcrt alleles in the Philippines. Antimicrobial Agents and Chemotherapy, *49*(5), 2102-2105. https://doi.org/10.1128/AAC.49.5.2102-2105.2005

[80] Cortese, J. F., Caraballo, A., Contreras, C. E., & Plowe, C. V. (2002). Origin and dissemination of plasmodium falciparum drug-resistance mutations in South America. Journal of Infectious Diseases, *186*(7), 999-1006. https://doi.org/10.1086/342946

[81] Vieira, P. P., Ferreira, M. U., Alecrim, M. D. G., Alecrim, W. D., Da Silva, L. H. P., Sihuincha, M. M., Joy, D. A., Mu, J., Su, X. Z., & Zalis, M. G.

(2004). Pfcrt polymorphism and the spread of chloroquine resistance in plasmodium falciparum populations across the Amazon Basin. Journal of Infectious Diseases, *190*(2), 417-424. https://doi.org/10.1086/422006

[82] Mita, T., Kaneko, A., Lum, J. K., Bwijo, B., Takechi, M., Zungu, I. L., Tsukahara, T., Tanabe, K., Kobayakawa, T., & Björkman, A. (2003). Recovery of chloroquine sensitivity and low prevalence of the plasmodium falciparum chloroquine resistance transporter gene mutation K76T following the discontinuance of chloroquine use in Malawi. American Journal of Tropical Medicine and Hygiene, *68*(4), 413-415. https://doi.org/10.4269/ajtmh.2003.68.413

[83] Takechi, M., Matsuo, M., Ziba, C., Macheso, A., Butao, D., Zungu, I. L., Chakanika, I., & Bustos, M. D. G. (2001). Therapeutic efficacy of sulphadoxine/pyrimethamine and susceptibility in vitro of P. falciparum isolates to sulphadoxine-pyremethamine and other antimalarial drugs in Malawian children. Tropical Medicine and International Health, *6*(6), 429-434. https://doi.org/10.1046/j.1365-3156.2001.00735.x

[84] Mita, T., Kaneko, A., Lum, J. K., Zungu, I. L., Tsukahara, T., Eto, H., Kobayakawa, T., Björkman, A., & Tanabe, K. (2004). Expansion of wild type allele rather than back mutation in pfcrt explains the recent recovery of chloroquine sensitivity of plasmodium falciparum in Malawi. Molecular and Biochemical Parasitology, *135*(1), 159-163. https://doi.org/10.1016/j.molbiopara.2004.01.011

[85] Liu, D. Q., Liu, R. J., Ren, D. X., Gao, D. Q., Zhang, C. Y., Qiu, C. P., Cai, X. Z., Ling, C. F., Song, A. H., & Tang, X. (1995). Changes in the resistance of plasmodium falciparum to chloroquine in Hainan, China. Bulletin of the World Health Organization, *73*(4), 483-486.

[86] Black, F., Bygbjerg, I., Effersoe, P., Gomme, G., Jepsen, S., & Axelgaard Jensen, G. (1981). Fansidar resistant falciparum malaria acquired in south east asia. Transactions of the Royal Society of Tropical Medicine and Hygiene, *75*(5), 715-716. https://doi.org/10.1016/0035-9203(81)90160-7

[87] Nair, S., Williams, J. T., Brockman, A., Paiphun, L., Mayxay, M., Newton, P. N., Guthmann, J. P., Smithuis, F. M., Hien, T. T., White, N. J., Nosten, F., & Anderson, T. J. C. (2003). A selective sweep driven by pyrimethamine treatment in southeast Asian malaria parasites. Molecular Biology and Evolution, *20*(9), 1526-1536. https://doi.org/10.1093/molbev/msg162

[88] Nash, D., Nair, S., Mayxay, M., Newton, P. N., Guthmann, J. P., Nosten, F., & Anderson, T. J. C. (2005). Selection strength and hitchhiking around two anti-malarial resistance genes. Proceedings of the Royal Society B: Biological Sciences, *272*(1568), 1153-1161. https://doi.org/10.1098/rspb.2004.3026

[89] Toma, H., Imada, Y., Vannachone, B., Miyagi, M., Kobayashi, J., Uechi, G., Pethuvang, R., Manivong, K., Phompida, S., Sato, Y., Station, M., Provincial, K., & Office, H. (2005). RESEARCH NOTE A MOLECULAR EPIDEMIOLOGIC STUDY OF POINT MUTATIONS FOR PYRIMETHAMINE-SULFADOXINE RESISTANCE OF *36*(3), 1-3.

[90] Maïga, O., Djimdé, A. A., Hubert, V., Renard, E., Aubouy, A., Kironde, F., Nsimba, B., Koram, K., Doumbo, O. K., Le Bras, J., & Clain, J. (2007). A shared asian origin of the triple-mutant dhfr allele in plasmodium falciparum from sites across Africa. Journal of Infectious Diseases, *196*(1), 165-172. https://doi.org/10.1086/518512

[91] Certain, L. K., Briceño, M., Kiara, S. M., Nzila, A. M., Watkins, W. M., &

Sibley, C. H. (2008). Characteristics of plasmodium falciparum dhfr haplotypes that confer pyrimethamine resistance, Kilifi, Kenya, 1987-2006. Journal of Infectious Diseases, *197*(12), 1743-1751. https://doi.org/10.1086/588198

[92] Mita, T., Tanabe, K., Takahashi, N., Tsukahara, T., Eto, H., Dysoley, L., Ohmae, H., Kita, K., Krudsood, S., Looareesuwan, S., Kaneko, A., Björkman, A., & Kobayakawa, T. (2007). Independent evolution of pyrimethamine resistance in plasmodium falciparum isolates in Melanesia. Antimicrobial Agents and Chemotherapy, *51*(3), 1071-1077. https://doi.org/10.1128/AAC.01186-06

[93] Walker, A. J., & Lopez-Antunano, F. J. (1968). Response to drugs of south american strains of plasmodium falciparum. Transactions of the Royal Society of Tropical Medicine and Hygiene, *62*(5), 654-667. https://doi.org/10.1016/0035-9203(68)90116-8

[94] Kremsner, P. G., Zotter, G. M., Feldmeier, H., Graninger, W., Kollaritsch, M., Wiedermann, G., Rocha, R. M., & Wernsdorfer, W. H. (1989). In vitro drug sensitivity of plasmodium falciparum in acre, Brazil. Bulletin of the World Health Organization, *67*(3), 289-293.

[95] McCollum, A. M., Mueller, K., Villegas, L., Udhayakumar, V., & Escalante, A. A. (2007). Common origin and fixation of plasmodium falciparum dhfr and dhps mutations associated with sulfadoxine-pyrimethamine resistance in a low-transmission area in South America. Antimicrobial Agents and Chemotherapy, *51*(6), 2085-2091. https://doi.org/10.1128/AAC.01228-06

[96] Cortese, J. F., & Plowe, C. V. (1998). Antifolate resistance due to new and known plasmodium falciparum dihydrofolate reductase mutations expressed in yeast. Molecular and Biochemical Parasitology, *94*(2), 205-214. https://doi.org/10.1016/S0166-6851(98)00075-9

[97] Vasconcelos, K. F., Plowe, C. V., Fontes, C. J., Kyle, D., Wirth, D. F., Pereira Da Silva, L. H., & Zalis, M. G. (2000). Mutations in plasmodium falciparum Dihydrofolate reductase and Dihydropteroate synthase of isolates from the Amazon region of Brazil. Memorias Do Instituto Oswaldo Cruz, *95*(5), 721-728. https://doi.org/10.1590/S0074-02762000000500020

[98] Zhou, Z., Griffing, S. M., De Oliveira, A. M., McCollum, A. M., Quezada, W. M., Arrospide, N., Escalante, A. A., & Udhayakumar, V. (2008). Decline in sulfadoxine-pyrimethamine-resistant alleles after change in drug policy in the Amazon region of Peru. Antimicrobial Agents and Chemotherapy, *52*(2), 739-741. https://doi.org/10.1128/AAC.00975-07

Chapter 7

A Double Line of Defense: Heat Shock Proteins and Polyamines Act as Contributing Factors to Drug Resistance of some *Plasmodium* Parasites

Xolani Henry Makhoba

Abstract

Malaria remains a threat to human life worldwide with children under the age of 5 being the most vulnerable. *Plasmodium falciparum*, known as the causative agent of the deadliest malaria, survives both in the mosquito vector and human host. The sudden temperature change seems to not affect the parasite's cellular system. Heat shock proteins and polyamines are the major house-keepers of the parasite's cellular system to remain viable, despite the temperature changes that the parasite gets exposed to. While heat shock proteins protect newly synthesized proteins until they are properly folded polyamines are needed for cell differentiation, proliferation, and cell growth. In plants for example, polyamines have been reported to act as molecular chaperones when cells are exposed to unfavorable conditions that could be detrimental to cells. In this review, the role of heat shock proteins and polyamines in plasmodium parasite drug resistance and their role in parasite survival are discussed. The current drugs against malaria as well as the alternative future approach towards malarial drug development are reviewed.

Keywords: heat shock proteins, polyamines, drug resistance, *Plasmodium falciparum*, drug development

1. Introduction

According to the world health organization, malarial cases are expected to double in recent times due to the much global focus to fight the covid-19 pandemic [1]. The global fight against the covid-19 pandemic slows down efforts to control or eliminate malaria as one of the life-threatening diseases worldwide. In 2018, 228 million cases of malaria were reported with 405 000 people died, and in Sub-Saharan Africa, 67% of children under the age of 5 prematurely succumbed to the disease [1, 2]. The currently available drugs in the market are not effective enough and there is a growing concern of reported cases of drug resistance in some parts of the world. These drugs include artemisinin combination therapy which was a promising treatment for malaria. Therefore, there is an urgent need for alternative drugs or vaccines for malaria. Among the six species of malaria causative agents namely,

Plasmodium vivax (*P. vivax*), *P. ovolae*, *P. malarae*, *P. yoelli*, and *P. falciparum*, *P. falciparum* is the causative agent of the deadliest form of malaria. *Plasmodium falciparum* parasites survive in the female anopheles mosquito and the human host. When the Anopheles mosquito bites a human during its blood meal, the parasite is then transferred to a human host. It is reported that the temperature in the mosquito vector is about 22°C, whereas in the human host the normal body temperature is 37°C, but when the malaria symptoms kick in, the temperature goes as high as 38°C and above [3–5]. However, these sudden temperature changes do not affect the parasite viability. The temperature changes put pressure on the physiology of the parasite because there is a group of proteins whose production increases when the parasite is exposed to human host temperature. These molecules or proteins are believed to be the housekeepers of the cellular system of the *P. falciparum* parasite. When the parasite enters the human host, it produces schizonts into the liver, they then matured into merozoite and rapture in the red blood cells, therefore invade red blood cells. This stage of the parasite life cycle is very important because this is when the parasite would then multiply, differentiate and produce more merozoite to invade red blood cells and malaria symptoms would then start to show and the human host temperature would increase above 38°C [6]. Therefore, the production of proteins called heat shock proteins steadily increases as means for parasite protection under harsh conditions or sudden change of temperature.

Heat shock proteins are ubiquitous, highly conserved molecules that occur in all recognized life forms. The constitutively expressed heat shock proteins are generally designated as 'heat shock cognate' (Hsc) forms to differentiate them from the inducible heat shock protein (Hsp) forms. The constitutively expressed forms play a housekeeping role, while the inducible forms are normally expressed in response to stress. The role of heat shock proteins is to protect the newly synthesized proteins from misfolding, which could result in the formation of inclusion bodies or truncated proteins that can be toxic to the cellular system of the parasite. On the other hand, a group of proteins known as polyamines is produced in the parasite for proliferation, differentiation, and growth. When merozoite invades red blood cells, polyamines are believed to be at the center of the parasite multiplication process and act as molecular chaperones. For example, when cells that lack polyamines are added with polyamines and exposed to a temperature above 37°C, the cells do survive [7], signifying that polyamines display chaperone activities. Wide studies conducted in plant biochemistry demonstrated that when plant cells are exposed to abiotic temperature, polyamines protect plant cells and improve growth and production [3]. In P. falciparum, it could be that polyamines do cooperate with heat shock proteins as means for the parasite to survive under harsh conditions. For example, Polyamines protected plasmid DNA strand breaks in vitro and aided the cell survival against irradiation in polyamine deficient *Escherichia coli* mutant strain [8]. It is shown that DNA strand breaks were prohibited 4–6 fold more by polyamines such as spermidine and spermine compared to putrescine and cadaverine in the dithiothreitol/Fe (III)/O_2 system [9]. After UV-irradiation, the protection of DNA strand disruptions by spermine and spermidine was twofold as effective as that by putrescine and cadaverine. To measure the viability of *Escherichia coli* cells lacking polyamines, they were grown in the medium containing putrescine and spermidine. They displayed increased survivability compared to polyamine-depleted medium at a dose of 60 and 40 J/m^2. After γ-irradiation to a dose of 80 Gy, cell survivals of a mutant strain were significantly increased to 7.7- and 23.8-fold by putrescine and spermidine, respectively. Taken together these results suggest the probability that polyamines play a powerful role in the protection of DNA or cell damage by radiation. Polyamines can play an essential role in cell growth and differentiation and are also involved in the protection of cell structures [10].

In addition, reports suggest that when polyamines metabolism is disrupted, several cellular processes are affected, including transcription, translation, gene expression regulation, autophagy, and stress resistance. Some studies reported that in fact, polyamines influence the production or synthesis of heat shock proteins, even though it is not clear how this process takes place. Heat shock proteins come in different sizes and activities, whereas polyamines include putrescine, spermidine, and spermine. With *P. falciparum* having a unique biosynthesis of polyamines, for example, S-Adenosylmethionine decarboxylase is connected to Ornithine decarboxylase (AdoMetDC/ODC) has been regarded as an ideal drug target [11]. Therefore, drug development starts at the protein level, where characteristics of proteins are examined, this unique arrangement of P. falciparum AdoMetDC/ODC is regarded as an ideal drug target for malaria due to its role in the biosynthesis of polyamines in the parasite [9, 12, 13]. On the other hand, heat shock proteins such as Hsp70/Hsp40 partnership, Hsp90, Hsp110, small heat shock proteins, have been extensively studied and they have been well documented on how they keep the parasite viable, but what we do not know is how the parasite cellular system brings together polyamines and heat shock proteins as its double line of defense as a survival strategy. This is protective system is especially vital during red blood cell merozoite invasion, which is a crucial stage for the parasite's survival. This, therefore, justifies the need to understand this mysterious partnership between these two molecules towards multidrug development. In our laboratory, we are currently interested in getting answers in that direction, intending to develop alternative drugs against malaria [8, 14–16].

2. The life cycle of *plasmodium falciparum* parasite

The parasite *Plasmodium falciparum* has a complex life cycle which includes anopheles' female mosquito and the human host. After parasites have been sucked up, Oocysts develop in the gut wall of the mosquito. Sporozoites then develop in the oocyte and the Sporozoites migrate to the salivary glands. When the mosquito bites, Sporozoites are injected into the human body, who then becomes the second host to the parasites (**Figure 1**). The Sporozoites enter the liver cells where they multiply for about 7 to 14 days, producing between 10,000 and 30,000 daughter cells called merozoites. These daughter cells then burst and invade the red blood cells. In the red blood cells, further multiplication occurs by asexual reproduction [9, 10]. Between 8 and 16 merozoites are produced every 48 or 72 hours, depending on the species of *Plasmodium*. Merozoites are then released through the bursting of red blood cells. This release of toxic substances causes febrile attacks of the disease. After several such cycles, male and female gametocytes are produced (the sexual stage) and taken up by a feeding mosquito. The *Plasmodium* life cycle is completed by sexual reproduction, resulting in new sporozoites.

Some of the symptoms of malaria include but not all, fever and headache, these normally display when merozoite invade red blood cells and this stage is essential for the parasite survival. Fever is shown by elevated temperature above 38°C in the human host system. This therefore, puts stress on the cellular system of the parasite thus results in increased production of heat shock proteins for cellular system protection (protein folding). On the other hand, the parasite proliferates when the merozoite invades the red blood cells. The primary role of polyamines includes cell proliferation, differentiation, and growth of which are what the parasite needs at the red blood cell stage in a human host. Therefore, both heat shock proteins and polyamines serve as a shield of the parasite in the human host when exposed to stress conditions [17–20]. A study reported that the chaperone activities of Hsp70

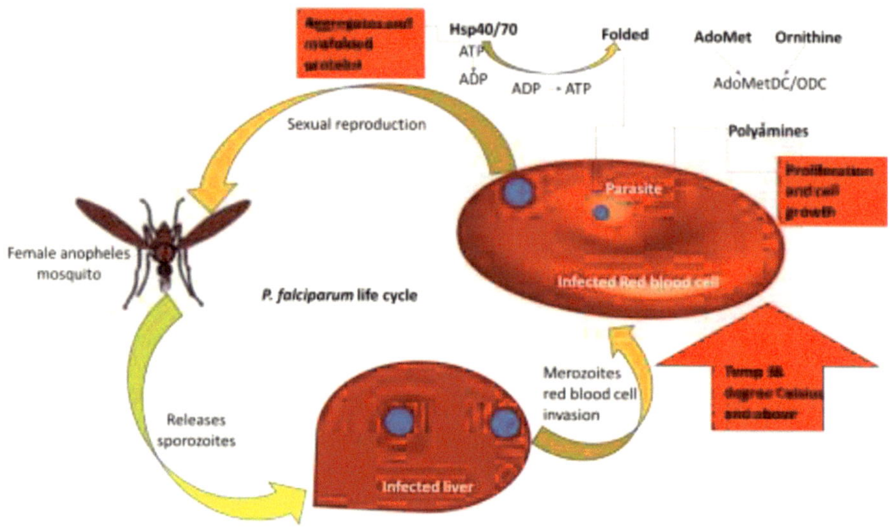

Figure 1.
Highlights of the plasmodium falciparum *life cycle and the synthesis of heat shock proteins and polyamines under stressful conditions for the parasite survival. Female mosquito bites during the blood meal release sporozoites to liver cells, where they undergo maturation stage and rapture to release matured merozoites to invade red blood cells. At this stage, the parasite undergoes heat shock and release stress proteins such as a heat shock proteins and polyamines so that the parasite proliferates and grow.*

sequester protein aggregates accumulated in bacteria during antibiotic treatment, therefore reducing the effect of the cure. Also, polyamines such as putrescine and spermidine have been suggested to exhibit chaperone activities when cells are exposed to stressful environments such as antibiotic therapies [21]. Taken together, the role polyamines and heat shock proteins play in a cellular system suggests that *Plasmodium falciparum* could apply similar methods to render current drugs ineffective by keeping the system's proteins in good shape (properly folded) during drug treatment [22]. In general, obligate human parasites depend upon a robust protein quality control system to ensure their survival, and hence, both employ a competent heat shock machinery and polyamines to this end.

3. Heat shock proteins

The outside milieu affects the in-house activity of the cellular system. If cells are exposed to stressful conditions, several molecular functions could be upset. For cells to remain functional active, the interior system should remain in good condition and if that is not the case, this could lead to cell death. Therefore, heat shock proteins of different sizes perform various functional activities to keep the cellular system in good condition. Molecular chaperone or heat shock proteins perform some activities as housekeepers of the cell, such as foldase, holdase, protein transportation, removal of inclusion bodies, modulation, and stabilization (**Table 1**). Whereas others are responsible for bringing the substrate for binding to reach a 3-dimensional structure. In *Plasmodium falciparum*, heat shock proteins have been regarded as ideal drug targets due to the aforementioned activities. Even though the role played by heat shock proteins favors the parasite viability, it is believed that their role in the parasite contributes to drug resistance. For example, when *E. coli* cells were exposed to some antibiotics, the production of Hsp70 chaperones was observed to have increased. It was then concluded that the cells developed resistance against antibiotics due to the

2HSPs	Role	Drugs	Refs
Hsp 40	Co-chaperone	Geldanamycin, radicicol, celastrol	[15, 23]
Hsp 70	Foldase, holdase, transportation	Geldanamycin	[24]
Hsp 90	Foldade and holdase	Geldanamycin, benzoquinone	[25, 26]
Hsp 110	Foldase	Geldanamycin	[16, 27]
Small Hsps	Modulation and stabilization		[19, 20, 22, 26]

Table 1.
Heat shock proteins and some compounds tested against them.

increased production of Hsp70 [16]. *Plasmodium falciparum* parasite is believed to use the same techniques when exposed to various drugs by increasing the production of heat shock proteins as a strategy to protect its internal environment, thus developing resistance to many drugs available in the market [28, 29].

Different kinds of compounds have been synthesized and their effectiveness against heat shock proteins was tested [17]. The complex nature of the *P. falciparum* makes it very difficult to develop effective drugs or vaccines. It is therefore, this reason why drug design and development against malaria has drawn so much research interest as matter of urgency.

4. The functional activities of Hsp70 in partnership with Hsp40

Both heat shock protein 70 and heat shock protein 40 were first discovered in bacteria that were exposed to stressful conditions, thus these proteins were overexpressed in response to the challenging conditions the bacteria organism was faced with [30]. As a result, the cellular protein structure and functional activities were

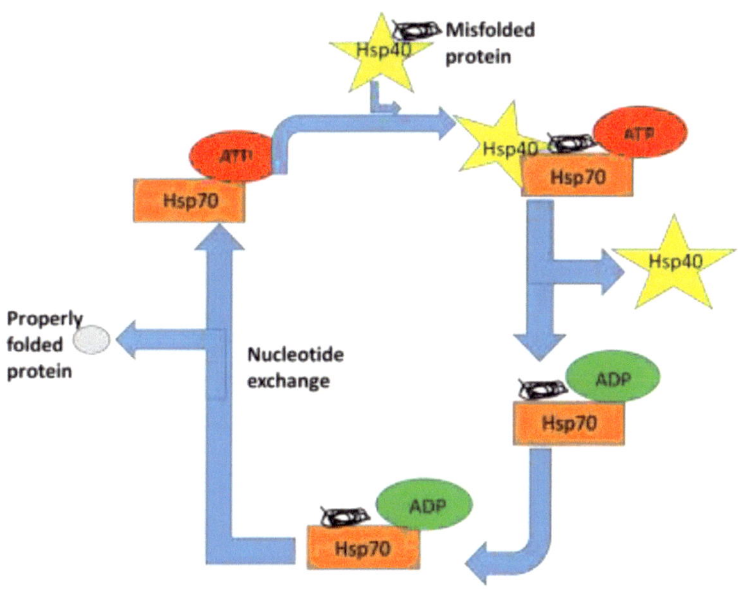

Figure 2.
Hsp70/Hsp40 partnership in folding process of newly synthesized proteins. Hsp40 hands over a newly synthesized protein to Hsp70 for proper folding with APT driven activity with help of nucleic exchange factor being at the Centre of the action. Unsuccessful protein folding are dealt with proteasome for degradation.

affected, Hsp70 was able to rescue aggregated and misfolded proteins (**Figure 2**). The partnership between Hsp70 and Hsp40 plays a major role in helping misfolded proteins to fold and gain their functional activities [31, 32]. To successfully assist misfolded proteins or substrates to fold properly, Hsp70 recognized and bind into the hydrophobic patches. The major role played by Hsp40 is to recognized and present misfolded proteins into an ATP Hsp70 for folding. The ATP is hydrolyzed to ADP, which then allows the substrate to bind to the ADP Hsp70 for folding. Once properly folded, the ADP is then converted to ATP thus releases the properly folded protein. Taken together, newly synthesized protein requires the assistance of heat shock proteins to fold properly, otherwise, they can be toxic to the cells if they are not properly folded.

5. Biosynthesis of polyamines

The synthesis of Polyamines such as putrescine, spermidine, and spermine is driven by *S-Adenosylmethionine decarboxylase* (AdoMetDC) and *Ornithine decarboxylase* (ODC). Both Adenosylmethionine and Ornithine function as precursors of polyamine biosynthesis [33, 34]. Unlike other species, *Plasmodium falciparum* AdoMetDC is connected to ODC which makes it an ideal drug target (**Figure 3**) [27]. These positively charged molecules are involved in various activities in the cellular system such as proliferation, differentiation, cell growth, protein synthesis, and RNA and DNA packaging [35]. In plants, polyamines have been reported to act as molecular chaperones or respond to heat shock to prevent plants. In addition to that, polyamines also prevent DNA damage of the cells exposed to UV radiation which could lead to cell death [35–37]. Taken together, this suggests that both polyamines and heat shock proteins are used by the parasite *Plasmodium falciparum*

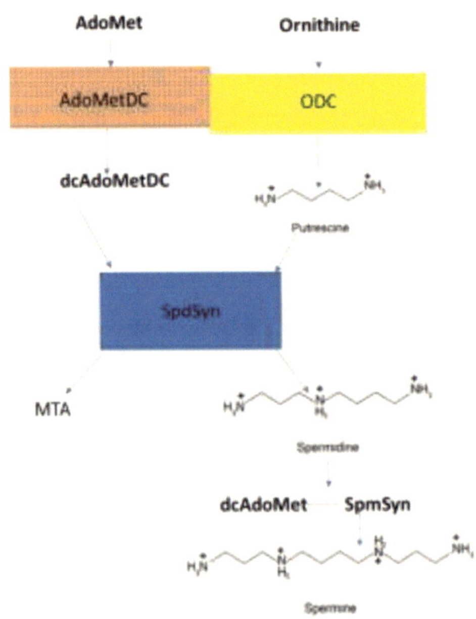

Figure 3.
Polyamines biosynthesis in plasmodium falciparum *parasite. Biosynthesis of polyamines in* P. falciparum *is driven by linked S-adenosylmethionine decarboxylase (AdoMetDC) and ornithine decarboxylase (ODC). Whereas in mammalian cells AdoMetDC and ODC are not joined together. Abreviations: SpdSyn, spermidine synthase; Spd, spermidine; dcAdoMet, decarboxylated S-adenosylmethionine; SpmSyn, spermidine synthase; Spm, spermine.*

as a strategy to survive under unfavorable conditions when it enters the human host (where it experiences a sudden change of temperature) from the mosquito [38–45]. It could be that both polyamines and heat shock proteins contribute a lot to drug resistance that the parasite has demonstrated to current drugs available in the market. Therefore, understanding how these two molecules cooperate in the parasite could lead to the right direction in the development of alternative malarial treatment [28, 29, 32].

6. Obligate parasites have many "talents" of survival

During their growth in the vertebrate host or mosquito vector, *Plasmodium* parasites undertake quick proliferation to yield a huge amount of offspring parasites. This speedy development depends sincerely on the effective achievement of vital nutrients such as purine nucleosides and nucleobases, amino acids, sugars, and vitamins from the host [46]. One of these vitamins, pantothenic acid (Vitamin B5), is a precursor of the important enzyme cofactor, CoA (**Figure 4**). As *Plasmodium* parasites cannot produce pantothenate *de novo*, the uptake and consumption of this precursor from the host are critical for existence. Studies in *P. falciparum* and *P. lophurae* have shown two diverse likely tactics used by malaria parasites in host erythrocytes to synthesize CoA [46]. While *P. falciparum* seems to use endogenous vitamin transporters to take up pantothenate from human plasma and a parasite-encoded transporter on the parasite plasma membrane to transport it from the erythrocyte cytoplasm into the parasite for the following employment, *P. lophurae* consumptions preformed CoA in its nucleated erythrocyte cytoplasm. The CoA transporter used by *P. lophurae* on its plasma membrane has not yet been identified.

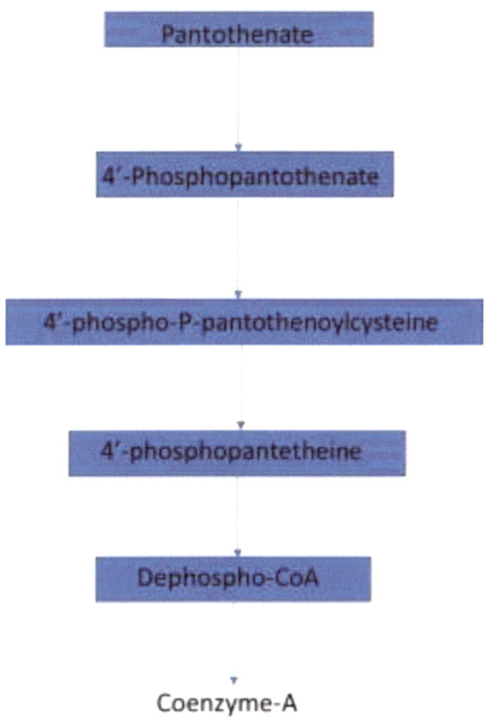

Figure 4.
Highlighting the role of panothenate in the synthesis of coenzyme-a in obligate parasites.

7. Current drugs are available in the market for malaria

Utmost of the antimalarial drugs aim at the asexual erythrocytic stages of the parasite, therefore named blood schizonticidal drugs. Tissue schizonticidal drugs mark the hypnozoites (dormant stage of the parasite) in the liver, while gametocytocidal drugs destroy sexual erythrocytic formulae of the parasite in the bloodstream and thus inhibit transmission of malaria to mosquito. Sporontocides stop or inhibit the formation of malarial oocysts and sporozoites in an infected mosquito. Chloroquine, quinine, and mefloquine are typically fast-acting schizonticidal drugs. Pyrimethamine, sulphonamides, and sulphone also possess schizonticidal activities, nevertheless, their action is dawdling (**Table 2**). Primaquine, Tafenoquine, and other novel kinase inhibitors have gametocidal activities. The main sporontocidal drugs are primaquine and praguanil. These antimalarial drugs were considered based on major metabolic differences of the malaria parasite with its host. Nucleic acid metabolism, heme toxification, oxidative stress, and fatty acid biosynthesis are some of the major pathways that were targeted mostly for antimalarial drug design. However, in the chemotherapy of malaria, the emergence of resistance to the available drugs is the major obstacle.

Furthermost of the existing antimalarial drugs have been used for decades and now their use is restricted by the emergence of drug resistance. According to various literature, there are no existing anti-malarial drugs that were developed in a fully rational manner, with a focused attempt to inhibit a known drug target [35, 36, 47]. Instead, in all cases, anti-malarial potency has been identified in animal or *in vitro* model studies. Consequently, the target of action for most existing agents inside the malaria parasite remains indeterminate.

8. Proposed drug candidate

There is an urgent need to develop new chemotherapeutic agents which display schizontocidal activity, thereby overcoming the making of merozoites from erythrocytes. The rise of drug resistance can be overcome by aiming the parasite transmission at the blood stage. Additionally, powerful drug candidates are vital to be explored. These should prove to be potent enough at a single dose to

Structural name	Types of compounds
(1) Aryl aminoalcohol compounds	• Quinine
	• Metfloquine
	• Halofantine
	• Lumafantine
(2) Antifolate compounds	• Proguanil
	• Pyrmethamine
	• Trimethopin
(3) Artemisinin compounds	• Artemisinin
	• Artesunate
	• Arthemether
	• Arteether

Table 2.
List of current malaria drugs in the market.

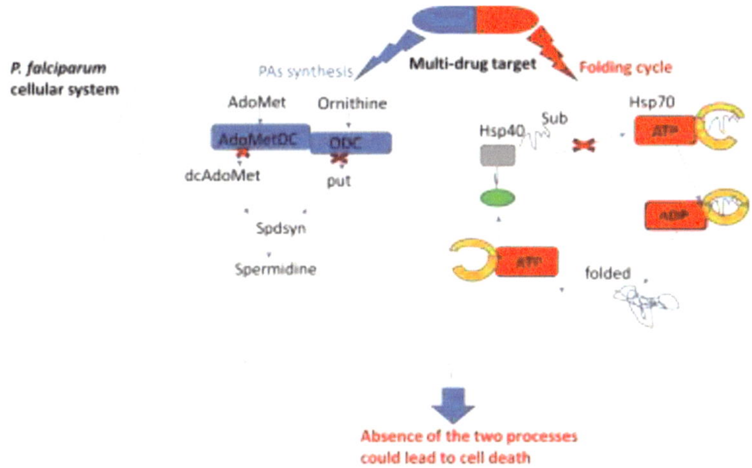

Figure 5.
Proposed drug candidate for plasmodium falciparum. *A multidrug target candidate that will inhibit polyamine biosynthesis and heat shock proteins could lead to dysfunctionality of the* plasmodium falciparum *parasite cellular system, which could lead to cell death.*

block the parasite transmission at the erythrocytic stage. Both safety and efficacy aspects of novel drug candidates also need distinct consideration to be a matter of great concern for antimalarial drug discovery. The medicinal chemist along with the pharmacologist necessities to work hard for the antimalarial drug development to achieve the desired safety, efficacy, and potency in a single dose molecule [30, 48, 49]. General, to decrease the present malaria load competently, more support is necessary in the long run. If the *P. falciparum* parasite uses polyamines and heat shock proteins as its shield under stressful conditions, these molecules could serve as an ideal drug target for malarial drug development [27]. The study to understand the mechanism behind this interplay is currently investigated in our laboratory and how this contributes to drug resistance. Below, we propose a drug candidate that will inhibit the biosynthesis of polyamines which could lead to reduced production of heat shock proteins if indeed polyamines influence the production of the former (**Figure 5**). Their essential role for pathogenic microorganisms growing in a host is of particular interest for drug discovery.

9. Conclusion and future perspectives

There has been regular work over the years for the radical treatment of malaria. Improvement of drug confrontation, existence the most problematic obstacle for the achievement of antimalarial therapy, most of the research is oriented towards overcoming the emergence and spread of resistance to existing drugs by one or the other means. Notwithstanding the pressing need, fewer energies have been absorbed in developing new drugs with new mechanism(s) of action. Now for the last periods, pharmaceutical consideration has on receiving more understandings into numerous metabolic or biochemical pathways of the parasite with the expectation to classify and exploit novel drug targets. The study is also underway to establish the mechanism of action of polyamines being influential in the synthesis of heat shock proteins and the role of polyamines being regarded or acting as chaperones in *P. falciparum* parasite during red blood cells merozoite invasion. This will lead to the development of new chemical compounds or specific inhibitors to act on these new targets.

Acknowledgements

The author wish to thank the University of Fort Hare for the support to this work. Lastly, wish to thank Dr. RA Mosa for his technical assistance.

Author details

Xolani Henry Makhoba
Department of Biochemistry and Microbiology, University of Fort Hare, Alice, South Africa

*Address all correspondence to: xmakhoba@ufh.ac.za

References

[1] World Health Organization (WHO), 2019.

[2] World Health Organization (WHO), 2020.

[3] Perdeh J, Berioso B, Love Q, LoGiudice N, Le TL, Harrelson JP, Roberts SC. (2020). Critical functions of the polyamine putrescine for proliferation and viability of *Leishmania donovani* parasites. Amino Acids 52:261-274.

[4] Vannier-Santosa MA and Suarez-Fontes AM. (2017). Role of polyamines in parasite cell architecture and function. Current Pharmaceutical Design 23:003.

[5] Niemand J, Birkholtz L, Louw AI, Kirk K. (2010). Polyamine uptake in the malaria parasite, *Plasmodium falciparum*, is dependent on the parasite's membrane potential. Malaria Journal 2010 9(Suppl 2):O24.

[6] Chattopadhyay MK, Tabor CW, and Tabor H. (2003). Polyamines protect *Escherichia coli* cells from the toxic effect of oxygen. PNAS 100(5):2261-2265.

[7] C. Hanfrey, S. Sommer, M.J. Mayer, D. Burtin, A.J. Michael. (2001). Arabidopsis polyamine biosynthesis: Absence of ornithine ecarboxylase and the mechanism of arginine decarboxylase activity. Plant J. 27:551-560.

[8] M.P. Hasne, I. Coppens, R. Soysa, B. Ullman (2010). A high-affinity putrescine-cadaverine transporter from *Trypanosoma cruzi*. Mol. Microbiol. 76:78-91.

[9] Ivanov IP, Shin B, Loughran G, Cao C, Tzani I, Young-Baird SK, Atkins JF, Dever TE. (2018). Polyamine control of translation elongation regulates start site selection on antizyme inhibitor mRNA via ribosome queuing. Molecular Cell 70:254-264.

[10] Oh TJ and Kim IG. (1998). Polyamines protect against DNA strand breaks and aid cell survival against irradiation in *Escherichia coli*. Biotechnology Techniques 12(10): 755-758.

[11] Miller-Fleming L, Olin-Sandoval V, Campbell K and Ralser M. (2015). Remaining mysteries of molecular biology: The role of polyamines in the cell. J Mol Biol 427:3389-3406.

[12] H.J. Rhee, E.-J. Kim, J.K. Lee (2007). Physiological polyamines: Simple primordial stress molecules. J. Cell. Mol. Med. 11:685-703.

[13] T. Kusano, T. Berberich, C. Tateda, Y. Takahashi (2008). Polyamines: Essential factors for growth and survival. Planta 228:367-381.

[14] S.A. Le Quesne, A.H. Fairlamb (1996). Regulation of a high-affinity diamine transport system in *Trypanosoma cruzi* epimastigotes. Biochem. J. 316:481-486.

[15] P.C. Tomar, N. Lakra, S.N. Mishra (2013). Cadaverine: A lysine catabolite involved in plant growth and development. Plant Signal Behav. 8:1-15.

[16] Y. Yamamoto, Y. Miwa, K. Miyoshi, J. Furuyama, H. Ohmori. The *Escherichia coli* ldcC gene encodes another lysine decarboxylase, probably a constitutive enzyme. Genes Genet. Syst. 72 (1997) 167-172.

[17] A. Romano, H. Trip, J.S. Lolkema, P.M. Lucas. Three component lysine/ornithine decarboxylation system in *Lactobacillus saerimneri* 30a. J. Bacteriol. 195 (2013) 1249-1254.

[18] Y. Tanaka, B. Kimura, H. Takahashi, T. Watanabe, H. Obata, A. Kai, et al.

Lysine decarboxylase of *Vibrio parahaemolyticus*: Kinetics of transcription and role in acid resistance. J. Appl. Microbiol. 104 (2008) 1283-1293.

[19] A.E. Pegg, S. McGill. Decarboxylation of ornithine and lysine in rat tissues. Biochim. Biophys. Acta 568 (1979) 416-427.

[20] P.A. Whitney, D.R. Morris. Polyamine auxotrophs of *Saccharomyces cerevisiae*. J. Bacteriol. 134 (1978) 214-220.

[21] Afanador, G.A., Tomchick, D.R., and Phillips, M.A. (2018). Trypanosomatid deoxyhypusine synthase activity is dependent on shared active-site complementation between pseudoenzyme paralogs. Structure 26(this issue):1499-1512.

[22] K. Kashiwagi, S. Miyamoto, E. Nukui, H. Kobayashi, K. Igarashi. Functions of PotA and PotD proteins in spermidine-preferential uptake system in *Escherichia coli*. J. Biol. Chem. 268 (1993) 19358-19363.

[23] C. Carrillo, S. Cejas, N.S. González, I.D. Algranati. (1999). *Trypanosoma cruzi* epimastigotes lack ornithine decarboxylase but can express a foreign gene encoding this enzyme. FEBS Lett. 454:192-196.

[24] Casero, R.A., Jr., Murray Stewart, T., and Pegg, A.E. (2018). Polyamine metabolism and cancer: Treatments, challenges and opportunities. Nat. Rev. Cancer 18:681-695.

[25] Geall AJ, Baugh JA, Loyevsky M, Gordeuk VR, Al-Abed Y, and Bucala R. (2004). Targeting malaria with polyamines. Bioconjugate Chem 15:1161–1165.

[26] K. Igarashi, K. Ito, K. Kashiwagi. Polyamine uptake systems in *Escherichia coli*. Res. Microbiol. 152 (2001) 271-278.

[27] Pegg, A.E. (2009). S-Adenosylmethionine decarboxylase. Essays Biochem. 46:25-45.

[28] Makhoba XH and Mthembu MS (2016). The role of small heat shock proteins on folding processes of PfAdoMetDC/ODC protein as a malarial drug target. Austin J Proteomics Bioinform and Genomics 3(1):1015.

[29] Makhoba XH and Mthembu MS (2017). Identification of possible binding sites on PfAdoMetDC by *E. coli* trigger factor using bioinformatics approach. Austin J Proteomic Bioinform and Genomics 4(1):1021.

[30] Nagai Y, Fujikake, N.H, Popiel A and Wada K. (2010). Induction of molecular chaperones as a therapeutic strategy for the polyglutamine diseases. Current Pharmaceutical Biotechnology 11:188-197.

[31] Charity Mekgwa Lebepe, Pearl Rutendo Matambanadzo, Xolani Henry Makhoba, Ikechukwu Achilonu, Tawanda Zininga, Addmore Shonhai (2020). Comparative characterisation of *Plasmodium falciparum* Hsp70-1 relative to *E. coli* DnaK reveals functional specificity of the parasite chaperone. Biomolecules 10:856. DOI:10.3390/biom10060856

[32] Xolani H. Makhoba, Claudio Viegas Jr., Rebamang A. Mosa, Flávia P. D. Viegas and Ofentse J. Pooe (2020). Potential impact of the multi-target drug approach in the treatment of some complex diseases. Drug Design, Development and Therapy 14:3235-3249.

[33] Kennedy, P.G. (2013). Clinical features, diagnosis, and treatment of human African trypanosomiasis (sleeping sickness). Lancet Neurol. 12:186-194.

[34] Park, M.H., and Wolff, E.C. (2018). Hypusine, a polyamine-derived amino acid critical for eukaryotic translation. J.

Biol. Chem. Published online on September 26, 2018. jbc.TM118.003341.

[35] Pegg, A.E., and McCann, P.P. (1982). Polyamine metabolism and function. Am. J. Physiol. 243:C212–C221.

[36] Pegg, A.E., and Michael, A.J. (2010). Spermine synthase. Cell. Mol. Life Sci. 67:113-121.

[37] Willert, E.K., Fitzpatrick, R., and Phillips, M.A. (2007). Allosteric regulation of an essential trypanosome polyamine biosynthetic enzyme by a catalytically dead homolog. Proc. Natl. Acad. Sci. USA 104:8275-8280.

[38] K. Igarashi, K. Kashiwagi. Characteristics of cellular polyamine transport in prokaryotes and eukaryotes. Plant Physiol. Biochem. 48 (2010) 506-512.

[39] K. Kashiwagi, S. Shibuya, H. Tomitori, A. Kuraishi, K. Igarashi. Excretion and uptake of putrescine by the PotE protein in *Escherichia coli*. J. Biol. Chem. 272 (1997) 6318-6323.

[40] W. Soksawatmaekhin, A. Kuraishi, K. Sakata, K. Kashiwagi, K. Igarashi. Excretion and uptake of cadaverine by CadB and its physiological functions in *Escherichia coli*. Mol. Microbiol. 51 (2004) 1401-1412.

[41] K. Higashi, H. Ishigure, R. Demizu, T. Uemura, K. Nishino, A. Yamaguchi, et al. Identification of a spermidine excretion protein complex (MdtJI) in *Escherichia coli*. J. Bacteriol. 190 (2008) 872-878.

[42] T. Uemura, K. Kashiwagi, K. Igarashi. Uptake of putrescine and spermidine by Gap1p on the plasma membrane in *Saccharomyces cerevisiae*. Biochem. Biophys. Res. Commun. 328 (2005) 1028-1033.

[43] Hesterberg RS, Cleveland JL and Epling-Burnette PK. (2018). Role of polyamines in immune cell functions. Med. Sci. 6:22. DOI:10.3390/medsci6010022

[44] Pendeville, H., Carpino, N., Marine, J.C., Takahashi, Y., Muller, M., Martial, J.A., Cleveland, J.L. The ornithine decarboxylase gene is essential for cell survival during early murine development. Mol. Cell. Biol. 2001; 21:6549-6558.

[45] Pegg, A.E. Regulation of ornithine decarboxylase. J. Biol. Chem. 2006;281:14529-14532.

[46] Hart RJ, Lawres L, Fritzen E, Mamoun CB, and Aly AIS (2014). *Plasmodium yoelii* vitamin B5 pantothenate transporter candidate is essential for parasite transmission to the mosquito. Scientific Reports 4:5665.

[47] Umland, T.C., Wolff, E.C., Park, M.H., and Davies, D.R. (2004). A new crystal structure of deoxyhypusine synthase reveals the configuration of the active enzyme and of an enzyme NAD inhibitor ternary complex. J. Biol. Chem. 279:28697-28705.

[48] Wu, H., Min, J., Zeng, H., McCloskey, D.E., Ikeguchi, Y., Loppnau, P., Michael, A.J., Pegg, A.E., and Plotnikov, A.N. (2008). Crystal structure of human spermine synthase: Implications of substrate binding and catalytic mechanism. J. Biol. Chem. 283:16135-16146.

[49] Kalia S. K, Kalia L.V and McLean P. J. (2010). Molecular chaperones as rational drug targets for Parkinson's disease therapeutics. CNS Neurol Disord Drug Targets 9(6):741-753.

Chapter 8

Molecular Approaches for Malaria Therapy

Mitali Mishra, Vikash Kumar Mishra, Varsha Kashaw and Sushil Kumar Kashaw

Abstract

Malaria is a potentially fatal blood disease spread by mosquitos. Malaria is preventable, but it is more prevalent in developing countries where prevention is difficult and prophylaxis is often inaccessible. Malaria remains one of the world's most serious public health problems, according to the World Health Organisation (WHO). The development of resistance is a current problem that poses a danger to the environment. Resistance is a current problem that could jeopardise the use of well-established and cost-effective antimalarials. The World Health Organisation recommends an artemisinin-based drug combination (ACT) to avoid or postpone the development of resistance. This book's chapter discusses current medicines as well as potential and rational possibilities for finding new drugs to treat malady. There were also WHO recommendations for both complicated and non-complicated malaria. Other preventive measures such as ITN and IPT are listed in the manuscript in addition to routine care. While a brief overview of the vaccine tested so far has been included, there is currently no vaccine available to treat malaria.

Keywords: Malaria, *Plasmodium falciparum*, artemisinin, drug repurposing, drug resistant malaria

1. Introduction

Malaria is a life-threatening disease spread by mosquito bites from infected female Anopheles mosquitos ("malaria vectors"). The Plasmodium parasite is borne by infected mosquitos. When an individual is bitten by this mosquito, the parasite is released into the bloodstream. Malaria is caused by a parasitic protozoan of the genus Plasmodium. *Plasmodium vivax*, *Plasmodium ovale*, *Plasmodium malariae,* and *Plasmodium falciparum* are the four types of malaria parasites that can infect humans. *Plasmodium falciparum* and *Plasmodium vivax* are the two most deadly species, responsible for more than 95 percent of all malaria cases worldwide. Each year, approximately 125 million pregnant women are at risk of infection; maternal malaria is linked to up to 200,000 reported child deaths in Sub-Saharan Africa. [1, 2] Maternal malaria is often linked to a number of negative outcomes for the mother, the foetus, and the infant.

The sporozoite form of the protozoan is preserved in the salivary glands of the mosquito. When a person is bitten by an infected female Anopheles mosquito, sporozoites are injected into the bloodstream and easily move into the human liver.

IntechOpen

The sporozoites replicate asexually in the liver cells for the next 7 to 10 days, causing no symptoms. The parasites are released in the form of merozoites from the liver cells and settle in the capillaries of the lungs. Merozoites are released from lung capillaries in the blood phase (also known as pathologic blood stages) of their growth, invading red blood cells (erythrocytes) and multiplying until the cells burst. This cycle continues forever, invading younger red blood cells. These infections in the blood can last for months. Some infected blood cells break the asexual multiplication cycle. Merozoites evolve into sexual forms of the parasite called gametocytes (precursors of male and female gametes) in these cells, which then circulate in the bloodstream. Malaria parasites will now abandon their human hosts and complete their life cycle in an insect vector. When a fertilised mosquito bites an infected individual, the gametocytes in the blood are swallowed by the mosquito, and the gametocytes mature in the mosquito gut. An ookinete is a fertilised, motile zygote produced when male and female gametocytes fuse. Ookinetes grow into new sporozoites, which migrate to the salivary glands of the bug, ready to infect a new host and restart the human infection cycle (**Figure 1**) [3].

Only certain species of mosquitoes of the Anopheles genus—and only females of those species—can transmit malaria. Chills, high fever, profuse sweating, headache, muscle pains, malaise, diarrhoea, and vomiting are all common symptoms of malaria. Malaria, on the other hand, is marked by occasional paroxysmal febrile episodes (i.e., a sudden recurrence or intensification of fever), and untreated infection results in spleen enlargement. *P. falciparum* can affect the lungs, liver, and kidneys, as well as cause extreme anaemia and coma in cerebral malaria, which sometimes leads to death. P. malariae infection can cause kidney damage, which can lead to nephrotic syndrome, which can be fatal. Malaria infections are highly debilitating and can render a person vulnerable to other diseases [4].

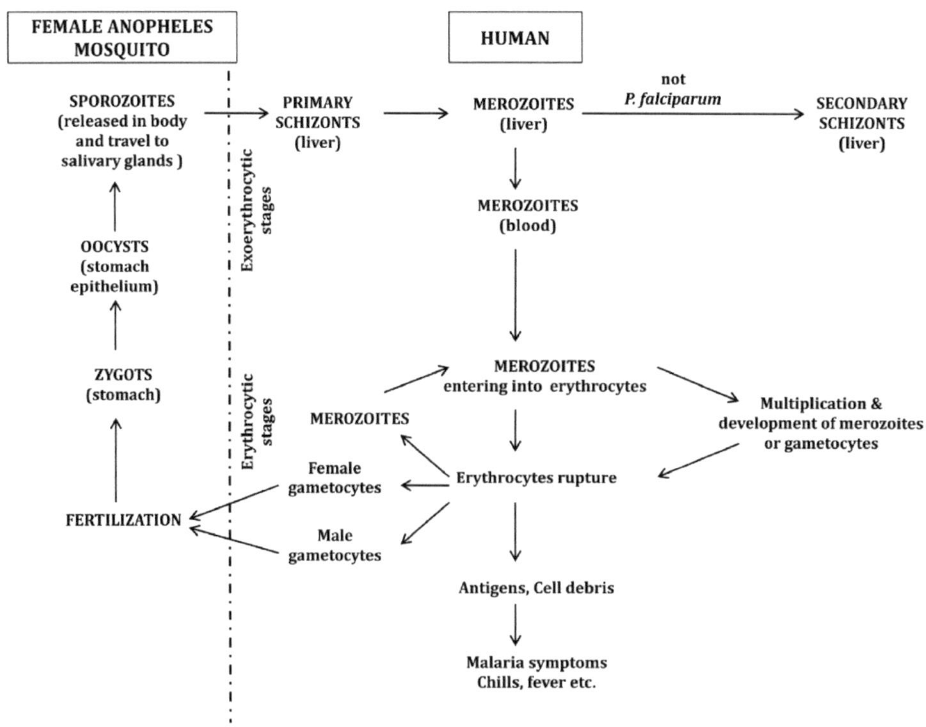

Figure 1.
Malaria parasite life cycle; outlines the steps of the parasite as it is injected into the human victim.

2. Prevention

The primary method for preventing and reducing malaria transmission is vector control. All people at risk of malaria should be covered with successful malaria vector control, according to the WHO. Insecticide-treated mosquito nets and indoor residual spraying are two types of vector control that are effective in a variety of situations [1].

2.1 Insecticide-treated mosquito nets

An insecticide-treated net (ITN) is a mosquito-blocking bed net that has been treated with a protected, residual insecticide for the purpose of killing and/or repelling mosquitoes. By providing both a physical barrier and an insecticidal effect, sleeping under an ITN may minimise mosquito-human interaction. Nets treated with insecticide have been shown to minimise infant mortality. Uncomplicated *P. falciparum* and *P. vixax* malaria episodes are also reduced by ITN [1, 2].

2.2 Indoor residual spraying (IRS)

Indoor residual spraying (IRS) consists of spraying a residual insecticide on the walls and other housing structures once or twice a year [1]. Mosquitoes and other insects that come into contact with these surfaces can be destroyed by the insecticide. Several pesticides have been used for IRS in the past, with DDT being the first and most well-known. Pyrethroids are also used in IRS, where they are sprayed on indoor surfaces.

3. Vaccines against malaria

Since there is currently no effective way to eradicate malaria, developing safe, effective, and cost-effective vaccines against the disease remains a top priority. The malaria vaccine RTS,S/AS01E (RTS,S; (brand name MosquirixTM) is the first and only vaccine to demonstrate that it can substantially reduce malaria in young African children, including life-threatening extreme malaria. RTS,S/AS01E is a candidate for a pre-erythrocytic *P. falciparum* vaccine. Over a four-year period, the vaccine prevented approximately 4 in 10 cases of malaria among children who received four doses in large-scale clinical trials [3]. A vaccine targeting the whole body, a live attenuated vaccine, a genetically modified vaccine, and a subunit vaccine are among the four alternatives to a malaria vaccine that have been studied. Preclinical and clinical studies have recently revealed that Pf sporozoite (SPZ) vaccines show great promise for human safety, but larger sample sizes are required to confirm their protective effects [3, 4].

4. Treatment

Malaria must be identified quickly in order to minimise infection spread in the population and avoid deaths. Before beginning care, the WHO suggests that all reported cases of malaria be confirmed using microscopy or a rapid diagnostic test.

4.1 Antimalarial drugs

Malaria-endemic areas are visited by an estimated 50 million tourists per year. Chemoprophylaxis, which suppresses the blood stage of malaria infections, may be used to avoid malaria in such travellers. WHO recommends at least three doses of sulfadoxine-pyrimethamin intermittent preventive treatment for pregnant women, particularly those living in moderate-to-high transmission areas. Similarly, for infants living in high-transmission areas of Africa, three doses of sulfadoxine-pyrimethamine intermittent preventive care are recommended. Seasonal malaria chemoprevention has been advised by the World Health Organisation (WHO) since 2012. It entails giving all children under the age of 5 months monthly courses of amodiaquine plus sulfadoxine-pyrimethamine [5].

5. Cinchona alkaloids

The medicinal use of the bark of the cinchona tree, which is native to South America, is the starting point for the discovery and synthesis of quinine and synthetic quinoline-containing antimalarial drugs. The quinoline derivatives quinine, quinidine, cinchonidine, and cinchonine are the four most abundant biologically active alkaloids found in the bark (**Figure 2**). The bark also includes quinoline derivatives such as quinicine (also known as quinotoxine) and indole-containing alkaloids including cinchonamine [6].

.

5.1 Quinine and quinidine

Quinine is the first example of a pure chemotherapeutic agent to be produced on an industrial scale and it was the only drug available for the treatment of malaria

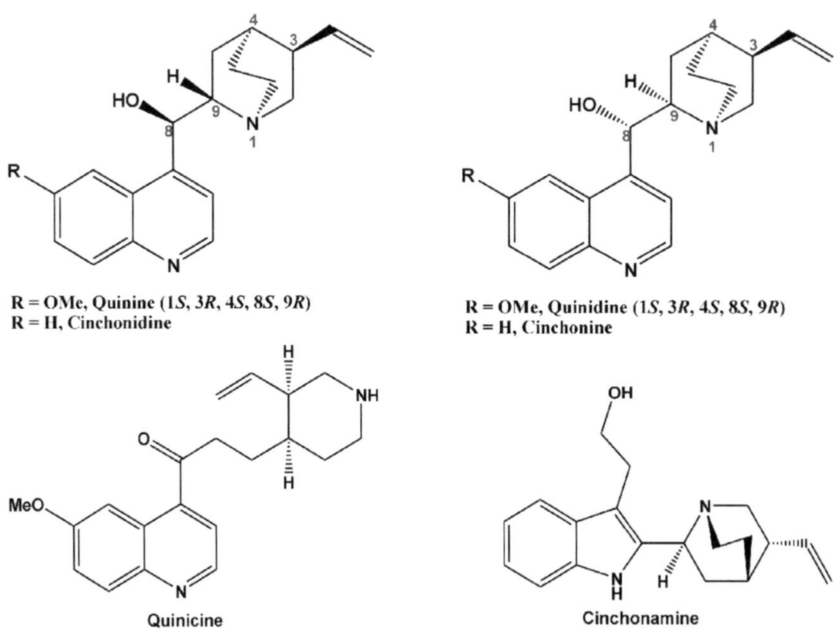

Figure 2.
Structures of the four major and two minor quinoline containing alkaloids obtained from the bark of the cinchona tree.

until the 1930s. Quinine has been used for "fevers" in South America since the 1600s. It is one of the major alkaloids was first used to treat malaria as early as the beginning of the 17th century, and became the standard therapy for malaria from the mid-19th century to the 1940s. The extraction of QN is still more economically viable than its synthetic production [6]. The pure alkaloids, quinine, and cinchonine were isolated in 1820. The stereoisomer, quinidine, is a more potent antimalarial, but it is also more toxic (less selectively toxic). Quinine is lethal for all *Plasmodium* schizonts and the gametocites from *P. vivax* and *P. malariae*, but not for *P. falciparum*. Today, quinine's spectrum of activity is considered too narrow for prophylactic use relative to the synthetic agents [7].

The emergence of resistant strains of *P. falciparum* was first reported in the 1980s [8] and as of 2006, quinine is no longer used as a front-line treatment for malaria but is still on the WHO's Model List of Essential Medicines (MLEM) [9] for the treatment of severe malaria in cases where artemisinins are not available. The mechanism of resistance to quinine is poorly understood and varies with the susceptibility of the parasite to other aminoquinoline antimalarial drugs. Quinine is the only treatment recommended for pregnant women in the first trimester3 and, until recently, it was the only clinical option for the treatment of severe malaria because it can be formulated for safe intravenous administration. However, intravenous artesunate is now preferred when available [10].

QN in clinical uses most often combined with a second agent to shorten the duration of therapy and thus minimise the adverse effects [11]. A toxic syndrome is referred to as cinchonism. Symptoms start with tinnitus, headache, nausea, and disturbed vision. If administration is not stopped, cinchonism can proceed to involvement of the gastrointestinal tract, nervous and cardiovascular system, and the skin. The stereoisomer, quinidine, is a schizonticide, but its primary indication is cardiac arrhythmias. It is a good example where stereochemistry is important because it provides a significantly different pharmacological spectrum [12].

6. 4-Aminoquinolines

4-aminoquinolines (4-AQ), 4-anilinoquinolines, 9-aminoacridines, and azaacridines are all members of this class. These groups are thought to have similar mechanisms of action, are successful on the same stage of the parasite, and may share similar mechanisms of resistance, in addition to their structural similarity (**Figures 3** and **4**).

4-Aminoquinoline is a type of aminoquinoline in which the amino group is located at the quinoline's 4-position. Antimalarial agents derived from 4-aminoquinoline can be used to treat erythrocytic plasmodial infections. Amodiaquine, chloroquine, and hydroxychloroquine are some examples [13].

Malaria is treated with 4-aminoquinolines (4-AQs) during the blood stage of the disease (the merozoites). The unprotonated form of these drugs is a weak base that can cross the food vacuolar membrane of parasites; however, once within the vacuole, both the quinoline nitrogen and the amino group of the side chain of 4-AQs become protonated species that is impermeable to the vacuolar membrane, causing ion-trapping inside the vacuole [14].

6.1 Chloroquine and hydroxychloroquine

Chloroquine, a 4-aminoquinoline, prevents ferriprotoporphyrin IX polymerisation, causing oxidative membrane damage and parasite death in infected erythrocytes. Because of widespread resistance, it's normally only used to treat malaria

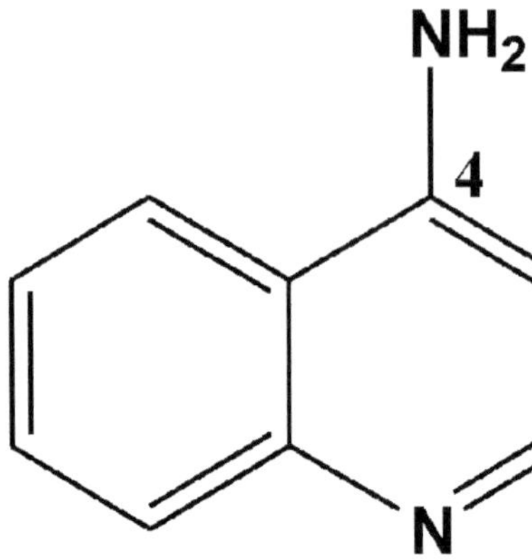

4-Aminoquinoline

Figure 3.
General chemical structure of 4-aminoquinoline.

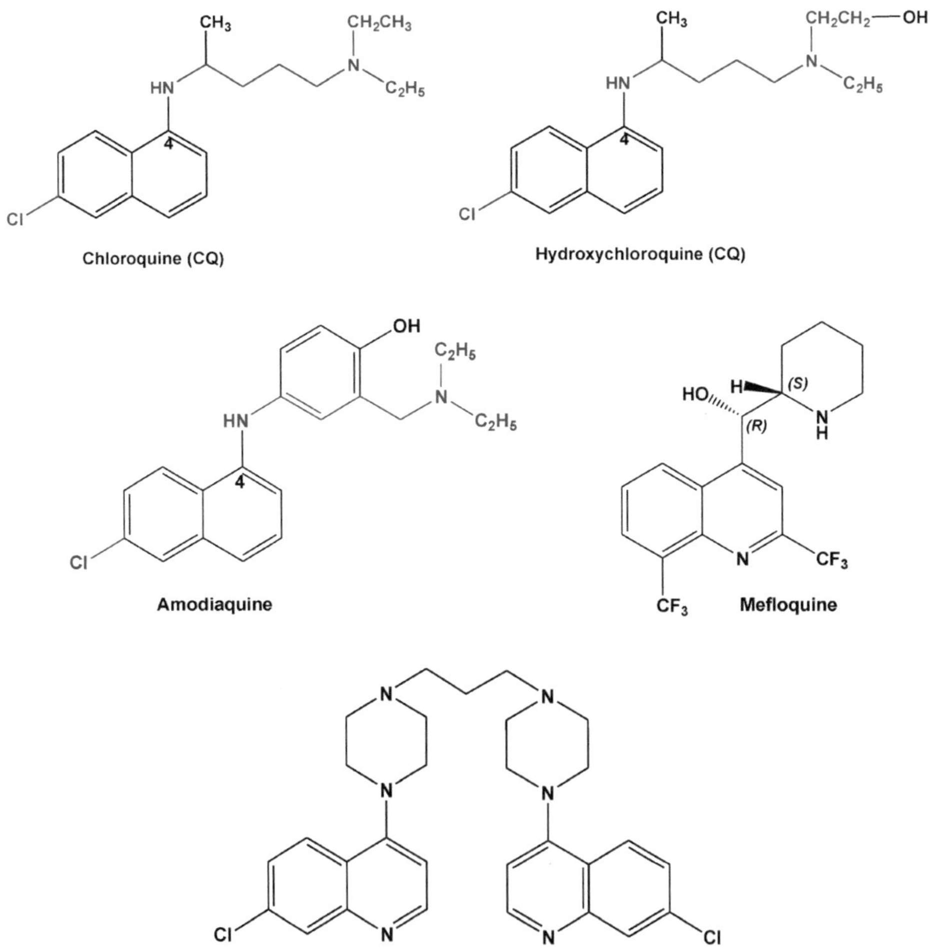

Figure 4.
Structures of some representative 4-aminoquinolines.

patients in situations where chloroquine susceptibility can be guaranteed. Malaria caused by *P. falciparum* is almost always immune to choloroquine, with the exception of cases acquired in Haiti.

Chloroquine is only effective against the parasite's erythrocytic stages; for the full cure of *P. vivax* and *P. ovale* infections, another agent (primaquine) is needed. Chloroquine has been used in conjunction with dehydroemetine to treat invasive amebiasis that has not responded to other treatments and to treat connective tissue autoimmune disorders that have not responded to other treatments.

Chloroquine is thought to get stuck in the parasite's food vacuole, where it prevents -hematin from crystallising. The acidic nature of the vacuole (pH 4.8–5.2) causes chloroquine to become 'trapped' in its membrane-impermeable doubly protonated shape, which is membrane-impermeable. Chloroquine then forms a complex with free heme, causing heme to accumulate and the parasite to die. *P. falciparum* resistant strains were discovered to have a mutation in the Pfcrt gene, which encodes the chloroquine resistance transporter (Pfcrt) protein [8, 9]. Because of changes in the membrane protein, this transporter protein induces reduced drug concentration inside the food vacuole, allowing chloroquine to disperse away from the vacuole. CQ-resistant parasite strains have a neutral threonine residue at position 76 of the Pfcrt protein in place of the positively charged lysine moiety, allowing chloroquine efflux from the digestive vacuole [15–17].

Within the parasite's food vacuole, the parasite catabolises the protein of the host cell haemoglobin, resulting in peptides, which are further degraded to produce amino acids, which are used by the parasite for survival and development. As a byproduct of haemoglobin degradation, free heme (iron (II) centred porphyrin) is produced, which quickly oxidises to hematin (iron (III) centred species). Heme and hematin are also extremely toxic to parasites. Heme may interfere with the parasite's organelles' various membranous structures, causing irreversible damage and disrupting transport processes and ion homeostasis. Multiple pathways result in parasite death. 25.19 Biomineralisation removes heme and hematin, resulting in hemozoin, a parasite-unfriendly substance. Hloroquine prevents or inhibits the parasite's ability to detoxify heme, resulting in parasite death [18–20].

Chloroquine tablets are bitter in taste and are available in the United States. Chloroquine suspensions are commonly available for paediatric use in other countries and are much more well tolerated. As a malaria chemoprophylactic, chloroquine may be used. Most people tolerate chloroquine well, even when used for long periods of time. Mild gastrointestinal symptoms (which are usually relieved if the medication is taken with food), intermittent headaches, blurred vision, dizziness, weakness, confusion, hair depigmentation, skin eruptions, corneal opacity, weight loss, and myalgias are all potential side effects. Antihistamines are commonly used to treat intense pruritus, which is a common problem among black Africans who take the medication. Patients with psoriasis, retinal disease, or porphyria should avoid chloroquine. In most respects, hydroxychloroquine is similar to chloroquine. The only structural difference is a hydroxy moiety on one of the N-ethyl groups. It stays in the body for over a month, much like chloroquine, and prophylactic dosing is once weekly. Children tolerate hydroxychloroquine better [21–24].

6.2 Amodiaquine

Amodiaquine was first documented to have antimalarial activity in 1946, but due to its toxicity, it was removed as a prescribed monotherapy in the early 1990s. It acts in a similar way to chloroquine and has some cross-resistance with CQ, but it does not have any advantages over other 4-aminoquinoline drugs [25] (**Figure 5**).

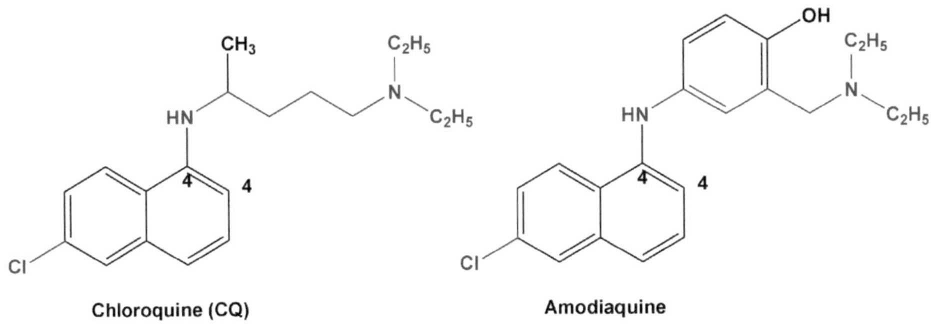

Figure 5.
The inter-nitrogen distance in the side chains of amodiaquine and CQ.

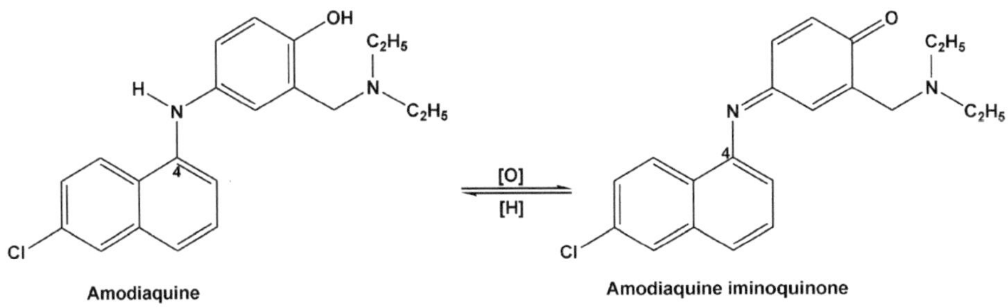

Figure 6.
Metabolic activation of amodiaquine to amodiaquine iminoquinone.

It had a higher rate of extreme hepatitis and agranulocytosis than chloroquine when used for malaria prophylaxis. The toxicity of amodiaquine is thought to be due to P450-mediated and/or autooxidation of the 1, 4-aminophenol group, which produces a quinone imine intermediate [26] (**Figure 6**).

Amodiaquine's efficacy against some chloroquine-resistant *Plasmodium falciparum* strains has led to a resurgence in its use, especially in combination therapy with artesunate. Although amodiaquine resistance in some parts of Africa can restrict the effectiveness of this combination in those areas, the artesunate–amodiaquine combination has proven to be very effective in areas where amodiaquine alone produces responses of more than 80% [27].

6.3 Mefloquine

The racemic form of mefloquine is the newest of the 4-aminoquinolines. The drug's optical isomers are all active in the same way. The US Army [28] built it in the 1970s. It was initially developed to treat chloroquine-resistant malaria, but it has since been used as a curative and prophylactic medication (travellers coming into regions of malaria) (**Figure 7**).

Mefloquine differs from other 4-aminoquinoline agents in that it has two trifluromethyl moieties at positions 2 and 8, and no electronegative substituents at positions 6 (quinine) or 7 (mefloquine) (chloroquine). Mefloquine is not schizonticidal, which distinguishes it from chloroquine and its analogues. Mefloquine is slowly metabolised to carboxymefloquine, its main inactive metabolite, through CYP3A4 oxidation. The majority of the parent compound is excreted in its natural state in the urine [29] (**Figure 8**).

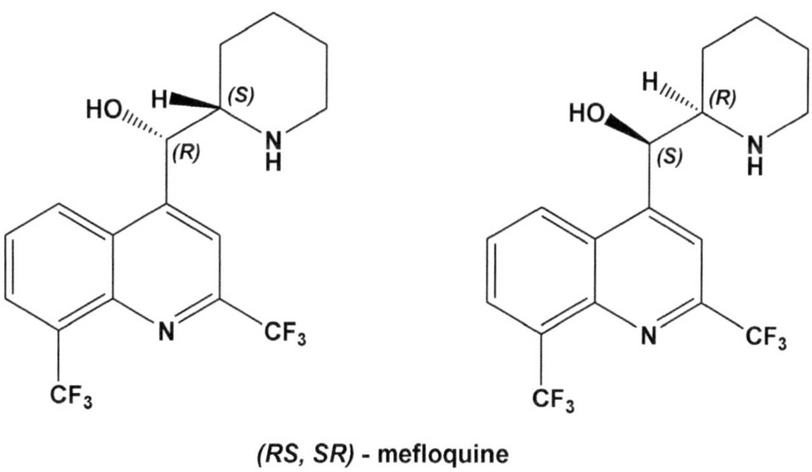

Figure 7.
Racemic forms (RS & SR) of mefloquine.

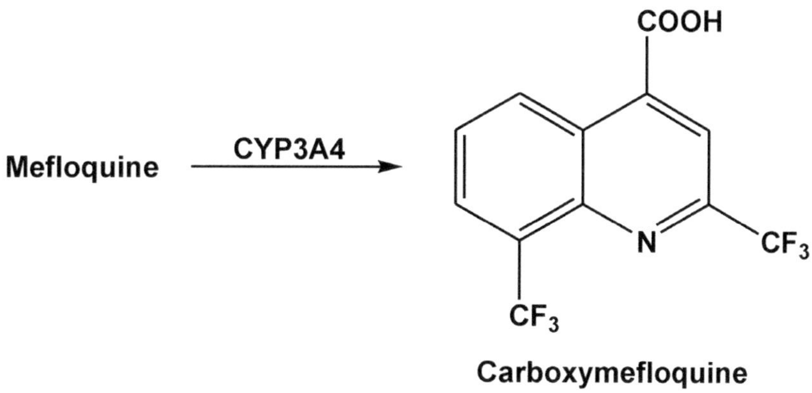

Figure 8.
Metabolic activation of mefloquine to carboxymefloquine.

P. falciparum mefloquine-resistant strains were first identified in 1986 [23]. In rats, rodents, and rabbits, mefloquine causes teratogenicity. This medication comes with an FDA-mandated warning that it can worsen mental illnesses, and the neuropsychiatric effects can be severe (e.g., suicidal impulses or seizures) or mild (e.g., headaches) (e.g., dizziness, vertigo, ataxia, and headaches). Bradycardia, arrhythmias, and extrasystoles are all possible cardiovascular side effects [30].

7. 8-Aminoquinolines

Another big class of antimalarial drugs based on the cinchona alkaloid quinoline moiety is substituted 8-aminoquinolines (**Figure 9**). The 8-aminoquinolines were the first synthetic antimalarial drugs approved by the FDA. The German researchers introduced pamaquine as the first compound in this sequence. Due to its high toxicity and restricted activity, pamaquine was no longer used in clinical trials [31]. In 1950, primaquine was introduced as a pamaquine analogue. It was the only approved treatment for removing the Plasmodium parasite from the liver and preventing malaria relapses caused by *P. ovale* and *P. vivax* until July 2018 [32].

In patients with erythrocytic glucose-6-phosphate dehydrogenase deficiency, all of the 8-aminoquinolines have been reported to cause hemolytic anaemia. This is a common genetic trait in people who live in malaria-endemic areas [33]. Since 4-AQs are active during the blood stages of the parasite life cycle, and the blood stages of *P. falciparum* can be cultured and thus studied relatively easily, the mechanism of action for 8-aminoquinolines (8-AQs) is less well known than for 4-aminoquinolines (4-AQs) [34, 35].

The mechanism of action for the 8-AQs cannot be inhibition of hemozoin formation because liver cells do not produce haemoglobin. Primaquine suggested an autoxidation of the 8-amino group to produce ROS. Augusto et al. [36] suggested the creation of a radical anion at the 8-amino group. Cell-destructive oxidants like hydrogen peroxide, superoxide, and the hydroxyl radical can form as a result, causing oxidative damage to essential cellular components.

The structure–activity relationships in this series display very little variance. The four agents in **Figure 9**, all have the same 6-methoxy moiety as quinine, but the substituent on quinoline are at position 8 rather than carbon-4, as they are on cinchona alkaloids. Between the two nitrogens, all of the agents in this sequence have a four to five carbon alkyl linkage or bridge. The other three 8-aminoquinolines, with the exception of pentaquine, all have one asymmetric carbon. Although there are some variations in the metabolism of each stereoisomer and the form of adverse reaction, there are little differences in antimalarial activity based on the stereochemistry of the compounds. In patients with a glucose-6-phosphate dehydrogenase deficiency, all of the 8-aminoquinolines can cause hemolytic anaemia (G6PD). This is a common genetic trait found in people who live in malaria-prone areas. The key clinical problems associated with primaquine are a short half-life (4–6 hours), which means it must be taken everyday for 14 days to be successful, and hemolysis [37–40].

7.1 Primaquine

Primaquine (PQ), an 8-aminoquinoline that has been clinically used since 1950, is still the only drug used worldwide to treat relapsing *P. vivax* malaria caused by

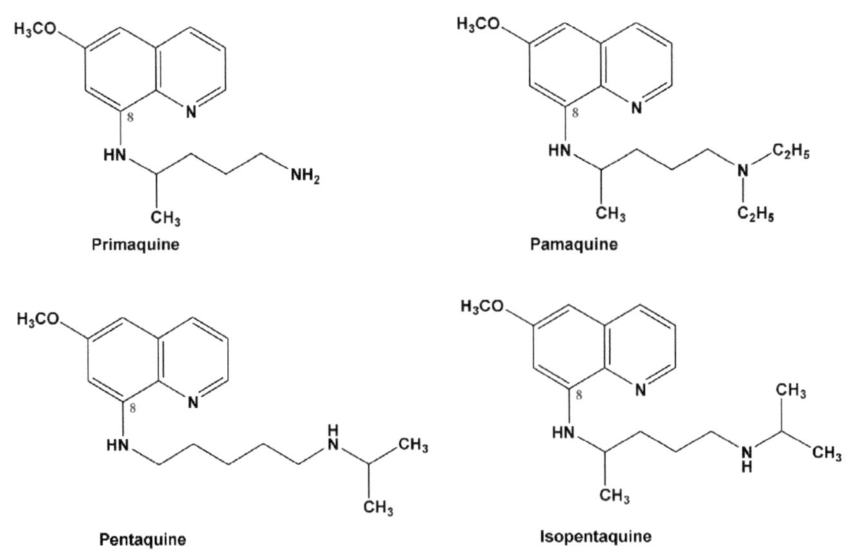

Figure 9.
Structures of some representative 8-aminoquinolines.

hypnozoites, and it inhibits gametocyte formation. It is not used in the prevention of disease. The only drug available for treating *P. vivax* and *P. ovale* latent hepatic life cycle forms is primaquine [41, 42]. Following the initiation of chloroquine treatment for the erythrocytic stages of infection, primaquine is recommended for the radical cure of these infections. It has one of the narrowest spectrums of activity of any currently used antimalarial drug, as it is only indicated for exoerythrocytic *P. vivax* malaria. Chloroquine or a drug prescribed for chloroquine-resistant *P. vivax* is combined with primaquine to treat endoerythrocytic *P. vivax*. It is also active against the exoerythrocytic stages of *P. ovale* and the main exoerythrocytic stages of *P. falciparum* [43], in addition to its accepted indication.

Primaquine is readily absorbed, widely spread, and cleared mainly by non-renal removal. Carboxyprimaquine is the primary metabolite. Primaquine is successful when administered once daily or even once weekly [44], despite the fact that the medication is quickly removed from the plasma. Except in people with G6PD deficiency, where administration can cause brisk hemolysis, primaquine is typically well tolerated. Prior to starting primaquine therapy, patients should be tested for G6PD deficiency. Regardless of G6PD status, primaquine should never be given to a pregnant woman. Neutropenia, gastrointestinal disturbances, and methemoglobinemia are rare side effects. *P. vivax* relapses after primaquine therapy have been treated with chloroquine and higher doses or longer courses of primaquine [45].

Primaquine is the most effective currently available prophylactic for *P. vivax* malaria and equivalent to such regimens as doxycycline, mefloquine, and atovaquone-proguanil for the prevention of *P. falciparum* malaria, according to a recent meta-analysis and systematic review [46, 47]. NPC1161B, a chiral 8-aminoquinoline derivative developed at the University of Mississippi, was still undergoing preclinical testing in 2014 [48–52].

8. Artemisinin and its derivatives

Artemisinin (ART), a sesquiterpene lactone[1], was discovered in 1971 by Tu Youyou, a Chinese scientist, in the plant *Artemisia annua* (a herbaceous plant in the Asteraceae family), which is widely used in Chinese traditional medicine [55]. Youyou shared the Nobel Prize in Physiology or Medicine in 2015 for "her findings concerning a novel therapy against malaria" [56], owing to the significant positive effect of ART in the fight against malaria.

Artemisinins are successful not only against multi-resistant strains of *Plasmodium falciparum*, but they also have strong stage specificity against the Plasmodium life cycle, including activity during the asexual blood stages [57] as well as the sexual gametocyte stages, which may help to minimise disease spread in low-transmission areas [58]. Artemisinin resistance was first recorded in western Cambodia in 2008 [59]. ART and its derivatives have been used as first-line drugs in the treatment of malaria since their antimalarial activity was discovered.

Since chemical synthesis of ART is considered to be costly, the key commercial sources of ART are field-grown leaves and flowering tops of *A. annua*. Since mature plants will lack the active drug, the plant must be grown from seed every year. To

[1] Sesquiterpene lactones (SLs) are a type of sesquiterpene with a lactone ring; a sesquiterpene has three isoprene (2-methyl-1,3-butadiene) units. Lactones are cyclic carboxylic esters with a 1-oxacycloalkan-2-one structure (C(=O)O); sesquiterpene lactones (SLs) are present primarily in Asteraceae plants (daisies, asters). Umbelliferae (celery, parsley, carrots) and Magnoliaceae (magnolias) are two other plant families with SLs [53, 54].

maximise artemisinin yield, the increasing conditions must be perfect. Plants grown in North Vietnam, China's Chongqing province, and Tanzania have recorded the highest yields so far [60].

As compared to other compounds historically and currently used, the artemisinin sequence is structurally distinct. The endoperoxide (C–O–O–C) and dioxepin oxygens tend to form a "trioxane," which appears to be the most significant structural element. Artemisinine, a sesquiterpene trioxane lactone with an endoperoxide bridge that is necessary for antimalarial activity, does indeed represent a new chemical class of antimalarial agents. It distinguishes artemisinins from other antimalarial drugs by limiting cross-resistance. Artemisinin derivatives such as artemether, artesunate, and arteether are the most common. These semi-synthetic derivatives are prodrugs that are converted to dihydroartemisinin, the active metabolite. Unlike quinine, artemisinin derivatives destroy young circulating parasites until they sequester in the deep microvasculature [61–65] (**Figure 10**).

Following oral administration, the artemisinins are rapidly absorbed, with maximum plasma concentrations occurring in 2 to 3 hours for artemisinin and artemether, and less than 1 hour for artesunate [66, 67]. Artemisinin is transformed to inactive metabolites in the liver, such as deoxyartemisinin, deoxydihydroartemisinin, and others, where the endoperoxide group is lost and the metabolites become ineffective. CYP2B6 is the enzyme that catalyses the reaction. Different artemisinin derivatives are metabolised. They're converted to dihydroartemisinin first (DHA). DHA is a potent antimalarial molecule that lasts for two to three hours in the bloodstream. Artesunate's antimalarial operation is mediated exclusively by DHA. (Direct antimalarials include artemisinin, arteether, artemether, and others.) Within a minute of absorption, artesunate is converted to DHA. DHA is converted to inactive metabolites in the liver by the cytochrome P450 enzyme system (which includes CYP2A6, CYP3A4, and CYP3A5). Both metabolites are glucuronidated before being excreted in the urine or faeces. Artemisinins are relatively safe drugs due to their quick metabolism [68–70].

Artesunate is a water-soluble semisynthetic form of artemisinin that can be taken orally or injected intravenously or intramuscularly. Artesunate is superior to artemisinin and other oil-based derivatives [71] due to its chemical property and pharmacokinetic profile, as it is almost instantly converted into dihydroartemisinin after ingestion, which accounts for the antimalarial activity. The endoperoxide pharmacophore alone has stimulated the production of many different groups of totally synthetic endoperoxides, including the trioxolane OZ277 [72] and the tetraoxane 3 [73], despite the fact that the exact mechanism of action is still highly debated [72] (**Figure 11**).

Although the exact mechanism of artemisinin is unknown, it is thought to be triggered by haem, which produces free radicals, which damage parasite survival proteins [74, 75]. The initial formation of highly reactive oxygen-centered radicals

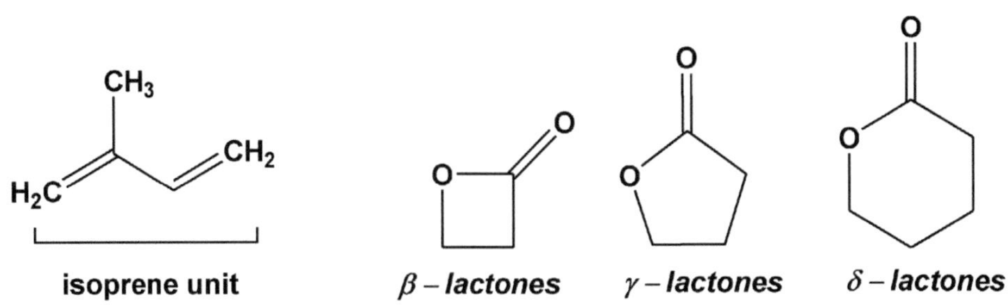

Figure 10.
Structural units of artemisinine family of compounds.

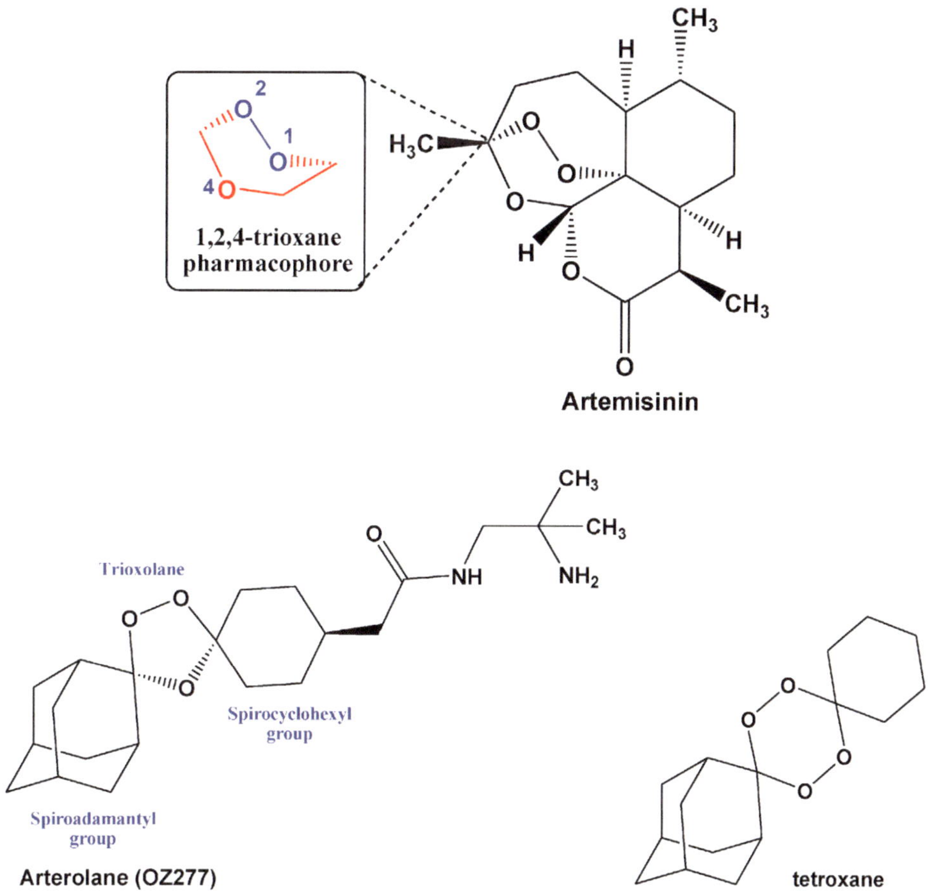

Figure 11.
Pharmacophoric structures of ART derivatives.

by iron(II)-catalysed homolytic cleavage of the peroxide bond is thought to result in rapid intramolecular rearrangement to give cytotoxic carbon-centered radical organisms, which then cause widespread damage to parasite biomolecules by alkylation or by initiating peroxidation (**Figure 12**).

9. Polycyclic antimalarial drugs

Three antimalarial drugs have polycyclic ring structures in common (**Figure 13**). Doxycycline, a popular tetracycline antibiotic, is the first. The second is halofantrine, and the third is quinacrine [76], a discontinued agent that was used in the South Pacific.

9.1 Halofantrine

The Walter Reed Army Institute of Research [77] developed halofantrine in the 1960s and 1970s. It is a phenanthrene-type compound that is structurally distinct from all other antimalarial drugs. The trifluromethyl moiety [78] is an excellent example of drug design that integrates bioisosteric concepts. Halofantrine is a synthetic antimalarial that functions as a blood schizonticide but has no effect on

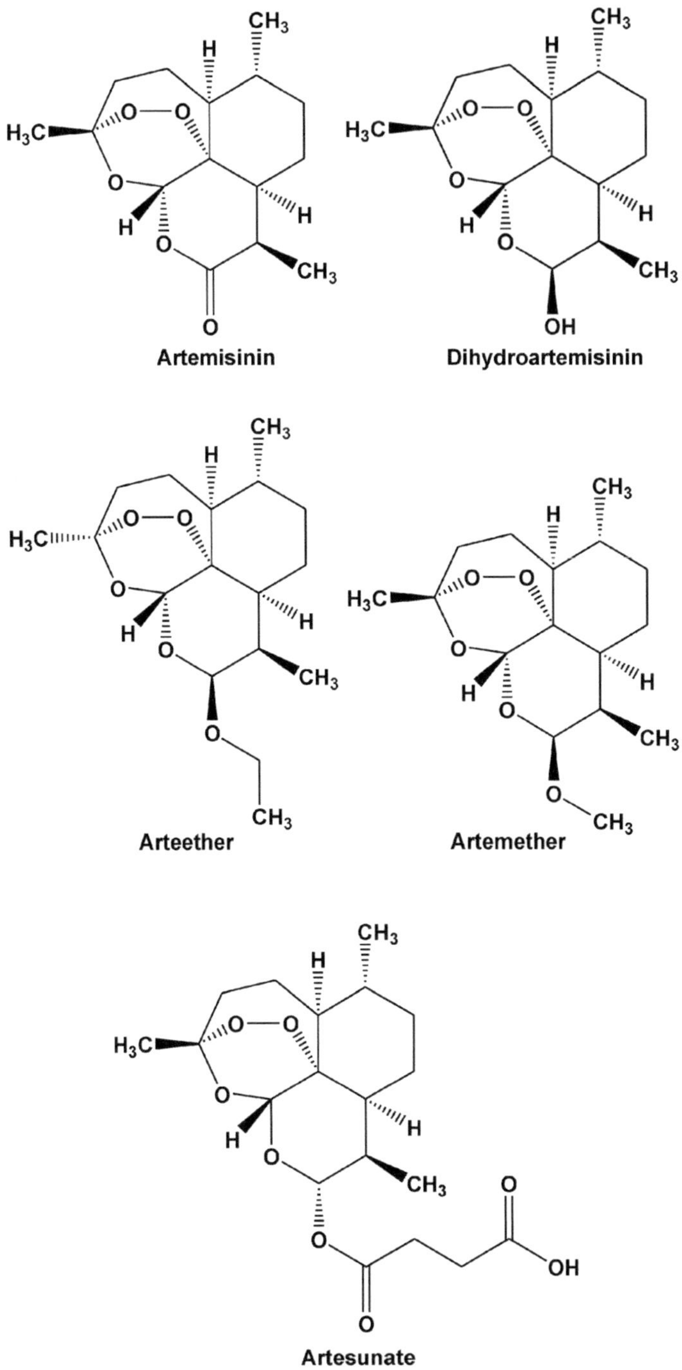

Figure 12.
Structures of ART derivatives.

the sporozoite, gametocyte, or hepatic stages of the parasite. It works against *P. falciparum* malaria that is immune to several drugs (including mefloquine).

The mechanism of action of halfantrine against the parasite is unknown. It tends to prevent heme molecules from polymerising (by the parasite enzyme "heme polymerase"), allowing the parasite to become infected by its own waste. CYP3A4 converts halofantrine to N-desbutyl-halofantrine, which is excreted primarily in the

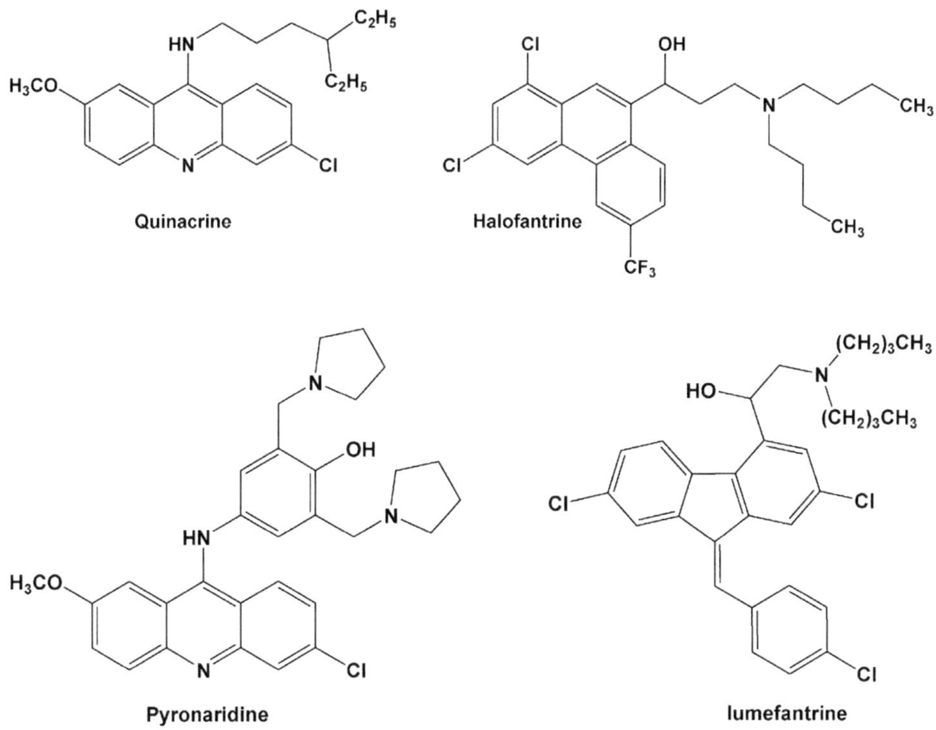

Figure 13.
Structures of some representative polycyclic antimalarial compounds.

faeces; both the parent compound and the N-desbutyl metabolite are involved in vitro.

Halofantrine is usually well tolerated, but consistent absorption requires that it be taken with a fatty meal. Halofantrine has been shown to block open and inactivated HERG channels preferentially, disrupting nerve conduction in cardiac tissue and inducing cardiotoxicity. Cardiac arrhythmias are the most dangerous side effect: halofantrine induces severe QT prolongation [79], which is seen even at normal doses.

9.2 Doxycycline

Doxycycline is a tetracycline derived from oxytetracycline that inhibits pathogen protein synthesis by reversibly inhibiting the 30S ribosomal subunit, preventing the 50s and 30s units from bonding. Since the ribosomal subunits of bacteria and Plasmodium differ significantly from mammalian ribosomes, this class of antibiotics does not readily bind to mammalian ribosomes and therefore has good selective toxicity [80].

Antimalarial doxycycline is mainly used for prophylaxis against *P. falciparum* strains immune to chloroquine and sulfadoxine–pyrimethamine. During malaria exposure, 100 mg (adult dose) of doxycycline should be given every day as prophylactic therapy. It can also be used in conjunction with quinine to treat resistant *P. falciparum* infections, although it has a slow onset of action in acute malaria and should not be used alone [81]. When treating acute cases, 100 mg of doxycycline per day for seven days should be given in accordance with quinine.

Doxycycline is well absorbed when taken orally (90–100% when fasting; decreased by 20% when taken with food or milk) and excreted partially in the faeces and partially in the urine. Since tetracyclines chelate calcium, they can interfere with the growth of permanent teeth in children. Doxycycline should only be used in children for a limited period. Tetracycline also increased photosensitivity, which is important because areas where malaria is endemic also have the most sunlight [82].

9.3 Pyronaridine

Pyronaridine was developed in 1970 at the Institute of Chinese Parasitic Disease [83, 84], and has been used in clinical trials in China since the 1980s. It is one of the components of the artemisinin combination therapy pyronaridine/artesunate and has been shown to be effective against chloroquine-resistant strains (Pyramax). It's also being investigated as a possible anticancer medication and Ebola treatment. Pyonaridine, like lumefantrine, tends to interfere with haematin, but it does not seem to share resistance mechanisms with chloroquine [85]. Pyronaridine is a form of pyronaridine that is The most common side effects of pyronaridine are headache, vomiting, stomach pain, bradycardia, and hypoglycemia.

9.4 Lumefantrine

Lumefantrine was first synthesised in China in 1976 and is now only used in conjunction with artemether. This mixture is often referred to as a "co-artemether" [86]. Lumefantrine is very lipophilic and has a much longer half-life than artemether, so it's thought to remove any lingering parasites after a combined injection. [No. 29] Lumefantrine has an uncertain molecular weight, but studies indicate that it inhibits the development of -hematin by forming a complex with hemin [87].

9.5 Quinacrine

Quinacrine (also known as mepacrine) was commonly used as a prophylactic during WWII, and was marketed under the brand name Atabrine [88]. Quinacrine is a derivative of methylene blue, a different anti-malarial discovered in 1891 [89, 90]. Quinacrine is no longer used because it has a high risk of harmful side effects, such as toxic psychosis [88]. It is one of the most dangerous antimalarial medications, despite the fact that it was once widely used (**Table 1**).

Intercalation of DNA strands, succinic dehydrogenase and mitochondrial electron transport, and cholinesterase are all sites where it functions within the cell. It

Drug	Original indications	Recent status as new potential anti-malarials
Methylene blue	In treatment of Methaemoglobinemia	Completed Phase II trials in 2017 (NCT02851108) as a combination with primaquine
Fosmidomycin	Antibiotic	Phase II trials in 2015 (NCT02198807) as a combination with piperaquine
Rosiglitazone	Antidiabetic drug	In clinical trials as an adjunctive therapy for severe malaria (NCT02694874)
Imatinib	In cancer treatment	In Phase II trials (NCT03697668) as a triple combination with dihydroartemisinin-piperaquine
Sevuparin	In treatment of sickle cell disease	Last in Phase I/II trials in 2014 (NCT01442168) as a combination with atovaquone-proguanil.

Table 1.
List of drugs repurposed in malaria treatment.

has been used as a sclerosing agent and may be tumorgenic and mutagenic. Quinacrine can cause yellow discoloration of the skin and urine because it is an acridine dye.

10. Fixed combinations

Resistance is a common concern in malaria prophylaxis and treatment; combination therapy seeks to minimise resistance through synergism and, when combined with longer-acting medications, improved therapy. Combination therapies have been developed that employ two distinct mechanisms.

10.1 Sulfadoxine and pyrimethamine

A sulfonamide antibacterial drug and a pyrimidinediamine similar to trimethoprim are used in this combination. Sulfonamides can be used in conjunction with pyrimethamine in a variety of ways. A sulfonamide with similar pharmacokinetic properties to the dihydrofolate reductase inhibitor is usually used (**Figure 14**).

Sulfadoxine, a sulfonamide with a structure identical to p-aminobenzoic acid (PABA), inhibits the parasite's ability to synthesise folic acid, whereas pyrimethamine, a pyrimidinediamine, prevents folic acid from being reduced to its active tetrahydrofolate coenzyme type. Sulfonamides avoid the production of dihydropteroic acid by preventing the incorporation of p-aminobenzoic acid (PABA). Since humans do not need to synthesise folic acid, sulfonamides have excellent selective toxicity. Nonetheless, sulfadoxine has been linked to serious to fatal cases of erythema multiforme, Stevens-Johnson syndrome, toxic epidermal necrolysis, and serum sickness syndromes. Pyrimethamine, first formulated in the 1950s, prevents the conversion of folic acid and dihydrofolic acid to the active tetrahydrofolate coenzyme form, which is required for amino acid and nucleic acid synthesis [91]. This combination is recommended for the prevention and treatment of *P. falciparum* chloroquine resistance and can be used in conjunction with quinine. Despite the fact that the combination is only suggested for *P. falciparum*, it is successful against all asexual erythocytic forms. It does not have any impact on the sexual gametocyte form [92].

10.2 Atovaquone and proguanil

Two separate and unrelated mechanisms of action against the parasite serve as the foundation for this combination. Atovaquone is a dihydrofolate reductase inhibitor, and cycloguanil is a selective inhibitor of the Plasmodium mitochondrial electron transport system. In a ratio of 2.5 atovaquone to 1 proguanil HCl calculated

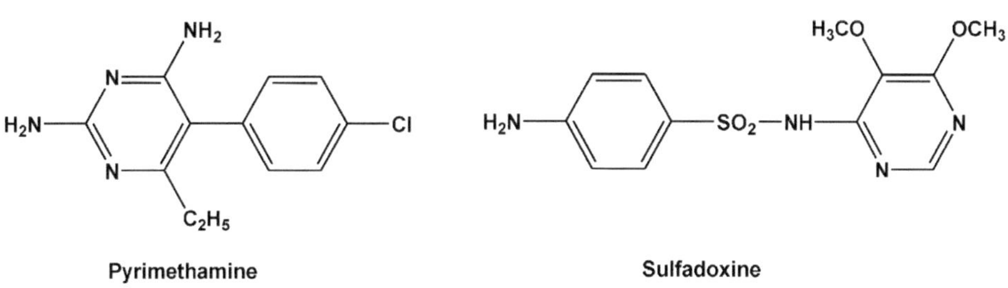

Figure 14.
Chemical structure of pyrimethamine and sulfadoxine in combination.

in mg (not mmoles), atovaquone and proguanil are given together [93]. The sporozoite stage is the primary focus of this mixture. Proguanil decreases the effective concentration of atovaquone needed to damage the mitochondrial membrane, while atovaquone increases the effectiveness of proguanil but not its active metabolite (Malarone) (**Figure 15**) [94–96].

Atovaquone was first formulated as an antimalarial, however due to its high failure rate (30%), it is no longer prescribed as a single chemical entity. However, atovaquone has been combined with proqanil to produce an effective prophylactic and therapeutic antimalarial [98]. Proguanil is an early example of a prodrug, having been produced in 1945. CYP2C19 is the enzyme that converts it to cycloguanil (**Figure 16**).

The chemistry of atovaquone is based on the fact that it is a naphthoquinone that participates in oxidation–reduction reactions as part of its quinonehydroquinone mechanism. The drug targets mitochondrial electron transport, specifically at the cytochrome bc1 site of the parasite. This deprives the cell of required ATP, potentially contributing to anaerobic conditions. A mutation in the parasite's cytochrome causes resistance to this drug, and a single-point mutation appears to be adequate [99]. The pharmacokinetics of atovaquone, when used as a monotherapy, are thought to be related to resistance. Since atovaquone is lipophilic and has a slow absorption rate, the pathogen is exposed to low concentrations of the medication for a prolonged period of time, which promotes resistance growth.

Cycloguanil (Proguanil) inhibits dihydrofolate reductase, which prevents deoxythymidylate synthesis. Amino acid shifts near the dihydrofolate reductase binding site are linked to resistance to proguanil/cycloguanil. Malaria immune to chloroquine, halofantrine, mefloquine, and amodiaquine is treated with this drug combination. To date, there has been no evidence of resistance to the combination [100].

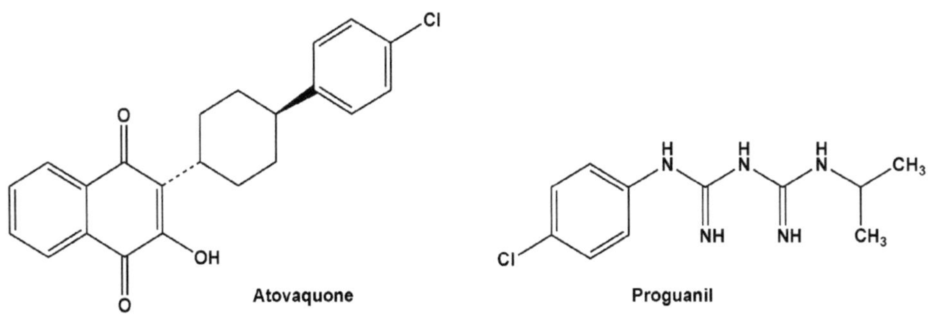

Figure 15.
Chemical structure of atovaquone and proguanil in combination. Sulfadoxine–pyrimethamine are among the other reportedly used combinations [97].

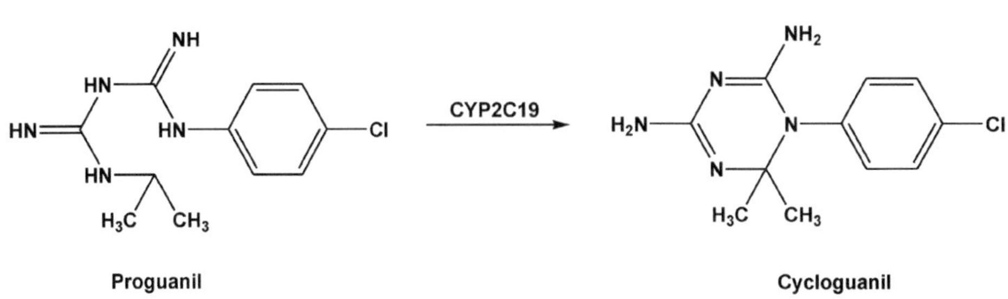

Figure 16.
Metabolic activation of proguanil to cycloguanil.

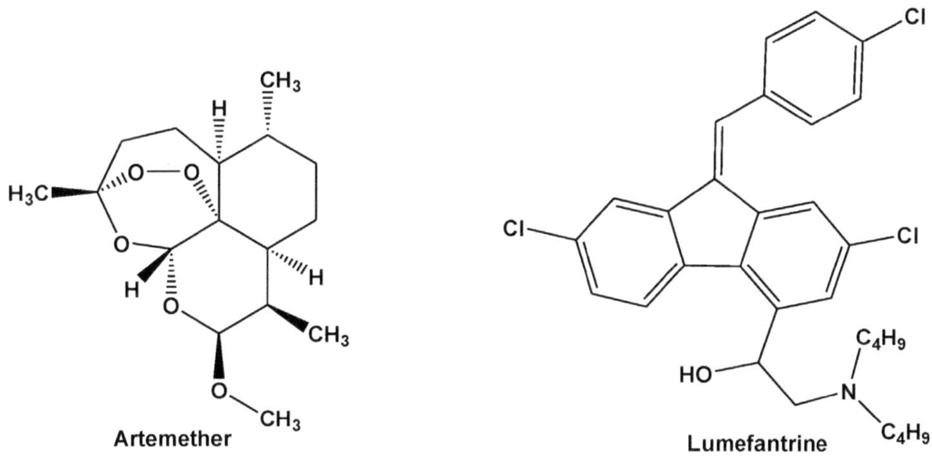

Figure 17.
Chemical structure of artemether and lumefantrine in combination.

10.3 Artemether and lumefantrine

Artemether–lumefantrine (Coartem) is one of the artemisinin-based combination therapy's fixed-dose formulations (ACT). The cure rates for these ACTs have been stated to be greater than 90%. Artesunate–fosmidomycin, amodiaquine–artesunate, chloroquine–artemisinin, and artesunate.

Artemether–lumefantrine interferes with heme metabolism, preventing development of parasite in erythrocyte states. Artemether acts oxidatively due to its endoperoxide, and lumefantrine can form a complex with hemin (**Figure 17**).

11. Future prospects of antimalarial drugs

With the recent emergence of resistance to existing frontline artemisinin-based combination therapy, the antimalarial drug pipeline is in dire need of newer lead molecules. The need for new anti-malarials that function through novel mechanisms of action has been moved to the forefront of the development agenda (**Figure 18**).

A variety of criteria are used to determine the ability of newer compounds to function as new anti-malarials: single-dose cures (artesunate and chloroquine are unable to do this); activity against both the asexual blood stages that trigger disease and the gametocytes that transmit the disease; compounds that avoid infection (chemoprotective agents); and compounds that clear *P. vivax* hypnozoites from the liver (anti-relapse agents) [101, 102].

Researchers can experiment with new combinations and formulations of currently available anti-malarial drugs. This may aid in the delivery of the drug, allowing it to be more successful, or it may help resolve issues with resistance to a specific component. The following are some recent methods used in the detection of new antimalarial agents:

1. Use of available antimalarial drugs to improve antimalarial therapy

2. Development of analogs of currently available medications.

3. Covalent bitherapy

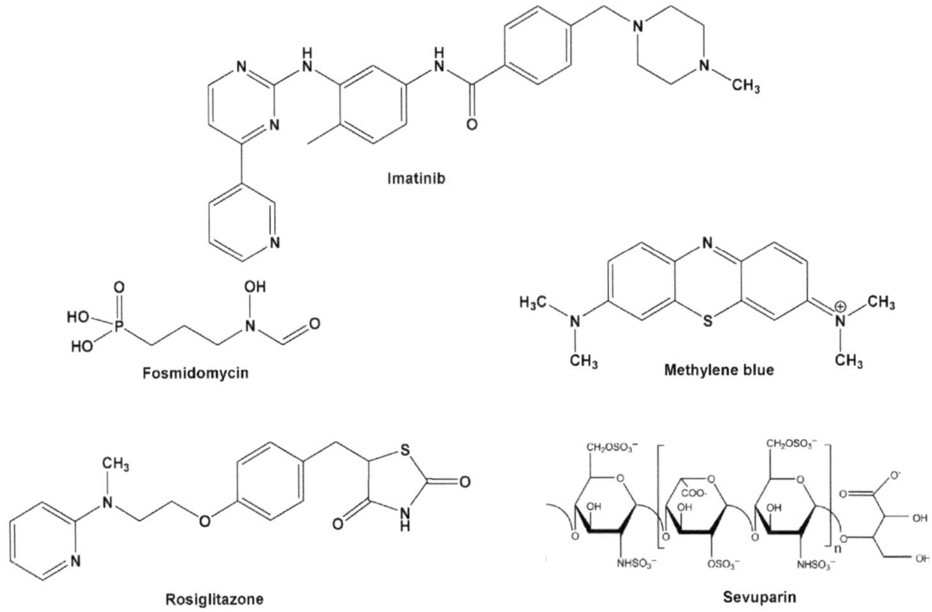

Figure 18.
Structures of some drugs repurposed for malaria therapy and are under various phases of clinical trials.

4. Exploitation of natural products and their derivatives.

5. Use of compounds that are effective against other diseases

6. Development of compounds that are active against novel targets.

7. Drug resistance reversers

8. Development of a malaria vaccine

11.1 Optimization of antimalarial therapy with available drugs

This technique involves mixing existing medications with new dosing regimens or formulations, as well as optimising treatment with currently available drugs. Other non-artemisinin-based combination therapies, in addition to the already proven and recommended artemisinin-based combination therapy, are intended to prevent the development of resistance, improve effectiveness, and tolerability. The idea is to combine two or more drugs with different mechanisms of action, resulting in different molecular targets in the parasite. In an area where *P. falciparum* transmission is endemic and Chloroquine resistance is high, chloroquine combined with sulfadoxine-pyrimethamine demonstrated a large therapeutic return over sulfadoxine-pyrimethamine alone.

11.2 Development of analogs of available drugs

This technique includes altering existing compounds chemically in order to produce newer compounds that are more potent, stronger, and cost-effective. The benefit of this strategy is that the biological target or mechanism of action of the lead compound is already known. Chemical modifications of quinine, for example, led to the discovery of chloroquine, halofantrine, and primaquine.

11.3 Covalent bitherapy

Covalent bitherapy entails the covalent bonding of two chemical moieties that act on different/same biological targets through different mechanisms of action [103–105]. Trioxaquine (SAR116242) is a synthetic hybrid compound with 1,2,4-trioxane and 4-aminoquinoline pharmacophores covalently related [106–108]. Since covalently linked pharmacophore is designed to target the parasite by: alkylation of heme with the trioxane moiety and binding of heme with the aminoquinoline moiety to inhibit hemozoin formation [109, 110], trioxaquine has been found to work on both asexual and sexual stages of malaria parasites.

11.4 Exploitation of natural products and their derivatives

Natural ingredients have long been a mainstay in drug production. The study of natural products, mostly by reverse pharmacology, yields useful knowledge about molecular models for the creation of new drugs. Natural molecular scaffolds including quinine, artemisinin, febrifugine, spiroindolone, and lapachol, for example, were discovered in herbal medicinal products [111].

11.5 Exploitation of compounds active against other diseases

This technique, also known as drug repurposing, could be used to combat malaria. Existing medicines that were previously used for other purposes could be found to be effective against malaria and repurposed as a new anti-malarial medication. N. M. Pazhayam et al. [112] looked at a variety of FDA-approved drugs that could be repurposed as antimalarials.

11.6 Development of compounds active against novel targets

The sixth strategy is the most clinically tested and appealing modern chemotherapy strategy. It requires knowledge of genomics and proteomics methods that have the potential to speed up the detection of new drug targets and the subsequent discovery of molecules that function on these targets. The identification and characterisation of putative targets in a particular biochemical pathway for parasite growth is an urgent need to combat the disease, given the rapid emergence of drug resistance to traditional therapeutics. Our fast advancement in the characterisation of the genomes of malaria parasites suggests that this strategy is plausible to identify important new antimalarial compounds in the future. Because of our rapid progress in sequencing the genomes of malaria parasites, we conclude that this approach will be useful in discovering essential new antimalarial compounds in the future.

11.7 Drug resistance reversers

The discovery and production of drug resistance reversers not only revitalises the use of chloroquine and other antimalarial drugs, but also offers a new way to keep existing drugs effective [113]. For example calcium channel blockers [114] like verapamil and diltiazem have been shown to reverse chloroquine resistance.

11.8 Development of a malaria vaccine

Vaccination of infectious diseases has a long history of success in curing disease. Similarly, malaria vaccination is being introduced to protect the vaccinated individual while also preventing malaria transmission in the environment. Malaria vaccines can prove to be a dynamic approach to malaria control and eradication. Malaria vaccines target three stages of the parasite's life cycle: (i) pre-erythrocytic (sporozoite/hepatic), (ii) erythrocytic (asexual), and (iii) reproductive (transmission blocking).

Author details

Mitali Mishra[1], Vikash Kumar Mishra[2], Varsha Kashaw[2] and Sushil Kumar Kashaw[1*]

1 Department of Pharmaceutical Sciences, Dr. Harisingh Gour University, Sagar, Madhya Pradesh, India

2 Sagar Institute of Pharmaceutical Sciences, Sagar, Madhya Pradesh, India

*Address all correspondence to: sushilkashaw@gmail.com

References

[1] World Health Organization. World Malaria Report 2019. Geneva.

[2] Cullen K. A; Mace K. E.; Arguin P. M. Centers for Disease C, Prevention. Malaria Surveillance—United States, **2013**, *MMWR Surveill Summ.* **20**[1] 16; 65 (2), 1. doi:10.15585/mmwr.ss6502a1.

[3] Ebstie Y. A.; Abay S. M.; Tadesse W. T.; Ejigu D. A. Tafenoquine and its potential in the treatment and relapse prevention of *Plasmodium vivax* malaria: the evidence to date. ***Drug** Des. Devel. Ther.* **2016,** *10*, 2387. doi:10.2147/DDDT.S61443.

[4] Rajapakse S.; Rodrigo C.; Fernando S. D. Tafenoquine for preventing relapse in people with *Plasmodium vivax* malaria. Cochrane Database *Syst. Rev.* **2015**, *(4)*:CD010458. doi:10.1002/14651858. CD010458.pub2.

[5] Ashley E. A; Dhorda M.; Fairhurst R. M. Amaratunga C.; Lim P.;, Suon S, et al. Spread of artemisinin resistance in *Plasmodium falciparum* malaria. *N. Engl. J. Med.* **2014**, *371(5)*, 411. doi:10.1056/NEJMoa1314981.

[6] Kacprzak, K. M. Chemistry and Biology of Cinchona Alkaloids. In Natural Products; Ramawat, K. G., Mérillon, *J. M., Eds.*, Springer: Berlin, **2013**; 605.

[7] Achan, J.; Talisuna, A. O.; Erhart, A.; Yeka, A.; Tibenderana, J. K.; Baliraine, F. N.; Rosenthal, P. J.; D'alessandro, U. Quinine, an Old Anti-Malarial Drug in a Modern World: Role in the Treatment of Malaria. *Mal. J.* **2011**, *10* (1), 144

[8] Song, C. E., Ed. An Overview of Cinchona Alkaloids in Chemistry. In Cinchona Alkaloids in Synthesis and Catalysis: Ligands, Immobilization and Organocatalysis; Wiley: Hoboken, N. J. **2009**; p. 1.

[9] Gildenhuys, J.; Sammy, C. J.; Müller, R.; Streltsov, V. A.; le Roex, T.; Kuter, D.; de Villiers, K. A. Alkoxide Coordination of Iron (III) Protoporphyrin IX by Antimalarial Quinoline Methanols: A Key Interaction Observed in the Solid-State and Solution. *Dalton Trans.* **2015**, *44 (38)*, 16767.

[10] Krishna, S.; White, N. J. Pharmacokinetics of Quinine, Chloroquine and Amodiaquine. Clinical Implications. *Clin. Pharmacokin.* **1996**, *30 (4)*, 263.

[11] Woodland, J. G.; Hunter, R.; Smith, P. J.; Egan, T. J. Shining New Light on Ancient Drugs: Preparation and Subcellular Localisation of Novel Fluorescent Analogues of Cinchona Alkaloids in Intraerythrocytic *Plasmodium falciparum*. *Org. Biomol. Chem.* **2017**, *15 (3)*, 589–597.

[12] Milner, E.; McCalmont, W.; Bhonsle, J.; Caridha, D.; Cobar, J.; Gardner, S.; Gerena, L.; Goodine, D.; Lanteri, C.; Melendez, V.; Roncal, N. Anti-Malarial Activity of a Non-Piperidine Library of Next-Generation Quinoline Methanols. *Mal. J.* **2010**, *9 (1)*, 51.

[13] Cheruku, S. R.; Maiti, S.; Dorn, A.; Scorneaux, B.; Bhattacharjee, A. K.; Ellis, W. Y.; Vennerstrom, J. L. Carbon Isosteres of the 4-Aminopyridine Substructure of Chloroquine: Effects on pKa, Hematin Binding, Inhibition of Hemozoin Formation, and Parasite Growth. *J. Med. Chem.* **2003**, *46 (14)*, 3166.

[14] Vippagunta, S. R.; Dorn, A.; Matile, H.; Bhattacharjee, A. K.; Karle, J. M.; Ellis, W. Y.; Ridley, R. G.; Vennerstrom, J. L. Structural Specificity of Chloroquine—Hematin Binding Related to Inhibition of Hematin Polymerization and Parasite Growth. *J. Med. Chem.* **1999**, *42 (22)*, 4630.

[15] Slater, A. F. G.; Cerami, A. Inhibition by Chloroquine of a Novel Haem Polymerase Enzyme Activity in Malaria Trophozoites. *Nature* **1992**, *355 (6356)*, 167.

[16] Pagola, S.; Stephens, P. W.; Bohle, D. S.; Kosar, A. D.; Madsen, S. K. The Structure of Malaria Pigment β-Haematin. *Nature* **2000**, *404 (6775)*, 307.

[17] Chugh, M.; Sundararaman, V.; Kumar, S.; Reddy, V. S.; Siddiqui, W. A.; Stuart, K. D.; Malhotra, P. Protein Complex Directs Hemoglobin-to-Hemozoin Formation in *Plasmodium falciparum*. *Proc. Nat. Acad. Sci.* **2013**, *110 (14)*, 5392.

[18] Kapishnikov, S.; Grolimund, D.; Schneider, G.; Pereiro, E.; McNally, J. G.; Als-Nielsen, J.; Leiserowitz, L. Unraveling Heme Detoxification in the Malaria Parasite by in situ Correlative X-Ray Fluorescence Microscopy and Soft X-Ray Tomography. *Sci. Rep.* **2017**, *7 (1)*, 7610.

[19] Fitch, C. D. Ferriprotoporphyrin IX, Phospholipids, and the Antimalarial actions of Quinoline Drugs. *Life Sci.* **2004**, *74 (16)*, 1957.

[20] Kuter, D.; Mohunlal, R.; Fitzroy, S. M.; Asher, C.; Smith, P. J.; Egan, T. J.; de Villiers, K. A. Insights into the Initial Stages of Lipid-Mediated Haemozoin Nucleation. *Cryst. Eng. Comm.* **2016**, *18 (27)*, 5177.

[21] Olafson, K. N.; Ketchum, M. A.; Rimer, J. D.; Vekilov, P. G. Mechanisms of Hematin Crystallization and Inhibition by the Antimalarial Drug Chloroquine. *Proceed. Nat. Acad. Sci.* **2015**, *112 (16)*, 4946.

[22] Olafson, K. N.; Nguyen, T. Q.; Rimer, J. D.; Vekilov, P. G. Antimalarials Inhibit Hematin Crystallization by Unique Drug–Surface Site Interactions. *Proc. Nat. Acad. Sci.* **2017**, *114 (29)*, 7531.

[23] Coronado, L. M.; Nadovich, C. T.; Spadafora, C. Malarial Hemozoin: From Target to Tool. *Biochimica et Biophysica Acta (BBA) Gen. Subj.* **2014**, *1840 (6)*, 2032.

[24] de Sousa, A. C. C.; Viana, G. M.; Diaz, N. C.; Rezende, M. G.; de Oliveira, F. F.; Nunes, R. P.; Pereira, M. F.; Areas, A. L. L.; Zalis, M. G.; da Silva Frutuoso, V.; de Castro Faria, H. C. Design, Synthesis and Evaluation of New Fluoroamodiaquine Analogues. *Chem. Pharmaceut. Bull.* **2016**, *64 (6)*, 594.

[25] O'Neill, P. M.; Barton, V. E.; Ward, S. A.; Chadwick, J. 4-Aminoquinolines: Chloroquine, Amodiaquine and Next-Generation Analogues. In Treatment and Prevention of Malaria; Springer Basel, **2011**, pp. 19.

[26] O'Neill, P. M.; Ward, S. A.; Berry, N. G.; Jeyadevan, J. P.; Biagini, G. A.; Asadollaly, E.; Park, B. K.; Bray, P. G. A Medicinal Chemistry Perspective on 4-Aminoquinoline Antimalarial Drugs. *Curr. Topics Med. Chem.* **2006**, *6 (5)*, 479.

[27] de Sousa, A. C. C.; Viana, G. M.; Diaz, N. C.; Rezende, M. G.; de Oliveira, F. F.; Nunes, R. P.; Pereira, M. F.; Areas, A. L. L.; Zalis, M. G.; da Silva Frutuoso, V.; de Castro Faria, H. C. Design, Synthesis and Evaluation of New Fluoroamodiaquine Analogues. *Chem. Pharmaceut. Bull.* **2016**, *64 (6)*, 594.

[28] Schlitzer, M. Malaria Chemotherapeutics Part I: History of Antimalarial Drug Development, Currently Used Therapeutics, and Drugs in Clinical Development. *Chem. Med. Chem.* **2007**, *2 (7)*, 944.

[29] Nosten, F.; Phillips-Howard, P. A.; ter Kuile, F. O. Other 4-Methanolquinolines, Amyl Alcohols and Phentathrenes: Mefloquine, Lumefantrine and Halofantrine. In Treatment and Prevention of Malaria; Springer Basel, **2011**; pp. 95.

[30] Dow, G. S.; Milner, E.; Bathurst, I.; Bhonsle, J.; Caridha, D.; Gardner, S.; Gerena, L.; Kozar, M.; Lanteri, C.; Mannila, A.; McCalmont, W. Central Nervous System Exposure of Next Generation Quinoline Methanols is Reduced Relative to Mefloquine After Intravenous Dosing in Mice. *Mal. J.* **2011**, *10* (1), 150.

[31] Kaur, K.; Jain, M.; Reddy, R. P.; Jain, R. Quinolines and Structurally Related Heterocycles as Antimalarials. *Eur. J. Med. Chem.* ***2010***, *45* (8), 3245–3264.

[32] Vale, N.; Moreira, R.; Gomes, P. Primaquine Revisited Six Decades After Its Discovery. *Euro. J. Med. Chem.* **2009**, *44 (3)*, 937.

[33] Greaves, J.; Evans, D. A.; Gilles, H. M.; Fletcher, K. A.; Bunnag, D.; Harinasuta, T. Plasma Kinetics and Urinary Excretion of Primaquine in Man. *British J. Clin. Pharmacol.* **1980**, *10 (4)*, 399.

[34] Davis, T. M.; Moore, B. R.; Salman, S.; Page-Sharp, M.; Batty, K. T.; Manning, L. Use of Quantitative Pharmacology Tools to Improve Malaria Treatments. *Expert Rev. Clin. Pharmacol.* **2016**, *9 (2)*, 303.

[35] Bennett, J. W.; Pybus, B. S.; Yadava, A.; Tosh, D.; Sousa, J. C.; McCarthy, W. F.; Deye, G.; Melendez, V.; Ockenhouse, C. F. Primaquine Failure and Cytochrome P-450 2D6 in *Plasmodium vivax* Malaria. *New England J. Med.* **2013**, *369 (14)*, 1381.

[36] Pybus, B. S.; Sousa, J. C.; Jin, X.; Ferguson, J. A.; Christian, R. E.; Barnhart, R.; Vuong, C.; Sciotti, R. J.; Reichard, G. A.; Kozar, M. P.; Walker, L. A. CYP450 Phenotyping and Accurate Mass Identification of Metabolites of the 8-Aminoquinoline, Anti-Malarial Drug Primaquine. *Mal. J.* **2012**, *11 (1)*, 259.

[37] Nodiff, E. A.; Chatterjee, S.; Musallam, H. A. Antimalarial Activity of the 8-Aminoquinolines. In Progress in Medicinal Chemistry, Vol. 28; Elsevier, **1991**, pp. 1–40.

[38] Sullivan, D. J. Cinchona Alkaloids: Quinine and Quinidine. In Treatment and Prevention of Malaria. Springer Basel, **2011**, pp. 45–68.

[39] Nosten, F.; Phillips-Howard, P. A.; ter Kuile, F. O. Other 4-Methanolquinolines, Amyl Alcohols and Phentathrenes: Mefloquine, Lumefantrine and Halofantrine. In Treatment and Prevention of Malaria; Springer Basel, **2011**, pp. 95–111.

[40] Dow, G. S.; Milner, E.; Bathurst, I.; Bhonsle, J.; Caridha, D.; Gardner, S.; Gerena, L.; Kozar, M.; Lanteri, C.; Mannila, A.; McCalmont, W. Central Nervous System Exposure of Next Generation Quinoline Methanols is Reduced Relative to Mefloquine After Intravenous Dosing in Mice. *Mal. J.* **2011**, *10 (1)*, 150.

[41] Wells, T. N. New Medicines to Combat Malaria: An Overview of the Global Pipeline of Therapeutics. In Treatment and Prevention of Malaria; Springer Basel, **2011**, 227–247.

[42] Campo, B.; Vandal, O.; Wesche, D. L.; Burrows, J. N. Killing the Hypnozoite—Drug Discovery Approaches to Prevent Relapse in *Plasmodium vivax*. *Pathogens Global Health* **2015**, *109* (3), 107–122.

[43] Diagana, T. T. Supporting Malaria Elimination with 21st Century Antimalarial Agent Drug Discovery. *Drug Discov. Today* **2015**, *20 (10)*, 1265.

[44] Mullard, A. Malaria Medicine Box Expands. *Nat. Rev. Drug Discov.* **2018**, *17*, 693–695.

[45] Held, J.; Jeyaraj, S.; Kreidenweiss, A. Antimalarial Compounds in Phase II Clinical Development. *Expert Opin. Invest. Drugs* **2015**, *24 (3)*, 363.

[46] Achan, J.; Talisuna, A. O.; Erhart, A.; Yeka, A.; Tibenderana, J. K.; Baliraine, F. N.; Rosenthal, P. J.; D'alessandro, U. Quinine, an Old Anti-Malarial Drug in a Modern World: Role in the Treatment of Malaria. *Mal. J.* **2011**, *10* (1), 144.

[47] Bunnag D.; Karbwang J.; Na-Bangchang K.; Thanavibul A.; Chittamas S.; Harinasuta T. Quinine-tetracycline for multidrug resistant *falciparum* malaria. *Southeast Asian J. Trop. Med. Public Health.* **1996**, *27*, 158.

[48] Model List of Essential Medicines. http://www.who.int/medicines/publications/essentialmedicines/en/.

[49] Vale, N.; Moreira, R.; Gomes, P. Primaquine Revisited Six Decades After Its Discovery. *Euro. J. Med. Chem.* **2009**, *44 (3)*, 937.

[50] Greaves, J.; Evans, D. A.; Gilles, H. M.; Fletcher, K. A.; Bunnag, D.; Harinasuta, T. Plasma Kinetics and Urinary Excretion of Primaquine in Man. *British J. Clin. Pharmacol.* **1980**, *10 (4)*, 399.

[51] Bennett, J. W.; Pybus, B. S.; Yadava, A.; Tosh, D.; Sousa, J. C.; McCarthy, W. F.; Deye, G.; Melendez, V.; Ockenhouse, C. F. Primaquine Failure and Cytochrome P-450 2D6 in *Plasmodium vivax* Malaria. *New England J. Med.* **2013**, *369 (14)*, 1381.

[52] Pybus, B. S.; Sousa, J. C.; Jin, X.; Ferguson, J. A.; Christian, R. E.; Barnhart, R.; Vuong, C.; Sciotti, R. J.; Reichard, G. A.; Kozar, M. P.; Walker, L. A. CYP450 Phenotyping and Accurate Mass Identification of Metabolites of the 8-Aminoquinoline, Anti-Malarial Drug Primaquine. *Mal. J.* **2012**, *11 (1)*, 259.

[53] Hien, T. T.; Turner, G. D. H.; Mai, N. T. H.; Phu, N. H.; Bethell, D.; Blakemore, W. F.; Cavanagh, J. B.; Dayan, A.; Medana, I.; Weller, R. O.; Day, N. P. J. Neuropathological assessment of artemether-treated severe malaria. *Lancet* ***2003***, *362 (9380)*, 295.

[54] O'Neill, P. M. The therapeutic potential of semi-synthetic artemisinin and synthetic endoperoxide antimalarial agents. *Expert Opin. Investig. Drugs* ***2005***, *14 (9)*, 1117.

[55] Liu, C. X. Discovery and development of artemisinin and related compounds. *Chinese Herbal Med.* ***2017***, *9 (2)*, 101.

[56] Golenser, J.; Waknine, J. H.; Krugliak, M.; Hunt, N. H.; Grau, G. E. Current perspectives on the mechanism of action of artemisinins. *Int. J. Parasitol.* ***2006***, *36 (14)*, 1427.

[57] Haynes, R. K.; Vonwiller, S. C. The behaviour of qinghaosu (artemisinin) in the presence of heme iron (II) and (III). *Tetrahedron Lett.* ***1996***, *37* (2), 253–256. 12. Olliaro, P. L.; Haynes, R. K.; Meunier, B.; Yuthavong, Y. Possible modes of action of the artemisinin-type compounds. *Trends Parasitol.* ***2001***, *17 (3)*, 122.

[58] Haynes, R. K.; Chan, W. C.; Lung, C. M.; Uhlemann, A. C.; Eckstein, U.; Taramelli, D.; Parapini, S.; Monti, D.; Krishna, S. The Fe2 + −mediated decomposition, PfATP6 binding, and antimalarial activities of artemisone and other artemisinins: the unlikelihood of C-Centered radicals as bioactive intermediates. *Chem. Med. Chem.* ***2007***, *2 (10)*, 1480.

[59] Haynes, R. K.; Chan, W. C.; Wong, H. N.; Li, K. Y.; Wu, W. K.; Fan, K. M.; Sung, H. H.; Williams, I. D.; Prosperi, D.; Melato, S.; Coghi, P. Facile oxidation of leucomethylene blue and dihydroflavins by artemisinins: relationship with flavoenzyme function and antimalarial mechanism of action. *Chem. Med. Chem.* ***2010***, *5 (8)*, 1282.

[60] Haynes, R. K.; Cheu, K. W.; Tang, M. M. K.; Chen, M. J.; Guo, Z. F.; Guo,

Z. H.; Coghi, P.; Monti, D. Reactions of antimalarial peroxides with each of leucomethylene blue and dihydroflavins: flavin reductase and the cofactor model exemplified. *Chem. Med. Chem.* ***2011***, *6 (2)*, 279.

[61] Haynes, R. K.; Cheu, K. W.; Chan, H. W.; Wong, H. N.; Li, K. Y.; Tang, M. M. K.; Chen, M. J.; Guo, Z. F.; Guo, Z. H.; Sinniah, K.; Witte, A. B. Interactions between artemisinins and other antimalarial drugs in relation to the cofactor model-a unifying proposal for drug action. *Chem. Med. Chem.* ***2012***, *7 (12)*, 2204–2226.

[62] Qinghaosu Antimalaria Coordinating Research Group. Antimalarial studies on Qinghaosu. *Chin. Med. J. (Engl).* **1979**, *92*, 811–6.

[63] The Nobel Prize in Physiology or Medicine 2015. https://www.nobelprize.org/nobel_prizes/medicine/laureates/2015/.

[64] Eastman R. T.; Fidock D. A. Artemisinin-based combination therapies: a vital tool in efforts to eliminate malaria. *Nat. Rev. Microbiol.* **2009**, *7*, 864–74.

[65] Noedl H.; Se Y.; Schaecher K.; Smith B. L.; Socheat D.; Fukuda M. M. Evidence of artemisinin-resistant aalaria in western Cambodia. *N. Engl. J. Med.* **2008**, *359*, 2619–20.

[66] Amato R.; Pearson R. D.; Almagro-Garcia J.; Amaratunga C.; Lim P.; Suon S.; et al. Origins of the current outbreak of multidrug-resistant malaria in southeast Asia: a retrospective genetic study. *Lancet Infect. Dis.* **2018**, *18*, 337–45.

[67] O'Neill P. M.; Barton V. E.; Ward S. A. The molecular mechanism of action of artemisinin—the debate continues. Molecules. **2010,** *15*, 1705.

[68] Wang, J.; Zhang, C. J.; Chia, W. N.; Loh, C. C.; Li, Z.; Lee, Y. M.; He, Y.; Yuan, L. X.; Lim, T. K.; Liu, M.; Liew, C. X. Haem-activated promiscuous targeting of artemisinin in *Plasmodium falciparum*. *Nat. Commun.***2015**, *6*, 10111.

[69] Tilley, L.; Straimer, J.; Gnädig, N. F.; Ralph, S. A.; Fidock, D. A. Artemisinin action and resistance in *Plasmodium falciparum*. *Trends Parasitol.* **2016**, *32* (9), 682–696.

[70] Shandilya A.; Chacko S.; Jayaram B.; Ghosh I. A plausible mechanism for the antimalarial activity of artemisinin: a computational approach. Sci Rep. **2013**, *3*, 2513.

[71] Yang, T.; Xie, S. C.; Cao, P.; Giannangelo, C.; McCaw, J.; Creek, D. J.; Charman, S. A.; Klonis, N.; Tilley, L. Comparison of the exposure time dependence of the activities of synthetic ozonide antimalarials and dihydroartemisinin against K13 wild-type and mutant *Plasmodium falciparum* strains. *Antimicrob. Agents Chemother.* **2016**, *60* (8), 4501–4510.

[72] Phyo, A. P.; Jittamala, P.; Nosten, F. H.; Pukrittayakamee, S.; Imwong, M.; White, N. J.; Duparc, S.; Macintyre, F.; Baker, M.; Möhrle, J. J. Antimalarial activity of artefenomel (OZ439), a novel synthetic antimalarial endoperoxide, in patients with *Plasmodium falciparum* and *Plasmodium vivax* malaria: an open-label phase 2 trial. *Lancet Infect. Dis.* **2016**, *16* (1), 61–69.

[73] Tripathi, R.; Jefford, C. W.; Dutta, G. P. Blood schizontocidal activity of selected 1, 2, 4-trioxanes (Fenozans) against the multidrug-resistant strain of *Plasmodium yoelii* nigeriensis (MDR) in vivo. *Parasitology* **2006**, *133* (1), 1–9.

[74] Shukla, K. L.; Gund, T. M.; Meshnick, S. R. Molecular modeling studies of the artemisinin (qinghaosu)-hemin interaction: docking between the antimalarial agent and its putative

receptor. *J. Mol. Graph.* **1995**, *13* (4), 215–222.

[75] Singh, C.; Gupta, N.; Puri, S. K. Photooxygenation of 3-aryl-2-cyclohexenols: synthesis of a new series of antimalarial 1, 2, 4-trioxanes. *Tetrahedron Lett.* **2005**, *46* (2), 205–207.

[76] Cosgriff T. M.; Desjardins R. E.; Pamplin C. L.; Canfield C. J.; Doberstyn E. B.; Boudreau E. F. Evaluation of the antimalarial activity of the phenanthrenemethanol halofantrine (WR 171,669)*. *Am. J. Trop. Med. Hyg.* 1982, *31*.1075.

[77] Croft A. M. A lesson learnt: the rise and fall of Lariam and Halfan. *J. R. Soc. Med.* **2007**, *100*, 170.

[78] Nosten, F.; Phillips-Howard, P. A.; ter Kuile, F. O. Other 4-Methanolquinolines, Amyl Alcohols and Phentathrenes: Mefloquine, Lumefantrine and Halofantrine. In Treatment and Prevention of Malaria; Springer Basel, 2011; pp. 95–111.

[79] Sanchez, C. P.; Dave, A.; Stein, W. D.; Lanzer, M. Transporters as Mediators of Drug Resistance in *Plasmodium falciparum*. *Int. J. Parasitol.* **2010**, *40* (10), 1109–1118.

[80] Lacy C. F.; Armstrong L. L.; Goldmann M. P.; Leonard L. L. *Lexi Comp's Drug Information Handbook.* Hudson, OH: Lexi Comp; **2006**.

[81] Andersen S. L.; Oloo A. J.; Gordon D. M.; Ragama O. B.; Aleman G. M.; Berman J. D.; Tang D. B.; Dunne M. W.; Shanks G. D. Successful double-blinded, randomized, placebo-controlled field trial of azithromycin and doxycycline as prophylaxis for malaria in western Kenya. *Clin. Infect. Dis.* **1998**, *26*, 146.

[82] Weiss W. R.; Oloo A. J.; Johnson A.; Koech D.; Hoffman S. L. Daily primaquine is effective for prophylaxis against falciparum malaria in Kenya: comparison with mefloquine, doxycycline, and chloroquine plus proguanil. *J. Infect. Dis.* **1995**, *171*, 1569.

[83] Zheng X. Y.; Xia Y.; Gao F. H.; Chen C. Synthesis of 7351, a new antimalarial drug. *Yao. Xue. Xue. Bao.* **1979**, *14*, 736.

[84] Chang C.; Lin-Hua T.; Jantanavivat C. Studies on a new antimalarial compound: pyronaridine. *Trans. R. Soc. Trop. Med. Hyg.* **1992**, *86*, 7.

[85] Croft S. L.; Duparc S.; Arbe-Barnes S. J.; Craft J.; Shin C. S.; Fleckenstein L.; et al. Review of pyronaridine anti-malarial properties and product characteristics. Malar. J. **2012,** *11*, 270.

[86] Nevin, R. L.; Croft, A. M. Psychiatric Effects of Malaria and Anti-Malarial Drugs: Historical and Modern Perspectives. *Mal. J.* **2016**, *15 (1)*, 332.

[87] Schmidt, M.; Sun, H.; Rogne, P.; Scriba, G. K.; Griesinger, C.; Kuhn, L. T.; Reinscheid, U. M. Determining the Absolute Configuration of (+)-Mefloquine HCl, the Side-Effect-Reducing Enantiomer of the Antimalaria Drug Lariam. *J. Am. Chem. Soc.* **2012**, *134 (6)*, 3080.

[88] Green R. A report on fifty cases of malaria treated with Atebrin. A new synthetic drug. *Lancet.* **1932,** *219*, 826.

[89] Guttman P.; Ehrlich P.; Ueber die wirkung des methylenblau bei malaria. *Berl Klin Wochenschr.* **1891**, *28*, 953.

[90] Schirmer R. H.; Coulibaly B.; Stich A.; Scheiwein M.; Merkle H.; Eubel J., et al. Methylene blue as an antimalarial agent. *Redox Rep.* **2003,** *8*, 272.

[91] Matar K. M.; Awad A. I.; Elamin S. B. Pharmacokinetics of artesunate alone and in combination with sulfadoxine/

pyrimethamine in healthy Sudanese volunteers. *Am. J. Trop. Med. Hyg.* **2014**, *90*, 1087.

[92] MMV - Medicines for Malaria Venture. 2017g. https://www.mmv.org/access/products-projects/spaqsulfadoxine-pyrimethamine-amodiaquine Accessed: 21 September 2017.

[93] Giao, P. T.; de Vries, P. J. Pharmacokinetic Interactions of Antimalarial Agents. *Clin. Pharmacokinetics* **2001**, *40* (5), 343–373.

[94] de Alencar F. E.; Cerutti C. Jr.; Durlacher R. R.; Boulos M.; Alves F. P.; Milhous W.; et al. Atovaquone and proguanil for the treatment of malaria in Brazil. *J. Infect. Dis.* **1997,** *175*, 1544.

[95] Looareesuwan S.; Wilairatana P.; Chalermarut K.; Rattanapong Y.; Canfield C. J.; Hutchinson D. B. Efficacy and safety of atovaquone/proguanil compared with mefloquine for treatment of acute *Plasmodium falciparum* malaria in Thailand. *Am. J. Trop. Med. Hyg.* **1999,** *60,* 526.

[96] Mulenga M., Sukwa T.Y., Canfield C.J., Hutchinson D.B. Atovaquone and proguanil versus pyrimethamine/sulfadoxine for the treatment of acute *falciparum* malaria in Zambia. *Clin. Ther.* **1999,** *21*, 841.

[97] Gautam A.; Ahmed T.; Sharma P.; Varshney B.; Kothari M.; Saha N.; et al. Pharmacokinetics and pharmacodynamics of arterolane maleate following multiple oral doses in adult patients with *P. falciparum* malaria. *J. Clin. Pharmacol.* **2011**, *51*, 1519.

[98] Anabwani G., Canfield C.J., Hutchinson D.B. Combination atovaquone and proguanil hydrochloride vs. halofantrine for treatment of acute *Plasmodium falciparum* malaria in children. *Pediatr. Infect. Dis. J.* **1999,** *18*, 456.

[99] Bustos D. G.; Canfield C. J.; Canete-Miguel E.; Hutchinson D. B. Atovaquone-proguanil compared with chloroquine and chloroquine–sulfadoxine–pyrimethamine for treatment of acute *Plasmodium falciparum* malaria in the Philippines. *J. Infect. Dis.* **1999,** *179*, 1587.

[100] Bouchaud O.; Monlun E.; Muanza K.; Fontanet A.; Scott T.; Goetschel A.; et al. Atovaquone plus proguanil versus halofantrine for the treatment of imported acute uncomplicated *Plasmodium falciparum* malaria in nonimmune adults: a randomized comparative trial. *Am. J. Trop. Med. Hyg.* **2000**, *63*, 274.

[101] Wells, T. N. New Medicines to Combat Malaria: An Overview of the Global Pipeline of Therapeutics. In Treatment and Prevention of Malaria; Springer Basel, 2011; 227–247.

[102] Burrows J. N.; Duparc S.; Gutteridge W. E.; van Huijsduijnen R. H.; Kaszubska W.; Macintyre F.; et al. New developments in anti-malarial target candidate and product profiles. *Malar. J.* **2017,** *16,* 26.

[103] B. Meunier, Hybrid molecules with a dual mode of action: dream or reality, Acc. Chem. Res. 41 (2008) 69-77. PMID: 17665872.

[104] F.W. Muregi, A. Ishih, Next-generation antimalarial drugs: hybrid molecules as a new strategy in drug design, Drug Dev. Res. 71 (2010) 20-32.

[105] A.C.C. Aguiar, E.M.M. da Rocha, N.B. de Souza, T.C.C. França, A.U. Krettli, New approaches in antimalarial drug discovery and development - a Review, Mem. Inst. 107 (2012) 831-845, http://dx.doi.org/10.1590/S0074-02762012000700001. Oswaldo. Cruz, Rio de Janeiro, l.

[106] O. Dechy-Cabaret, F. Benoit-Vical, A. Robert, B. Meunier, Preparation and

antimalarial activities of "trioxaquines," new modular molecules with a trioxane skeleton linked to a 4-aminoquinoline, Chem. Biol. Chem. 1 (2000) 281-283.

[107] O. Dechy-Cabaret, F. Benoit-Vical, C. Loup, et al., Synthesis and antimalarial activity of trioxaquine derivatives, Chem. Eur. J. 10 (2004) 1625-1636, http://dx.doi.org/10.1002/chem.200305576.

[108] F. Benoit-Vical, J. Lelievre, A. Berry, et al., Trioxaquines are new antimalarial agents active on all erythrocytic forms, including gametocytes, Antimicrob. Agents Chemother. 51 (2007) 1463-1472, http://dx.doi.org/10.1128/AAC.00967-06.

[109] F. Bousejra-EI Garah, C. Claparols, F. Benoit-Vical, B. Meunier, A. Robert, The antimalarial trioxaquine DU1301 alkylates heme in malaria-infected mice, Antimicrob. Agents Chemother. 52 (2008) 2966-2969, http://dx.doi.org/10.1128/AAC.00165-08.

[110] S.A.L. Laurent, C. Loup, S. Mourgues, A. Robert, B. Meunier, Heme alkylation by the antimalarial endoperoxides artesunate and trioxaquine, Chem. Biol. Chem. 6 (2005) 653-658.

[111] E. Fernandez- Alvaro, W.D. Hong, G.L. Nixon, P.M. O'Neill, F. Calderon, Anti-malarial chemotherapy: natural product inspired development of preclinical and clinical candidates with diverse mechanisms of action, J. Med. Chem. (2016), http://dx.doi.org/10.1021/acs.jmedchem.5b01485. Article ASAP.

[112] Pazhayam, N. M.; Chhibber-Goel, J.; Sharma, A. New leads for drug repurposing against malaria. *Drug Discov. Today*. **2019,** *24 (1)*, 263. https://doi.org/10.1016/j.drudis.2018.08.006.

[113] D.H. Peyton, Reversed chloroquine molecules as a strategy to overcome resistance in malaria, Curr. Top. Med. Chem. 12 (2012) 400-407, http://dx.doi.org/10.2174/156802612799362968.

[114] J.A. Martiney, A. Cerami, A.F.G. Slater, Verapamil reversal of chloroquine resistance in the malaria parasite *Plasmodium falciparum* is specific for resistant parasites and independent of the weak base effect, J. Biol. Chem. 270 (1995) 22393-22398, http://dx.doi.org/10.1074/jbc.270.38.22393.

Chapter 9

Regulation of T-reg/Th-17 Balance: One Step Closer Towards Immunotherapy Against Malaria Infection

Saikat Mukherjee, Soubhik Ghosh and Arindam Bhattacharyya

Abstract

According to World Malaria Report 2020, the rate of decline in malaria case incidence and deaths caused by malaria has ceased in latter half of the past decade. Though Artemisinin Combination Therapy (ACT) is still the major therapeutic approach globally to treat malaria patients, increased resistance of *Plasmodium* sp. to artemisinin can be looked upon as a major factor responsible for the rate of decline. In the present world, immunotherapeutic approaches are in the limelight to treat several infections, autoimmune disorders, cancers but application of such therapeutic measures in case of malaria are yet not available. Among different immune cells, T-regulatory cells (T-reg) and Th-17 cells and the balance between them, helps in determining the outcome of the immune response in host during both lethal and non-lethal malaria. TGFβ and IL-6 are two major cytokines that play important role in fine tuning the Treg/Th-17 balance by modulating dendritic cell responses, specially by regulating the ratio between myeloid DC and plasmacytoid DC (mDC/pDC). Studies in rodent malaria models have revealed that neutralization of IL-6 by using anti IL-6 monoclonal antibodies *in-vivo* has been found effective in declining the parasitemia, malaria induced deaths and also in reverting back the altered T-reg/Th-17 balance to normal levels. Apart from these, autophagy is one of the major factors which also contributes to regulate the T-reg/Th-17 balance. In malaria infected mice, autophagy induction has been found to normalise the dysregulated T-reg/Th-17 ratio and promote anti-inflammatory Th-2 pathway by supressing pro-inflammatory Th-1 pathway. So, Treg/Th-17 balance and its associated regulators can be important immunotherapeutic targets for malaria prevention in near future.

Keywords: Malaria, drug resistance, immunotherapy, T regulatory cells, Th-17, IL-6, TGFβ, dendritic cells, autophagy

1. Introduction

World Malaria Report 2020 published by World Health Organization estimated 229 million cases of malaria infection around the world in 2019 among which 94%

IntechOpen

of the cases were reported from the WHO African region. The number of estimated cases globally in 2019 was 1 million more than that of the previous year. But in the context of last 20 years, the number of the existing malaria cases has declined from 238 million in 2000. Besides, the total number of estimated cases globally, another parameter that has been in the centre of studying the impact of this disease is, malaria case incidence (cases per 1000 population at risk). Malaria case incidence reduced from 80 in 2000 to 57 in 2019 globally but the rate of decline has ceased in the latter half of the past decade. The deaccelerating rate of decline has also been found in case of malaria mortality rate (i.e. deaths per 100000 population at risk). Despite the steady reduction in number of malaria induced deaths in the past two decades, more than 400 thousand malaria deaths have been reported in 2019. Children aged below 5 years account for 67% of the total malaria deaths, which is a major concern [1].

Among various *Plasmodium* strains that can infect human beings, cerebral malaria causing *Plasmodium falciparum* bring about majority of malaria deaths in Africa and parts of Asia. Apart from *Plasmodium falciparum*, another strain, *Plasmodium vivax* also cause malaria deaths in various other parts of the world [2, 3]. Among several available therapeutic and controlling measures, Artemisinin based Combination Therapy (ACT) is being used worldwide and has been of great success in combating this disease [4–6]. But in recent times, the use of ACT got a major setback due to emergence of Artemisinin resistant *Plasmodium* strains [7, 8]. It may be one of the plausible causes behind the diminishing rate of decline in the rate of malaria case incidence and malaria mortality rate since 2015. Researchers worldwide are putting up constant efforts on making ACT more effective and finding other therapeutic strategies to combat this disease in order to eradicate it in near future. Among other therapeutic measures, immunotherapy has been the prime focus of study over the past decade. Nowadays immunotherapy is being used for various infectious diseases and cancer therapy and the success rate of such therapies are quite promising [9–11]. In case of malaria, immunotherapeutic strategies are not yet available for use. This compels researchers worldwide to find various molecules or cells that can be targeted for effective therapeutic measures in malaria infection [12].

In malaria different stages of the parasitic life cycle can trigger both the innate and adaptive immune response within the host. It is quite difficult to study whether the immune cells play protective or pathogenic or dual roles, especially in human [13]. Still, long-term research reveals specific roles of antibodies and B cells in protection of the host body against the malaria parasite. Besides, several other immune cells like inflammatory cytokines (TNF α, TGFβ, IFN-γ etc.), different subsets of T cells (T-helper cells and Cytotoxic T cells), NK cells and Macrophages also play their part in protection or pathogenesis or both depending on the type of malaria parasite and the stage of life cycle they are in [14]. During life cycle of *Plasmodium* sp. within the host, several major organs and the immune environment within those organs show changes due to presence of parasite factors. Spleen, being a major lymphoid organ and the main blood filtration unit, harbours most of these immune cells [15, 16]. In presence of *Plasmodium* sp. in host body, the immune environment changes rapidly in a day specific manner post infection. Investigation of the changes and regulatory mechanisms within splenic compartment during infections in humans is difficult for several reasons. Most of the study is restricted to observations of clinical symptoms and analysis of tissue sections that are available only after post-mortem. So, there is always lack of enough samples available to investigate the changes and their associated mechanisms in spleen and other lymphoid organs properly [17, 18]. To overcome this, researchers worldwide have focused on studying the major changes in rodent models of malaria. Murine malaria models are very much in use for their ready availability. Various rodent specific parasite strains like *Plasmodium berghei* ANKA, *Plasmodium yoelii*, *Plasmodium chabaudi* are constantly used in laboratories and they almost resemble different parameters (i.e. anaemia, body temperature changes, loss of weight, and occasional death) shown by human during malaria infection. Apart from these basic parameters, several immune parameters like changes in T helper cell and Cytotoxic T cell percentages in lymphoid organs, activities of B cell, concentration of antibodies, disruption of blood brain barrier and migration of immune cells in the brain during cerebral malaria infection also show resemblance to that of human malaria infections. *Plasmodium berghei* ANKA and *Plasmodium chabaudi* infections show similar symptoms, immunological changes as discussed with that of *Plasmodium falciparum* infection in human which might be due to similarities in infective strategies. Both these rodent and human strains can disrupt the blood brain barrier in a similar manner and immune cells (majorly T cells) infiltrate in the brain which can be lethal to the respective hosts. Another rodent specific non-lethal strain *Plasmodium yoelii* has similar effect on the host immune system to that of *Plasmodium vivax* infection in humans [19]. Working with these rodent strains of *Plasmodium* sp. has been found effective in inferring how the immune system is being regulated during malaria and the elaborated regulatory mechanisms that controls the inflammatory balance that occurs. The balance between pro-inflammatory and regulatory immune responses determines the outcome of malaria infection [20]. The balance is maintained by various cytokines, chemokines, several immune cells (macrophages, dendritic cells) and processes like autophagy. The role of CD4+ T helper cells and CD8+ cytotoxic T cells has been found important in regulating the immune response during malaria infection using both rodent models and human samples. The focus has now been shifted to find out the exact role of different subsets of CD4+ T helper cells and how the balance between them defines the outcome of malaria infection. Among these subsets, Th1/Th2 balance and the cytokines regulating this balance has been found crucial for monitoring the immune homeostasis [21, 22]. But recently, balance between two other subsets of T helper cells was found to be important in regulation of immune responses in various infections, autoimmunity and also cancer immunology. These are termed as T regulatory cells that regulates immune-tolerance by secretion of IL-10 and Th17 cells which inflicts inflammatory responses by secreting IL-17, IL-22, IL-23. Naïve CD4+ T cells differentiate into T-regulatory cells (T-reg) in presence of TGFβ and into Th-17 in presence of TGFβ and IL-6. Majority of functions executed by these cells are regulated by their major transcription factors FOXP3 and RORγT for T-reg and Th17 cells respectively [23–25]. As discussed, the differentiation of Treg and Th17 cells is reciprocally regulated by shared and different cytokines and recent studies even show the plasticity of these cells which states that each subset can convert itself to the other one under different inflammatory stimuli [26–28]. These stimuli modulates the cytokine environment of the host and also changes the homeostatic balance between pro-inflammatory and anti-inflammatory cytokines that culminates into Treg/Th17 disbalance. So, T-reg/Th17 balance and regulation of factors that influence this balance has been found to be pivotal in several viral, bacterial and parasitic infections. In case of several autoimmune disorders like rheumatoid arthritis (RA), psoriasis, inflammatory bowel disease (IBD), multiple sclerosis (MS), Th-17 is the major role player and the T-reg/Th-17 balance skews towards pro-inflammatory Th-17 mediated response. Therapeutic approaches which target Th-17 cells and its functional transcription factor RORγT has been successful in reverting the T-reg/Th-17 cell ratio to normal levels [29]. Monoclonal antibodies designed against the human IL-6R, and drugs like sarilumab and tocilizumab can reduce Th-17 cells and increase T-reg cells that helps in amelioration of RA in humans [30]. In malaria, the T-reg cells has been found to help the malaria parasite to evade the immune response [31]. Apart from T-regs, Th-17 cells have been also known to play an important role in blood brain barrier disruption, which is a prime reason behind deaths due to cerebral malaria. This article summarizes the recent advancements on understanding Treg/Th-17 balance with respect to malaria [32].

2. Differential role of T-regulatory cells and Th-17 cells in malaria

During malaria, failure in development of an effective pro-inflammatory and anti-inflammatory balance has been found to contribute towards unrestricted replication of parasite and severe immunopathology [31, 33]. Several subsets of T cells (Th-1, Th-2, NKT cells) are involved in controlling the lethal and non-lethal malaria infection [34]. T-reg cells have been primarily found to control the immune evading mechanism of the *Plasmodium* sp. in both mouse and human [35]. A number of other studies have also reported that T-regs may play an important part in facilitating parasite clearance and enhance parasite burden [36, 37]. However, in a separate study, depletion of Foxp3+ T-regs failed to provide protection against experimental cerebral malaria (ECM), which questions the actual role of T-regs in lethal and non-lethal malaria [38]. Augmented generation of Th-17 cells and quick death due to high inflammation in several organs in adult healthy mice upon ablation of T-reg cells, point towards a counter regulatory pathway that might control the pathogenic Th-17 pathway [39]. Th-17 cell itself and cytokines associated with its differentiation from naïve CD4+ T cells has been found to play a role in blood brain barrier (BBB) disruption and cooperate with each other to allow migration of T cells into the brain [40]. As BBB disruption is a salient feature of lethal cerebral malaria, Th-17 pathway and its probable counter regulatory pathway controlled by T-regulatory cells is thought to be important in depicting the probable outcome of the immune response elicited by the host against the malaria parasite. In malaria, the balance between pro-inflammatory and anti-inflammatory factors was found to be important when we reported differential expressions of anti-inflammatory TGFβ and pro-inflammatory TNFα and their role in regulation of splenocyte apoptosis [41]. Keeping the outcome of evaluation of TGFβ and TNFα in context to splenocyte apoptosis and shared requirements of TGFβ during differentiation of T-regs and Th-17 cells, we checked whether the balance between anti-inflammatory T regulatory cells and pro-inflammatory Th-17 cells (T-reg/Th-17) is important in malaria immunology in both spleen and brain. T regulatory cells were found to increase in spleen of non-lethal *P. yoelii* infection at 8 days post infection (dpi) in a day specific manner but in case of lethal *P. berghei* ANKA infection, it decreased with an increase in the infection and the percentage of T-regs in spleen was lowest at 8 dpi. Not only Tregs but the transcription factors, specially FOXP3 also showed similar trend in spleen of lethal and non-lethal malaria infection. In contrast to the T-regulatory cells, Th-17 cells increased significantly at 8 dpi in lethal *P. berghei* ANKA infection but decreased optimally at 8 dpi after an initial surge at 2 dpi. The major transcription factor of Th-17 cells shows the similar trend in both lethal and non-lethal malaria infection as does Th-17 cells [42]. Not only in spleen but also in cerebral cortex and cerebellum of the *P. berghei* ANKA infected mice, differential expression of FOXP3 and RORγT has been found to be critical in regulating the glial cell mediated neuro-inflammation and neuronal cell death [43]. So, the contrasting behaviour shown by these two cells and their transcription factors highlights the importance of T-reg/Th-17 balance and their regulators in malaria.

3. Role of cytokines (TGFβ and IL-6) in regulation of T-reg/Th-17 balance in malaria

TGFβ and IL-6 are cytokines that play major roles in the regulation of innate and adaptive immune responses in different viral (viz. influenza A, Respiratory Syncytical virus etc.), bacterial (viz. *Streptococcus, Mycobacterium* etc), parasitic (viz. *Leishmania*, *Trypanosoma*, *Toxoplasma* etc.) infections, cancers and autoimmune disorders [44–47]. In malaria, IL-6 is found in circulation of patients infected with *Plasmodium vivax* and *Plasmodium falciparum* and it plays a major role in host response [48–50]. There are reports stating that decreased IL-6 levels upon treatment with anti-malarial compounds is associated with decreased parasitaemia [51–53]. However, several reports raise question on actual involvement of IL-6 in the pathogenesis of cerebral malaria [54–56]. In case of TGFβ, we have found that low concentration of TGFβ was found to be pro-inflammatory where high concentration of TGFβ have anti-inflammatory effects [41]. So, as factors responsible for disease outcome in malaria, both of these cytokines and their regulatory effect on T-reg/Th-17 balance seem to be important. We neutralized TGFβ and IL-6 by administration of neutralizing antibodies *in-vivo* at specific concentration. Parasitaemia was highest in TGFβ neutralized group than any other groups whereas parasitaemia was lowest in IL-6 neutralized group. This has been supported by the results of survival percentages of mice, where TGFβ neutralized group showed lowest survival percentage and IL-6 neutralized group showed the highest survival percentage of mice. Thus, it is quite evident that TGFβ and IL-6 directly affects the outcome of the immune response elicited by the host in malaria. Focusing on the effect of these two cytokines on the T-reg/Th-17 balance, it is found that neutralization of TGFβ results in significant induction of Th-17 cells at 8 dpi than control and infected ones. Whereas neutralization of IL-6 causes reduction in percentage and number of Th-17 cells than *Plasmodium berghei* ANKA infected group. Analysis of percentage and number of T regulatory cells in spleen show the reverse phenomenon to that of Th-17 cells upon neutralization of TGFβ and IL-6. Thus T-reg/Th-17 balance, which is skewed towards Th-17 in *Plasmodium berghei* ANKA infection is dependent on fine tuning maintained by TGFβ and IL-6. IL-6 neutralization reverts the dysregulated T-reg/Th-17 balance to homeostatic levels by inhibiting Th17 induction, but neutralization of TGFβ has opposing effect and causes the balance to skew more towards Th17. These changes in T-reg/Th17 balance by regulatory effects of TGFβ and IL-6 is mainly maintained by expression of STAT3 and STAT5, which are the major signalling molecules that take part in the signalling mechanism of these two cytokines [57]. Neutralization of TGFβ and IL-6 not only have its impact on splenic T-reg/Th-17, but also in that of cerebral cortex and cerebellum. In Anti-IL-6 treated *Plasmodium berghei* ANKA infected mice, glial cell mediated neuroinflammation is reduced whereas the anti-TGFβ treated mice upon infection show similar level of neuroinflammation as that of only infected mice. Consistent to that, astrocyte and microglia activation levels show similar changes in IL-6 and TGFβ neutralized groups. Regarding T-reg/Th-17, the major transcription factor of T-reg cells, FOXP3 expression was significantly higher in Anti-IL-6 treated infected group and significantly lower in Anti-TGFβ treated infected mice. The expression of IL-17, a major cytokine secreted by Th-17 cells, show the opposite result to that of FOXP3 in both the groups than the only

Plasmodium berghei ANKA infected ones [43]. But the actual percentages of the T-reg and Th-17 in cerebral cortex and cerebellum and their changes upon neutralization of these two cytokines is not yet investigated. Though there are few reports that cerebral malaria development is independent of IL-17 [58], several other reports shows that significant amount of IL-17 is found in circulation of malaria infected mice and human patients [59–61]. Genetic variants of IL-17 and its receptor IL-17RA increase the risk of malaria as investigated in African population [62]. Protective role of IL-17 during malaria pathogenesis has been found by working with IL-17RA deficient mice, in which IL-17 doesn't function in a proper way. These IL-17RA deficient mice show increased parasitemia, earlier onset of malaria, increased mortality during acute stage than the wild type mice [63]. So, it can be summarised that IL-17 itself and IL-17 expressing CD4+ T helper cells (Th17 cells) is of pivotal importance during malaria but the actual outcome of the immune response against the malaria parasite is dependent on the Treg/Th-17 balance, which is maintained majorly by TGFβ and IL-6.

4. Role of plasmacytoid dendritic cells (pDC) and myeloid dendritic cells (mDC) in regulation of Treg/Th-17 balance in malaria

Dendritic cells (DC), a professional antigen presenting cell, function as a bridge between innate and adaptive immune responses. In various infections, including malaria, different subsets of dendritic cells and co-stimulatory molecules (CD40, CD80, CD86, MHC-II etc.) expressed by them show significant changes which indicates that dendritic cells play a major role in the regulation of T cell differentiation and function [64]. Among different subsets, plasmacytoid DC (pDC), specially the tolerogenic pDCs induces and regulates the function of T regulatory cells [65]. Myeloid DC (mDC), on the other hand mainly secretes factors which are important for differentiation of Th-17 cells from naïve CD4+ T cells in several inflammatory disorders. Regulation of mDC function by several microRNA or other factors has its effect on Th-17 induction and function [66, 67]. In malaria, it has already been reported that mDC/pDC ratio has an impact on host immune response against *Plasmodium* sp. and disease pathogenesis [68, 69]. Analysis of splenic mDC/pDC ratio in *Plasmodium berghei* ANKA infection has shown that the ratio is increased significantly and the result is consistent with Th-17 mediated response against the murine cerebral malaria. This increased mDC/pDC ratio has been shown to revert back to homeostatic levels upon neutralization of IL-6, which also has its impact on Th-17 cells and functions in controlling the disease progression as discussed earlier [57]. Thus mDC/pDC ratio may be crucial in serving as a mediator that regulates the T-reg/Th-17 ratio in malaria. However, further investigation is still required to actually find out how exactly mDC/pDC ratio regulates the T-reg/Th-17 balance and how it influences the outcome of the immune response against malaria parasite.

5. Role of autophagy in the regulation of T-reg/Th17 balance in malaria infection

Autophagy is a well-known process which plays a beneficial role against infectious disease not only by degrading pathogens but also by activating host immune system. Autophagy plays an important role in multiple aspects of immune system like cytokine balance, modulation of immune cells, innate and adaptive immunity and antigen presentation [70]. In our study we have found increased expression of all five major markers of autophagy pathway viz. BECLIN1, ATG3, ATG5, ATG7, p62 with the progression of disease and the expressions were highest at 8 dpi *Plasmodium berghei* ANKA infection. An increase in the expression of LC3B has also been found. Simultaneously, the ratio of LC3B:LC3A increased at 8 dpi *Plasmodium berghei* ANKA infection which indicates the conversion of LC3A to LC3B and an upregulation of autophagic flux [71]. It has been reported that pDC harbours live *Plasmodium* parasite which have the ability to cause malaria symptoms when transferred to naïve mice [72]. Rapamycin (known autophagy inducer) treatment reduces the plasmodium load in splenic pDC. Autophagic induction increases the expression of CD205 and MHC I on pDC which stimulates antigen processing and antigen presentation respectively as compared to non-treated PbA infected group. Relative downregulation of proinflammatory cytokines like IL-6 and TNFα and positive induction of anti-inflammatory cytokines like IL10 was observed in autophagy induced mice. A tilt towards low Treg/Th-17 and high mDC/pDC ratio have been observed during malaria infection which induce Th1 pathway mediated immune regulation and poor prognosis for host. But autophagy induction can shift the Treg/Th17 balance towards increased T-reg population along with increased pDC population which can alter the mDC/pDC ratio, suppress the proinflammatory response and promote Th2 pathway [73]. Autophagic regulation of splenic red pulp macrophages show similar results in context to Treg/Th-17 balance [74]. Upregulation of proinflammatory cytokines production and alteration of Treg/Th-17 balance towards increased population of Th17 is a major cause for poor prognosis of malaria. Autophagy induction can revert the imbalance and help in betterment of host immune response.

6. Conclusion and future perspectives

Despite of continuous efforts towards invention of a proper and effective vaccines for malaria prevention, very few of them have their impact on reducing the number of malaria cases and malaria induced mortality. ACT still is the major therapeutic strategy in combating this disease, although emergence of Artemisinin resistance has been a major worry for the effectiveness of ACT during treatment of malaria patients. Immunotherapeutic strategies have been quite promising in several inflammatory disorders, cancers, autoimmune disorders and other infections. In case of malaria, although immunomodulation is very effective in murine studies, causing declination of parasitemia and increasing the survival percentages, application of those immunotherapeutic strategies in human is still awaiting. The balance between two T helper cell subsets i.e. T regulatory cells and Th-17 cells has been found to be important in both lethal and non-lethal malaria and factors which regulate this balance seems to play a pivotal role in disease manifestation. Studies using murine models has been quite effective in determining the factors and how they influence the disease outcome by regulating the Treg/Th-17 balance. Among those factors, TGFβ and IL-6 directly regulate the percentage of cells, expression of their characteristic transcription factors and functional cytokines secreted by Treg and Th-17 cells. Neutralization of IL-6 has direct effect on parasitaemia and survival percentages of mice infected with *Plasmodium* sp. It also reverses the dysregulated Treg/Th-17 ratio to optimal levels and can be a target for future therapeutic interventions against malaria infection. mDC/pDC ratio also play the role of a regulator and as a bridge to control Treg/Th-17 ratio. IL-6 neutralization can also bring the altered mDC/pDC ratio to normal levels. Apart from these, autophagic regulation of dendritic cells and macrophages in the spleen has its effect on Treg/Th-17 balance. Though, use of T-regulatory cells and drugs that directly regulate the altered ratio is regarded as a potentially attractive therapeutic strategy in autoimmune disorders, application of these approaches in malaria and other parasitic infections needs more attention and caution. Further investigations are still required to achieve the goal of a malaria free world.

Acknowledgements

The authors are thankful to the Department of Zoology, University of Calcutta for their support and research scholars of the Immunology Laboratory for their generous help for completing this research work. We also like to acknowledge Department of Science and Technology, Govt. of India (SB/SO/HS-106/2013, dated November 21, 2014), Department of Atomic Energy -BRNS: (37(1)/14/54/2014-BRNS/1740 dated October 28, 2014), West Bengal Department of Biotechnology (22(Sanc)/BT (Estt)/RD-20/2013 dated January 07, 2015) for their financial support to carry out these works. Fellowship support from Council of Scientific and Industrial Research (CSIR), India (for SM, SG) and University Grants Commission (UGC), India is also hereby acknowledged.

Conflict of interest

The authors declare no conflict of interest.

Author details

Saikat Mukherjee, Soubhik Ghosh and Arindam Bhattacharyya*
Immunology Laboratory, Department of Zoology, University of Calcutta, Kolkata, West Bengal, India

*Address all correspondence to: arindam19@yahoo.com

References

[1] World malaria report 2020, World Health Organization.

[2] Institute of Medicine (US) Committee on the Economics of Antimalarial Drugs; Arrow KJ, Panosian C, Gelband H, editors. Saving Lives, Buying Time: Economics of Malaria Drugs in an Age of Resistance. Washington (DC): National Academies Press (US); 2004. 6, The Parasite, the Mosquito, and the Disease. Available from: https://www.ncbi.nlm.nih.gov/books/NBK215619/

[3] Kwiatkowski DP. How malaria has affected the human genome and what human genetics can teach us about malaria. Am J Hum Genet. 2005 Aug;77(2):171-92. doi: 10.1086/432519. Epub 2005 Jul 6. PMID: 16001361; PMCID: PMC1224522.

[4] Eastman RT, Fidock DA. Artemisinin-based combination therapies: a vital tool in efforts to eliminate malaria. Nat Rev Microbiol. 2009 Dec;7(12):864-74. doi: 10.1038/nrmicro2239. Epub 2009 Nov 2. PMID: 19881520; PMCID: PMC2901398.

[5] Lalloo DG, Shingadia D, Bell DJ, Beeching NJ, Whitty CJM, Chiodini PL; PHE Advisory Committee on Malaria Prevention in UK Travellers. UK malaria treatment guidelines 2016. J Infect. 2016 Jun;72(6):635-649. doi: 10.1016/j.jinf.2016.02.001. Epub 2016 Feb 12. PMID: 26880088; PMCID: PMC7132403.

[6] Tse EG, Korsik M, Todd MH. The past, present and future of anti-malarial medicines. Malar J. 2019 Mar 22;18(1):93. doi: 10.1186/s12936-019-2724-z. PMID: 30902052; PMCID: PMC6431062.

[7] Talman AM, Clain J, Duval R, Ménard R, Ariey F. Artemisinin Bioactivity and Resistance in Malaria Parasites. Trends Parasitol. 2019 Dec;35(12):953-963. doi: 10.1016/j.pt.2019.09.005. Epub 2019 Nov 4. PMID: 31699532.

[8] Lu F, He XL, Richard C, Cao J. A brief history of artemisinin: Modes of action and mechanisms of resistance. Chin J Nat Med. 2019 May 20;17(5):331-336. doi: 10.1016/S1875-5364(19)30038-X. PMID: 31171267.

[9] Rosenberg SA. Decade in review-cancer immunotherapy: entering the mainstream of cancer treatment. Nat Rev Clin Oncol. 2014 Nov;11(11):630-2. doi: 10.1038/nrclinonc.2014.174. Epub 2014 Oct 14. PMID: 25311350; PMCID: PMC6310157.

[10] Ramamurthy D, Nundalall T, Cingo S, Mungra N, Karaan M, Naran K, Barth S. Recent advances in immunotherapies against infectious diseases. Immunotherapy Advances. 2021 Jan;1(1):ltaa007.

[11] Naran K, Nundalall T, Chetty S, Barth S. Principles of immunotherapy: implications for treatment strategies in cancer and infectious diseases. Frontiers in microbiology. 2018 Dec 21;9:3158.

[12] Cabral-Miranda G, Heath MD, Gomes AC, Mohsen MO, Montoya-Diaz E, Salman AM, Atcheson E, Skinner MA, Kramer MF, Reyes-Sandoval A, Bachmann MF. Microcrystalline Tyrosine (MCT®): A Depot Adjuvant in Licensed Allergy Immunotherapy Offers New Opportunities in Malaria. Vaccines. 2017; 5(4):32. https://doi.org/10.3390/vaccines5040032

[13] Belachew EB. Immune Response and Evasion Mechanisms of *Plasmodium falciparum* Parasites. J Immunol Res. 2018 Mar 25;2018:6529681. doi: 10.1155/2018/6529681. PMID: 29765991; PMCID: PMC5889876.

[14] Long CA, Zavala F. Immune Responses in Malaria. Cold Spring Harb Perspect Med. 2017 Aug 1;7(8):a025577. doi: 10.1101/cshperspect.a025577. PMID: 28389518; PMCID: PMC5538407.

[15] Del Portillo HA, Ferrer M, Brugat T, Martin-Jaular L, Langhorne J, Lacerda MV. The role of the spleen in malaria. Cell Microbiol. 2012 Mar;14(3):343-355. doi: 10.1111/j.1462-5822.2011.01741.x. Epub 2012 Feb 2. PMID: 22188297.

[16] Henry B, Roussel C, Carucci M, Brousse V, Ndour PA, Buffet P. The Human Spleen in Malaria: Filter or Shelter? Trends Parasitol. 2020 May;36(5):435-446. doi: 10.1016/j.pt.2020.03.001. Epub 2020 Mar 30. PMID: 32298631.

[17] Dinis-Oliveira RJ, Vieira DN, Magalhães T. Guidelines for Collection of Biological Samples for Clinical and Forensic Toxicological Analysis. Forensic Sci Res. 2017 Jan 16;1(1):42-51. doi: 10.1080/20961790.2016.1271098. PMID: 30483610; PMCID: PMC6197137.

[18] Tashjian RS, Williams RR, Vinters HV, Yong WH. Autopsy Biobanking: Biospecimen Procurement, Integrity, Storage, and Utilization. Methods Mol Biol. 2019;1897:77-87. doi: 10.1007/978-1-4939-8935-5_8. PMID: 30539436; PMCID: PMC6777723.

[19] White NJ, Turner GD, Medana IM, Dondorp AM, Day NP. The murine cerebral malaria phenomenon. Trends Parasitol. 2010 Jan;26(1):11-5. doi: 10.1016/j.pt.2009.10.007. Epub 2009 Nov 22. PMID: 19932638; PMCID: PMC2807032.

[20] Gonçalves RM, Lima NF, Ferreira MU. Parasite virulence, co-infections and cytokine balance in malaria. Pathog Glob Health. 2014 Jun;108(4):173-8. doi: 10.1179/2047773214Y.0000000139. Epub 2014 May 23. PMID: 24854175; PMCID: PMC4069333.

[21] Kurup SP, Butler NS, Harty JT. T cell-mediated immunity to malaria. Nat Rev Immunol. 2019 Jul;19(7):457-471. doi: 10.1038/s41577-019-0158-z. PMID: 30940932; PMCID: PMC6599480.

[22] Perez-Mazliah D, Langhorne J. CD4 T-cell subsets in malaria: TH1/TH2 revisited. Frontiers in immunology. 2015 Jan 12;5:671.

[23] Lee GR. The Balance of Th17 versus Treg Cells in Autoimmunity. Int J Mol Sci. 2018 Mar 3;19(3):730. doi: 10.3390/ijms19030730. PMID: 29510522; PMCID: PMC5877591.

[24] Eisenstein, E., Williams, C. The T_{reg}/Th17 Cell Balance: A New Paradigm for Autoimmunity. Pediatr Res **65**, 26-31 (2009). https://doi.org/10.1203/PDR.0b013e31819e76c7

[25] Knochelmann, H.M., Dwyer, C.J., Bailey, S.R. *et al.* When worlds collide: Th17 and Treg cells in cancer and autoimmunity. Cell Mol Immunol **15**, 458-469 (2018). https://doi.org/10.1038/s41423-018-0004-4

[26] Omenetti S, Pizarro TT. The Treg/Th17 Axis: A Dynamic Balance Regulated by the Gut Microbiome. Front Immunol. 2015 Dec 17;6:639. doi: 10.3389/fimmu.2015.00639. PMID: 26734006; PMCID: PMC4681807.

[27] Kleinewietfeld M, Hafler DA. The plasticity of human Treg and Th17 cells and its role in autoimmunity. Semin Immunol. 2013 Nov 15;25(4):305-12. doi: 10.1016/j.smim.2013.10.009. Epub 2013 Nov 5. PMID: 24211039; PMCID: PMC3905679.

[28] Lee YK, Mukasa R, Hatton RD, Weaver CT. Developmental plasticity of Th17 and Treg cells. Current opinion in immunology. 2009 Jun 1;21(3):274-280.

[29] Fasching P, Stradner M, Graninger W, Dejaco C, Fessler J. Therapeutic Potential of Targeting the Th17/Treg Axis in Autoimmune Disorders. Molecules. 2017 Jan 14;22(1):134. doi: 10.3390/molecules22010134. PMID: 28098832; PMCID: PMC6155880.

[30] Raimondo MG, Biggioggero M, Crotti C, Becciolini A, Favalli EG. Profile of sarilumab and its potential in the treatment of rheumatoid arthritis. Drug Des Devel Ther. 2017 May 24;11:1593-1603. doi: 10.2147/DDDT.S100302. PMID: 28579757; PMCID: PMC5447699.

[31] Hansen DS, Schofield L. Natural regulatory T cells in malaria: host or parasite allies? PLoS Pathog. 2010 Apr 29;6(4):e1000771. doi: 10.1371/journal.ppat.1000771. PMID: 20442856; PMCID: PMC2861684.

[32] Balasa R, Barcutean L, Balasa A, Motataianu A, Roman-Filip C, Manu D. The action of TH17 cells on blood brain barrier in multiple sclerosis and experimental autoimmune encephalomyelitis. Human immunology. 2020 May 1;81(5):237-243.

[33] Couper KN, Blount DG, Wilson MS, Hafalla JC, Belkaid Y, Kamanaka M, Flavell RA, de Souza JB, Riley EM. IL-10 from CD4CD25Foxp3CD127 adaptive regulatory T cells modulates parasite clearance and pathology during malaria infection. PLoS Pathog. 2008 Feb 29;4(2):e1000004. doi: 10.1371/journal.ppat.1000004. PMID: 18401464; PMCID: PMC2291447.

[34] Rouse BT, Suvas S. Regulatory cells and infectious agents: detentes cordiale and contraire. J Immunol. 2004 Aug 15;173(4):2211-2215. doi: 10.4049/jimmunol.173.4.2211. PMID: 15294929.

[35] Walther M, Jeffries D, Finney OC, NjieM, EbonyiA, DeiningerS, LawrenceE, Ngwa-Amambua A, Jayasooriya S, Cheeseman IH, Gomez-Escobar N, Okebe J, Conway DJ, Riley EM. Distinct roles for FOXP3 and FOXP3 CD4 T cells in regulating cellular immunity to uncomplicated and severe *Plasmodium falciparum* malaria. PLoS Pathog. 2009 Apr;5(4):e1000364. doi: 10.1371/journal.ppat.1000364. Epub 2009 Apr 3. PMID: 19343213; PMCID: PMC2658808.

[36] Feng H, Zhu XT, Qi ZM, Wang QH, Wang GG, Pan YY, Li Y, Zheng L, Jiang YJ, Shang H, Cui L, Cao YM. Transient attenuated Foxp3 expression on $CD4^+$ T cells treated with 7D4 mAb contributes to the control of parasite burden in DBA/2 mice infected with lethal Plasmodium chabaudi chabaudi AS. Scand J Immunol. 2012 Jan;75(1):46-53. doi: 10.1111/j.1365-3083.2011.02622.x. PMID: 21916916.

[37] Haque A, Best SE, Amante FH, Mustafah S, Desbarrieres L, de Labastida F, Sparwasser T, Hill GR, Engwerda CR. CD4+ natural regulatory T cells prevent experimental cerebral malaria via CTLA-4 when expanded in vivo. PLoS Pathog. 2010 Dec 9;6(12):e1001221. doi: 10.1371/journal.ppat.1001221. PMID: 21170302; PMCID: PMC3000360.

[38] Steeg C, Adler G, Sparwasser T, Fleischer B, Jacobs T. Limited role of CD4+Foxp3+ regulatory T cells in the control of experimental cerebral malaria. J Immunol. 2009 Dec 1;183(11):7014-7022. doi: 10.4049/jimmunol.0901422. Epub 2009 Nov 4. PMID: 19890049.

[39] Veldhoen M, Hocking RJ, Atkins CJ, Locksley RM, Stockinger B. TGFbeta in the context of an inflammatory cytokine milieu supports de novo differentiation of IL-17-producing T cells. Immunity. 2006 Feb;24(2):179-189. doi: 10.1016/j.immuni.2006.01.001. PMID: 16473830.

[40] Cipollini V, Anrather J, Orzi F, Iadecola C. Th17 and Cognitive

Impairment: Possible Mechanisms of Action. Front Neuroanat. 2019 Nov 19;13:95. doi: 10.3389/fnana.2019.00095. PMID: 31803028; PMCID: PMC6877481.

[41] Keswani T, Bhattacharyya A. Splenocyte apoptosis in Plasmodium berghei ANKA infection: possible role of TNF-α and TGF-β. Parasite Immunol. 2013 Feb;35(2):73-90. doi: 10.1111/pim.12005. PMID: 23009201.

[42] Keswani T, Bhattacharyya A. Differential role of T regulatory and Th17 in Swiss mice infected with Plasmodium berghei ANKA and Plasmodium yoelii. Exp Parasitol. 2014 Jun;141:82-92. doi: 10.1016/j.exppara.2014.03.003. Epub 2014 Mar 24. PMID: 24675415.

[43] Sarkar S, Keswani T, Sengupta A, Mitra S, Bhattacharyya A. Differential modulation of glial cell mediated neuroinflammation in Plasmodium berghei ANKA infection by TGF β and IL 6. Cytokine. 2017 Nov;99:249-259. doi: 10.1016/j.cyto.2017.07.026. Epub 2017 Aug 10. PMID: 28803696.

[44] Gough NR. Enhancing and Inhibiting TGF-β Signaling in Infection. Science Signaling. 2015 Jan 13;8(359):ec9-.

[45] Massagué J. TGFbeta in Cancer. Cell. 2008 Jul 25;134(2):215-30. doi: 10.1016/j.cell.2008.07.001. PMID: 18662538; PMCID: PMC3512574.

[46] Kumari N, Dwarakanath BS, Das A, Bhatt AN. Role of interleukin-6 in cancer progression and therapeutic resistance. Tumour Biol. 2016 Sep;37(9):11553-11572. doi: 10.1007/s13277-016-5098-7. Epub 2016 Jun 3. PMID: 27260630.

[47] Tanaka T, Narazaki M, Kishimoto T. IL-6 in inflammation, immunity, and disease. Cold Spring Harb Perspect Biol. 2014 Sep 4;6(10):a016295. doi: 10.1101/cshperspect.a016295. PMID: 25190079; PMCID: PMC4176007.

[48] J. Scheller, A. Chalaris, D. Schmidt-Arras, S. Rose-John, The pro- and antiinflammatory properties of the cytokine interleukin-6, Biochim. Biophys. Acta 1813 (2011) 878-888.

[49] L.J. Robinson, M.C. D'Ombrain, D.I. Stanisic, J. Taraika, N. Bernard, J.S. Richards, et al., Cellular tumor necrosis factor, gamma interferon, and interleukin-6 responses as correlates of immunity and risk of clinical Plasmodium falciparum malaria in children from Papua New Guinea, Infect. Immunol. 77 (2009) 3033-3043.

[50] J. Jason, L.K. Archibald, O.C. Nwanyanwu, M. Bell, I. Buchanan, J. Larned, et al., Cytokines and malaria parasitemia, Clin. Immunol. 100 (2001) 208-218.

[51] E. Hugosson, S.M. Montgomery, Z. Premji, M. Troye-Blomberg, A. Björkman, Relationship between antipyretic effects and cytokine levels in uncomplicated falciparum malaria during different treatment regimes, Acta Trop. 99 (2006) 75-82.

[52] J.Y. Seoh, M. Khan, S.H. Park, H.K. Park, M.H. Shin, E.H. Ha, et al., Serum cytokine profiles in patients with Plasmodium vivax malaria: a comparison between those who presented with and without hyperpyrexia, Am. J. Trop. Med. Hyg. 68 (2003) 102-106.

[53] J.L. Sarthou, G. Angel, G. Aribot, C. Rogier, A. Dieye, A. Toure Balde, et al., Prognostic value of anti-Plasmodium falciparum-specific immunoglobulin G3, cytokines, and their soluble receptors in West African patients with severe malaria, Infect. Immun. 65 (1997) 3271-3276.

[54] I.M. Medana, N.H. Hunt, G. Chaudhri, Tumor necrosis factor alpha

expression in the brain during fatal murine cerebral malaria: evidence for production by microglia and astrocytes, Am. J. Pathol. 150 (1997) 1473-1486.

[55] G.E. Grau, S. de Kossodo, Cerebral malaria: mediators, mechanical obstruction or more?, Parasitol Today 10 (1994) 408-409.

[56] G.E. Grau, G. Bieler, P. Pointaire, S. De Kossodo, F. Tacchini-Cotier, P. Vassalli, et al., Significance of cytokine production and adhesion molecules in malarial immunopathology, Immunol. Lett. 25 (1990) 189-194.

[57] Keswani T, Sarkar S, Sengupta A, Bhattacharyya A. Role of TGF-β and IL-6 in dendritic cells, Treg and Th17 mediated immune response during experimental cerebral malaria. Cytokine. 2016 Dec;88:154-166. doi: 10.1016/j.cyto.2016.08.034. Epub 2016 Sep 12. PMID: 27632786.

[58] Ishida H, Matsuzaki-Moriya C, Imai T, Yanagisawa K, Nojima Y, Suzue K, Hirai M, Iwakura Y, Yoshimura A, Hamano S, Shimokawa C. Development of experimental cerebral malaria is independent of IL-23 and IL-17. Biochemical and biophysical research communications. 2010 Nov 26;402(4):790-795.

[59] Helegbe GK, Huy NT, Yanagi T, Shuaibu MN, Kikuchi M, Cherif MS, Hirayama K. Elevated IL-17 levels in semi-immune anaemic mice infected with Plasmodium berghei ANKA. Malar J. 2018 Apr 17;17(1):169. doi: 10.1186/s12936-018-2257-x. PMID: 29665817; PMCID: PMC5905139.

[60] Raballah E, Kempaiah P, Karim Z, Orinda GO, Otieno MF, Perkins DJ, Ong'echa JM. CD4 T-cell expression of IFN-γ and IL-17 in pediatric malarial anemia. PloS one. 2017 Apr 20;12(4):e0175864.

[61] Bueno LL, Morais CG, Lacerda MV, Fujiwara RT, Braga EM. Interleukin-17 producing T helper cells are increased during natural Plasmodium vivax infection. Acta Trop. 2012 Jul;123(1):53-57. doi: 10.1016/j.actatropica.2012.02.071. Epub 2012 Mar 27. PMID: 22476130.

[62] Marquet S, Conte I, Poudiougou B, Argiro L, Cabantous S, Dessein H, Burté F, Oumar AA, Brown BJ, Traore A, Afolabi NK. The IL17F and IL17RA genetic variants increase risk of cerebral malaria in two African populations. Infection and immunity. 2016 Feb 1;84(2):590-597.

[63] Ghosh D, Brown SL, Stumhofer JS. IL-17 Promotes Differentiation of Splenic LSK⁻ Lymphoid Progenitors into B Cells following *Plasmodium yoelii* Infection. J Immunol. 2017 Sep 1;199(5):1783-1795. doi: 10.4049/jimmunol.1601972. Epub 2017 Jul 21. PMID: 28733485; PMCID: PMC5585076.

[64] Yap XZ, Lundie RJ, Beeson JG, O'Keeffe M. Dendritic Cell Responses and Function in Malaria. Front Immunol. 2019 Mar 4;10:357. doi: 10.3389/fimmu.2019.00357. PMID: 30886619; PMCID: PMC6409297.

[65] Matta BM, Castellaneta A, Thomson AW. Tolerogenic plasmacytoid DC. Eur J Immunol. 2010 Oct;40(10):2667-76. doi: 10.1002/eji.201040839. PMID: 20821731; PMCID: PMC3974856.

[66] Terhune J, Berk E, Czerniecki BJ. Dendritic Cell-Induced Th1 and Th17 Cell Differentiation for Cancer Therapy. Vaccines (Basel). 2013 Nov 21;1(4):527-49. doi: 10.3390/vaccines1040527. PMID: 26344346; PMCID: PMC4494209.

[67] Ifergan I, Chen S, Zhang B, Miller SD. Cutting Edge: MicroRNA-223 Regulates Myeloid Dendritic Cell-Driven Th17 Responses in Experimental Autoimmune Encephalomyelitis. J Immunol. 2016 Feb 15;196(4):1455-1459. doi: 10.4049/jimmunol.1501965. Epub

2016 Jan 18. PMID: 26783338; PMCID: PMC4744529.

[68] Turner, T.C., Arama, C., Ongoiba, A. *et al.* Dendritic cell responses to *Plasmodium falciparum* in a malaria-endemic setting. Malar J **20,** 9 (2021).

[69] Keswani T, Sengupta A, Sarkar S, Bhattacharyya A. Dendritic cells subsets mediated immune response during Plasmodium berghei ANKA and Plasmodium yoelii infection. Cytokine. 2015 Jun;73(2):198-206. doi: 10.1016/j.cyto.2015.02.023. Epub 2015 Mar 16. PMID: 25792277.

[70] Deretic V, Saitoh T, Akira S. Autophagy in infection, inflammation and immunity. Nature Reviews Immunology. 2013 Oct;13(10):722-737.

[71] Sengupta A, Mukherjee S, Ghosh S, Keswani T, Sarkar S, Majumdar G, Das M, Bhattacharyya A. Partial impairment of late-stage autophagic flux in murine splenocytes leads to sqstm1/p62 mediated nrf2-keap1 antioxidant pathway activation and induced proteasome-mediated degradation in malaria. Microb Pathog. 2020 Oct;147:104289. doi: 10.1016/j.micpath.2020.104289. Epub 2020 Jul 18. PMID: 32693118.

[72] Wykes MN, Kay JG, Manderson A, Liu XQ, Brown DL, Richard DJ, et al. Rodent blood-stage Plasmodium survive in dendritic cells that infect naive mice. Proc Natl Acad Sci U S A 2011;108:11205e10.

[73] Sengupta A, Keswani T, Sarkar S, Ghosh S, Mukherjee S, Bhattacharyya A. Autophagic induction modulates splenic plasmacytoid dendritic cell mediated immune response in cerebral malarial infection model. Microbes Infect. 2019 Dec;21(10):475-484. doi: 10.1016/j.micinf.2019.05.004. Epub 2019 Jun 8. PMID: 31185303.

[74] Sengupta A, Sarkar S, Keswani T, Mukherjee S, Ghosh S, Bhattacharyya A. Impact of autophagic regulation on splenic red pulp macrophages during cerebral malarial infection. Parasitol Int. 2019 Aug;71:18-26. doi: 10.1016/j.parint.2019.03.008. Epub 2019 Mar 11. PMID: 30872003.

Chapter 10

A Comprehensive Review of 4(1*H*)-Quinolones and 4(1*H*)-Pyridones for the Development of an Effective Antimalarial

Ami H. Asakawa and Roman Manetsch

Abstract

Malaria is a global public health issue. Despite the efforts in malaria prevention, nearly half the world's population is at risk of infection. Until present-day, researchers are struggling to design and discover an efficacious antimalarial. In comparison to most common antimalarial chemotypes that eliminate erythrocytic stages of *P. falciparum*, 4(1*H*)-quinolones and 4(1*H*)-pyridones exhibit antimalarial activity against multiple stages of the parasite. They have potential to treat blood stages of multidrug resistant *P. falciparum* malaria, eradicate dormant exoerythro stages of relapsing malaria species (*P. vivax*), and prevent transmission of infectious gametocytes to mosquitoes. However, thus far, the advancement of these chemotypes towards pre-clinical and clinical development has been impeded due to poor physicochemical properties, poor oral bioavailability, and poor dose-proportionality limiting preclinical safety and toxicity studies. Despite all these challenges, 4(1*H*)-quinolones and 4(1*H*)-pyridones continue to be at the forefront for the development of the next-generation antimalarials as they would have tremendous global public health impact and could significantly enhance current malaria elimination efforts.

Keywords: 4(1*H*)-quinolones, 4(1*H*)-pyridones, malaria, resistance, plasmodium, antimalarials

1. Introduction

1.1 Malaria

Malaria is a global, mosquito-borne, parasitic disease that is serious and fatal, putting people of 87 countries at risk. The population with the highest risk of infection are young children under the age of five and pregnant women living in the sub-Saharan Africa. In 2020, the World Health Organization (WHO) reported an estimate of 229 million malaria cases, with approximately 409,000 deaths in 2019 alone [1]. This is a significant decrease from that of ten years ago, where the global number of malaria cases and deaths were 243 million and 863,000, respectively. The increased efforts in malaria prevention had led to these decreases in cases [2].

Malaria is a disease caused by a protozoan parasite of the genus *Plasmodium*. These species are *P. falciparum*, *P. vivax*, *P. knowlesi*, *P. malariae*, and *P. ovale*, of which *P. falciparum* is the most common species of transmission [3, 4].

To develop efficacious antimalarial drugs, it is important to understand the *Plasmodium* lifecycle via its route of infection. Initially, the disease is transmitted into the host via a pregnant, female *Anopheles* mosquito when it takes a bloodmeal to feed her eggs by simultaneously injecting sporozoites and an anticoagulant to prevent blood clotting. Those that penetrate the blood vessels enter the bloodstream and head to the hepatocytes. The parasites entry point to the hepatocytes requires the penetration of the liver sinusoidal barrier, consisting of sentinel Kupffer cells [4].

Once *Plasmodium* sporozoites invade the hepatocytes, they do not mature immediately within the first invaded hepatocyte. They migrate through several hepatocytes, causing necrosis. When the parasite settles, these develop into the liver schizont form. Liver schizont is a multinucleate state of the cell during asexual reproduction called schizogony. One infected liver cell can develop into thousands of merozoites. These merozoites are released into the bloodstream when the hepatocytes bursts. Once these merozoites are released into the bloodstream, they will invade the erythrocytes through specific ligand-receptor interactions mediated by the proteins on the surfaces of the parasite and the erythrocyte [3, 5, 6].

Once inside the erythrocytes, the parasites can hide from the hosts' immune response. These merozoites begins to enlarge and become a uninucleate cell termed trophozoite. The nucleus of the trophozoites divides asexually to produce a schizont. The schizont then divides and produces merozoites. These merozoites can invade other erythrocytes and continue replicating. The clinical symptoms of malaria appear when these erythrocytes rupture and releases merozoites [3].

After many rounds of schizogony in the erythrocyte, some merozoites, rather than replicating, enter a sexual phase, where they develop into male and female gametocytes. Erythrocytes containing gametocytes do not rupture. Gametocytes are incapable of forming gametes within their hosts and form only when they are taken up by a mosquito. The importance of sexual differentiation is that it is responsible for the transmission from host to the *Anopheles* mosquito. The male and female gametocytes fuse within the mosquito, which forms a diploid zygote that becomes an ookinete. These ookinetes migrate to the midgut of the mosquito, pass through the gut wall, and form oocysts. The meiotic division of the oocysts occur and form sporozoites, which migrate to the salivary glands of the mosquito. This mosquito then injects these sporozoites to the next host, completing the transmission cycle [3].

Opposed to the common *P. falciparum* infection, *P. vivax* can infect the liver cells and remain dormant for as long as several years by remaining in the hepatocytes as hypnozoites, rather than developing into liver schizonts. This is the cause of malaria relapse (**Figure 1**) [7].

Unfortunately, this infection follows a vicious, never-ending cycle between human and mosquito, if a cure is not discovered for all forms of the parasite. Hence, the life cycle dictates design consideration from the onset of the discovery, optimization, and development of a new antimalarial agent.

1.2 Past and present antimalarial drugs

Decline in malaria cases are being observed due to the increased efforts in preventing, controlling, and treating malaria [8]. Still, chemotherapy is the most common method of prevention and treatment utilized for this infection. Of course, given the complex nature of the parasite, these drugs act differently towards

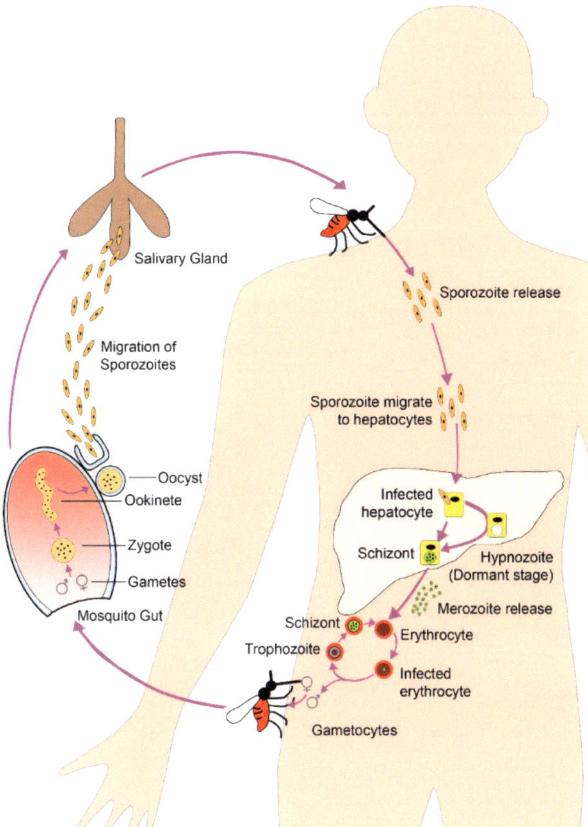

Figure 1.
Schematic representation of the malaria life cycle.

different stages of the parasite. For this reason, antimalarials are categorized by their activity – blood schizonticidal, tissue schizonticidal, gametocytocidal, and sporontocidal drugs. Blood schizonticidal drugs are antimalarials that target the asexual erythrocytic stages of the parasite. Tissue schizonticidal drugs are antimalarials that target hypnozoites. Gametocytocidal drug are antimalarials that targets the sexual erythrocytic forms of the parasite in the blood. Lastly, sporontocidal drugs are antimalarials that prevent formation of malarial oocytes and sporozoites in infected mosquito (**Table 1**) [9, 10].

Quinine (**1**), the first medicine to treat malaria, is an alkaloid isolated from the bark of *Cinchona* trees, which targets the asexual and sexual blood stage (**Figure 2**). This initial discovery in the 17th century of a natural product with antimalarial activity was revolutionary, as it was the first successful use of a chemical compound to treat an infectious disease. Unfortunately, due to its toxic nature and its rise of resistant *P. falciparum* strain, **1** was abandoned [11, 12]. However, its structure became the inspiration for the development of current antimalarials [13].

Currently, the majority of drugs target the asexual blood stages of the parasite. The most utilized drugs are chloroquine (**2**), artemisinin (**3**), and mefloquine (**4**) (**Figure 2**). Mefloquine (**4**), discovered during World War II, is a highly effective against blood stages of all *Plasmodium spp.* that affects humans [14, 15]. Chloroquine (**2**), initially discovered during the 1930s, was deemed toxic. However, with re-evaluation in the 1940s, chloroquine (**2**) became the standard medication for the treatment of malaria. Given its many advantages, such as excellent bioavailability, low cost, low toxicity, and effectiveness, chloroquine (**2**) was predominately

	Classification via Activity			
	Blood Schizonticidal	**Tissue Schizonticidal**	**Gametocytocidal**	**Sporontocidal**
Chloroquine	(+)	(−)	(−)	(−)
Quinine	(+)	(−)	(+)	(−)
Primaquine	(−)	(+)	(+)	(+)
Artemisinin	(+)	(−)	(+)	(−)
Atovaquone	(+)	(+)	(−)	(−)
Mefloquine	(+)	(−)	(−)	(−)

Table 1.
Antimalarials targeting different forms of parasite.

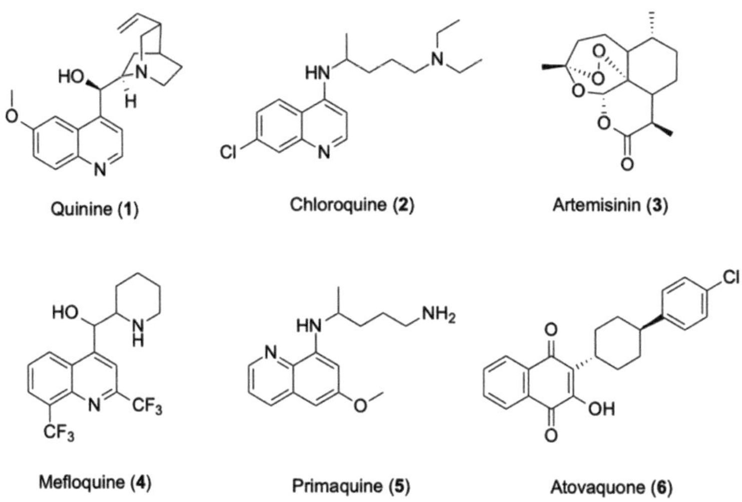

Figure 2.
Past and present antimalarial drugs.

used for at least two decades [15, 16]. Artemisinin (**3**), discovered in 1972, is a natural product isolated from *Artemisia annua* (sweet wormwood) and has been used as an antimalarial drug in China [15]. However, our supply of varying antimalarial is very limited, where we do not have many that target beyond the blood stage. Primaquine (**5**) and atovaquone (**6**) are the commonly utilized drug against liver stage parasites (**Figure 2**). Primaquine (**5**) has restricted use because it poses a major health concern, as it causes haemolysis for those with glucose-6-phosphate dehydrogenase (G6PD) deficiency. G6PD deficiency is an X-linked abnormality that is very common in tropical areas, where malaria is most prevalent [17].

Not only is the inadequate number of antimalarials that are active against the different life stages of parasite an issue, the development of resistance towards currently available drugs is a major concern. Resistance towards current antimalarial drugs are usually a result of a point mutation that can decrease drug accumulation through altered influx/efflux mechanism or change the affinity of the drug to its' validated targets [18, 19]. Actions have been taken by the WHO to act against resistance. Originally, artemisinin (**3**) was used as a monotherapy; however, given the relatively high recrudescence rate of approximately ten percent and the need for a seven-day course, this drug is now recommended by the WHO to be used in combination with another antimalarial. This is known as artemisinin combination therapy (ACT). With the ACT, the treatment length is three days, which prevents the emergence of resistant strains [20, 21]. ACTs are a combination of drugs that have separate mechanism of action against the same stage of the parasite. In other words, ACTs would combine fast-acting artemisinin derivative antimalarial with a slow-acting, structurally different antimalarial. This enables the fast-acting antimalarial to quickly reduce the parasite burden as the slow-acting antimalarial will completely eliminate the remaining parasite population [22].

Despite these efforts, increased resistance from mutant strains of *Plasmodium spp.* and inadequate number of antimalarials have urged the need of novel antimalarials that are active against multi-drug resistant strains for different forms of the parasite.

1.3 Recommended candidate profiles for the next generation of antimalarials

We are currently facing issues with current antimalarials due to resistant strains and lack of antimalarials to combat this problem. To develop the next generation of antimalarials, a description of the desired drug profile has been summarized in a Target Product Profile (TPP). TPPs are divided into different target candidate profiles (TCPs) since malaria chemotherapies will exist as combination therapy, containing more than one active ingredient. The main considerations across all TCPs are that these drugs are safe, affordable, and efficacious against multi-drug resistant *Plasmodium spp.* [23, 24].

2. Development of 4(1*H*)-quinolones and 4(1*H*)-pyridones

Abiding to the TCPs to develop a novel class of antimalarials is the current measure taken to assist in the eradication of malaria. 4(1*H*)-quinolones and 4(1*H*)-pyridones are a promising class of antimalarials, exhibiting potent activity [25, 26]. Structurally, 4(1*H*)-quinolones and 4(1*H*)-pyridones are synthetic compounds that contain the common ring, making them distinctive (**Figure 3**).

Previously discovered 4(1*H*)-quinolones and 4(1*H*)-pyridones with antimalarial activity in either avian, rodent, or primate were quickly abandoned without adequate evaluation. Recently, various research groups re-evaluated these older antimalarial 4(1*H*)-quinolones, 4(1*H*)-pyridones, and its' derivatives – endochin (7), clopidol (**8**), ICI56,780 (**9**), and floxacrine (**10**) – which shed light to the possibility that they can be viable leads if improvements to their physicochemical properties are successfully accomplished (**Figure 4**).

To improve physicochemical properties, it is necessary to scrutinize the properties, such as molecular weight, polar surface area, rotatable bonds, hydrogen bond acceptors and hydrogen bond donors as introduced in Lipinski's paper introducing Rule of Five and other subsequent papers [27, 28]. Another key feature to consider is the complexity of the molecule via Fsp^3, which measures saturation of the

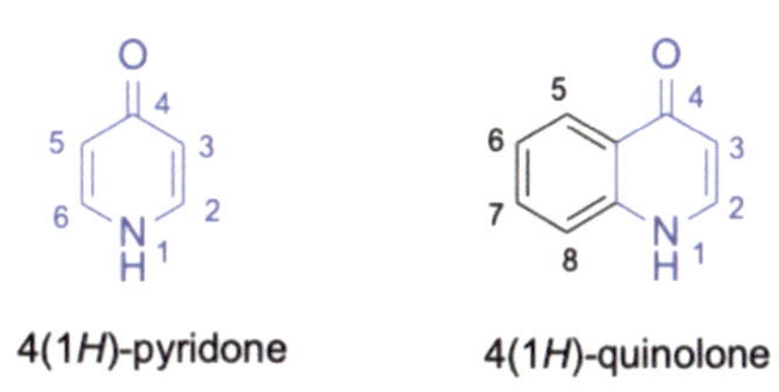

Figure 3.
4(1H)-quinolone and 4(1H)-pyridone scaffold.

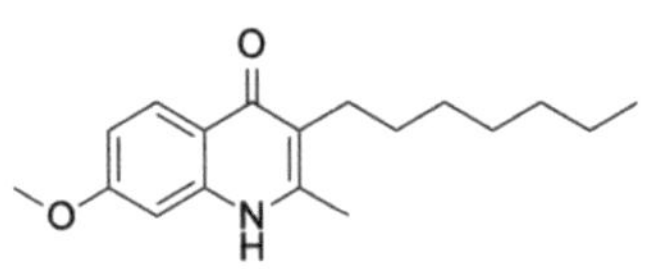

endochin (**7**)

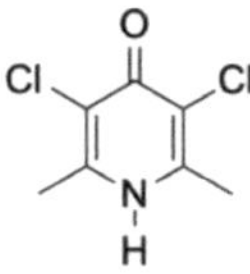

clopidol (**8**)

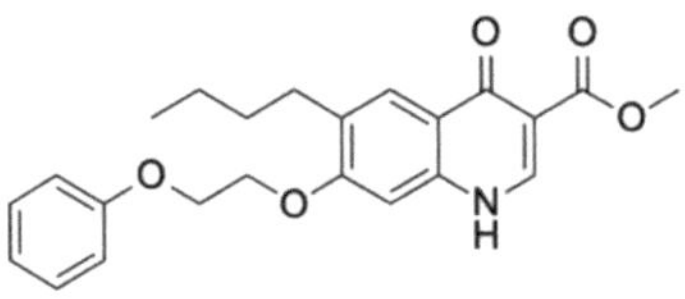

ICI56,780 (**9**)

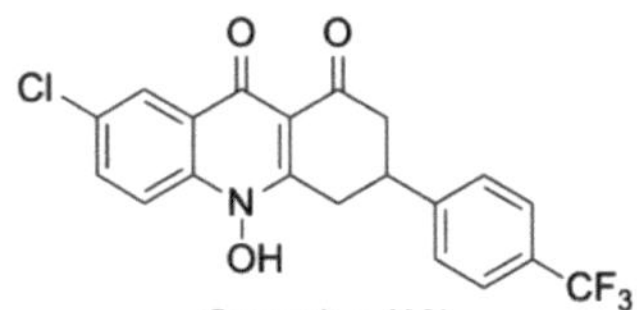

floxacrine (**10**)

Figure 4.
Original 4(1H)-pyridones, 4(1H)-quinolones, and its' derivatives with antimalarial activity.

compound. It has been observed that increase saturated carbons leads to higher aqueous solubility – a major downfall in 4(1*H*)-quinolone and 4(1*H*)-pyridone type molecules [29].

2.1 4(1*H*)-pyridones

2.1.1 Optimization of clopidol

An anticoccidial drug clopidal (**8**) was discovered to possess antimalarial activity in the 1960s by the Walter Reed Army Institute of Research. Assays presented activity towards four strains of *Plasmodium spp. – P. berghei*, *P. gallinaceum*, *P. cynomologi*, and *P. falciparum* [25, 30].

After several decades, scientists at GlaxoSmithKline (GSK) exerts efforts to optimize clopidal (**8**) due to emerging evidence that **8** may employ similar cytochrome bc_1 inhibition, like atovaquone (**6**) [31]. They hypothesize that clopidal (**8**) acts as a ubiquinone-mimic; therefore, replacing C-3 chlorine with a lipophilic sidechain. Installing an *n*-octyl chain improved *in vitro* activity (IC_{50} = 4 μM) but diminished *in vivo* activity ($ED_{50} \geq 60$ mg/kg). They hypothesized that the difference in activity may be due to metabolic degradation of the alkyl chain. To resolve this issue regarding the chemically labile sidechain, they installed the *trans*-(4-chlorophenyl) cyclohexyl sidechain of atovaquone (**6**), known to be resistant to metabolism, which significantly increased both *in vitro* and *in vivo* activity (IC_{50} = 0.05 μM; ED_{50} = 0.6 mg/kg). This led to the study of biaryl analogues, where 4-phenoxyphenyl sidechain also exhibited similar *in vitro* and *in vivo* activity. More in-depth SAR study was performed on 5-(phenoxyphenyl)-4(1*H*)-pyridones (**Figure 5**) [32].

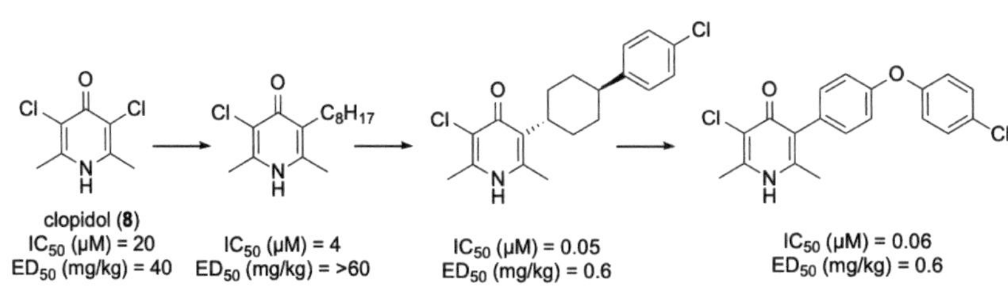

Figure 5.
Initial optimization of clopidol.

Variations to the C-2, C-3, and C-6 position were made and further improvements could not be observed (**Figure 6**). Variations on the aryl group made a major impact on the *in vitro* activity. This led to GW308678 (**11**) and GW844520 (**12**), where **12** entered preclinical trials [32]. However, after observing mild and reversible histopathological findings in skeletal and cardiac muscles, this study was abandoned. They hypothesized that these findings were due to its high lipophilic nature and long half-life. Therefore, they sought to improve the physicochemical properties [25].

To improve the physicochemical properties of GW844520 (**12**), the scientists at GSK introduced a hydroxymethyl group on C-2 position that significantly diminished the activity (IC_{50} = 0.13 μM). Interestingly, its isomer with the hydroxymethyl group on the C-6 position maintained high level of antimalarial activity (IC_{50} = 0.005 μM) with improved solubility. Simultaneously, a prodrug approach was introduced to optimize solubility. The newly introduced hydroxy group offered more chemically stable prodrugs than previous attempts utilizing the C4-OH. This led to GSK932121 (**13**) and a phosphate ester prodrug of **13**, where it was selected to enter human trials. Regrettably, this study was terminated due to toxicological findings from lack of species-specific target selectivity of the parent drug (**Figure 7**) [25, 33].

Recently, various linkers and heteroaromatic rings have been investigated. Compounds with rigid linker (alkyne) are still active; however, relative to their

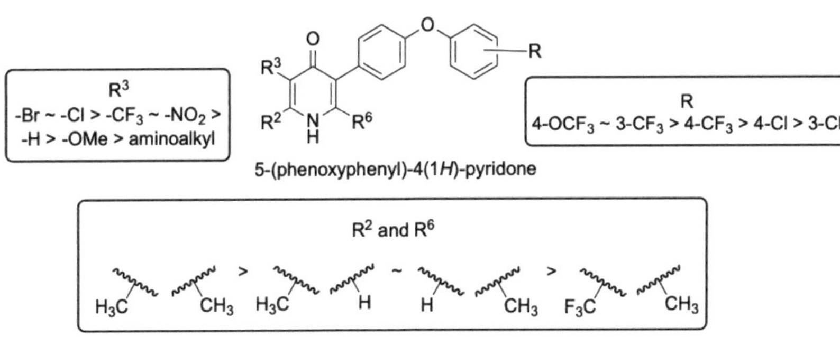

Figure 6.
SAR of 5-(phenoxyphenyl)-4(1H)-pyridones.

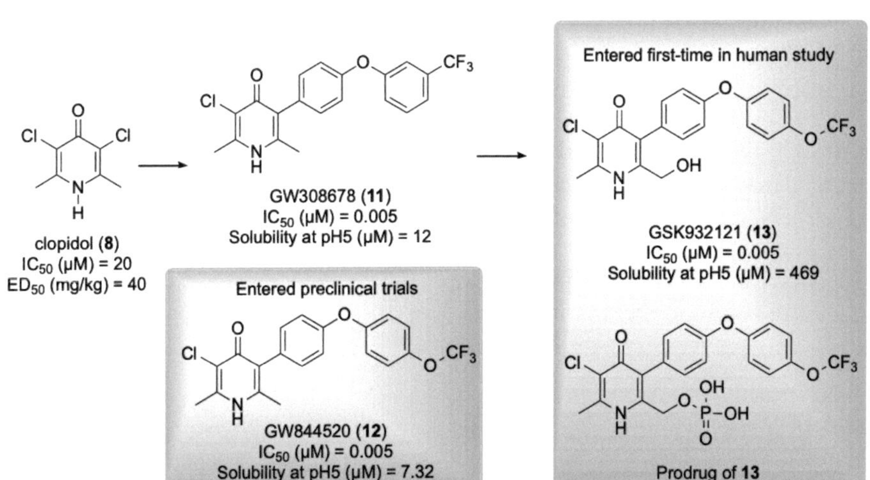

Figure 7.
Overall optimization scheme of clopidol.

flexible linker (ether and alkane) counterparts, their potency decreases by a ten-fold. They anticipate that the flexibility allows the compound to mold into the active site with correct hydrophobic interactions. Another observation was that replacing the proximal phenyl ring with a pyridine ring maintains the activity and improves pharmacokinetic profiles. This demonstrates the potential of analogues of **13** in hopes of improving pharmacokinetic and toxicology profiles of 4(1*H*)-pyridones [34].

2.2 4(1*H*)-quinolones

With renewed efforts to optimize 4(1*H*)-quinolones, three main factors are considered –aqueous solubility, resistance index (RI), and potency. Aqueous solubility is essential in developing a dose-proportional pharmacokinetic profile for orally administered drugs. The RI is the ratio of the effective concentration to kill 50% of the parasite population of two clinically relevant malaria strains, where one is the parent or sensitive strain. For instance, W2 and TM90-C2B are frequently used, where W2 is the multi-drug resistant strain that is atovaquone-sensitive and TM90-C2B is atovaquone-resistant due to a point mutation in cytochrome *b*. Given this, RI would be the EC_{50} of TM90-C2B divided by the EC_{50} of W2 [35]. Ideally, this value is 1, which demonstrates that the drug is equally potent against both malaria strains; values between 0.3 and 3.0 are acceptable. Finally, low nanomolar potency of both strains is preferred.

The balance amongst these three qualities are necessary for the development of a potent, orally bioavailable antimalarial quinolones.

2.2.1 Optimized of floxacrine

In 1974, an evaluation of floxacrine (**10**) for antimalarial activity was performed. It was discovered that **10** exhibited casual prophylactic activity. However, it had several liabilities – cardiovascular toxicity, parasite drug resistance, and poor aqueous solubility [36, 37]. Efforts have been made to synthesize analogous compounds devoid of these drawbacks. In the 1990s, WR243251 (**14**), a 1,2,3,4-tetrahydroacridin-9(10*H*)-ones (THAs), was discovered and did not display any cardiovascular toxicity (**Figure 8**) [37]. However, it still displayed resistance and had poor aqueous solubility [37, 38].

Due to limited exploration of THAs since the discovery of WR243251, Manetsch and Kyle initiated a structure–activity relationship (SAR) and a structure–property relationship (SPR) studies to better understand THAs and its ability to exert activity towards both the blood and liver stage of the parasite.

Altering the number of carbons on the saturated ring system significantly reduced the activity and the aqueous solubility. Here on out, the scientists modified the 5-, 6-, 7-, and 8- position of the benzenoid ring with the 6-membered saturated

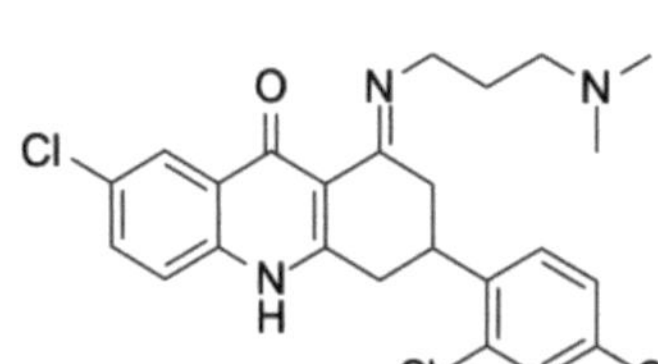

WR234251 (**14**)

Figure 8.
Structure of WR243251.

ring. It became evident that the 6- and 7-position are key positions for antimalarial activity, which also affected the RI. The electronics on the 6-position did not significantly alter the activity. However, the 7-position was more sensitive, as it displayed preference for electron donating groups to retain potency and maintain the RI between 0.3 and 3. Furthermore, an inverse relationship was observed between potency and aqueous solubility. Substituting either or both the 5-position and 8-position, decreased activity and increased solubility. With this, THA-114 (**15**) and THA-115 (**16**) were found to exhibit nanomolar antimalarial activity with an acceptable RI that lacks toxicity. However, its solubility did not fall within the acceptable range of 40 μM or greater (**Figure 9**). Developing a candidate that is both active and has optimal physicochemical properties is difficult; nonetheless, it is necessary. The inability to develop such molecules leads to issues with *in vivo* efficacy studies and hinders with safety assessment studies [39].

2.2.2 Optimization of ICI56,780

Scientists at Imperial Chemical Industries (ICI) developed ICI56,780 (**9**) as an antimalarial agent. What was striking about this compound series was its activity against blood stage and liver stage parasites in *P. cynomolgi* in rhesus monkeys and *P. berghei* in mice. However, disappointingly, resistance was developed in *P. berghei* after one passage [40, 41].

Manetsch and Kyle initiated work on SAR to optimize **9**. ICI56,780 (**9**) was utilized as the reference molecule, where they observed excellent potency for both W2 and TM90-C2B and *in vitro* liver stage activity; however, the potential to observe cross–resistance with atovaquone was high. Examination of the 2-, 3-, 6-, and 7-position concluded that the original 6- and 7- substituents are optimal. 3-position was rather interesting. Alteration significantly decreased the activity; however, remained within acceptable range. Interestingly, the RI fell into an appropriate range. Finally, the 2-position was examined with and without a methyl group, where the analogue with the methyl group displayed higher potency. This led to PEQ-1020 (**17**) an PEQ-437 (**18**). With promising *in vitro* blood stage data, compound **17** were tested *in vivo*. The insoluble nature of the compound **17** hindered *in vivo* testing and displayed poor activity (61% inhibition at day 6) (**Figure 10**) [42, 43].

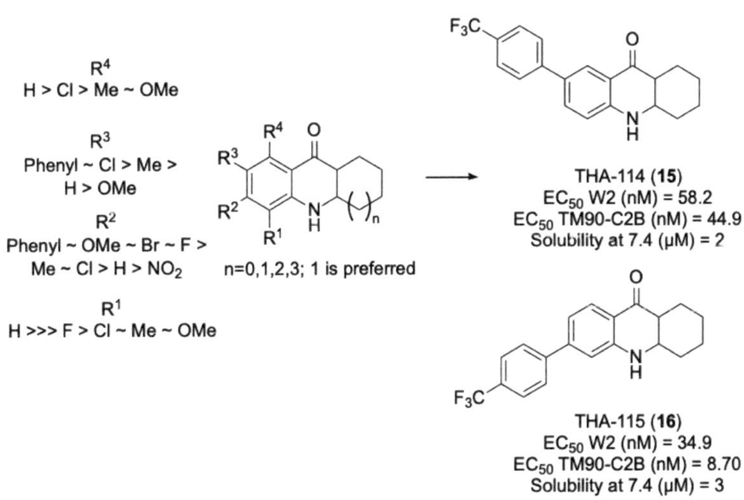

Figure 9.
Optimization of floxacrine.

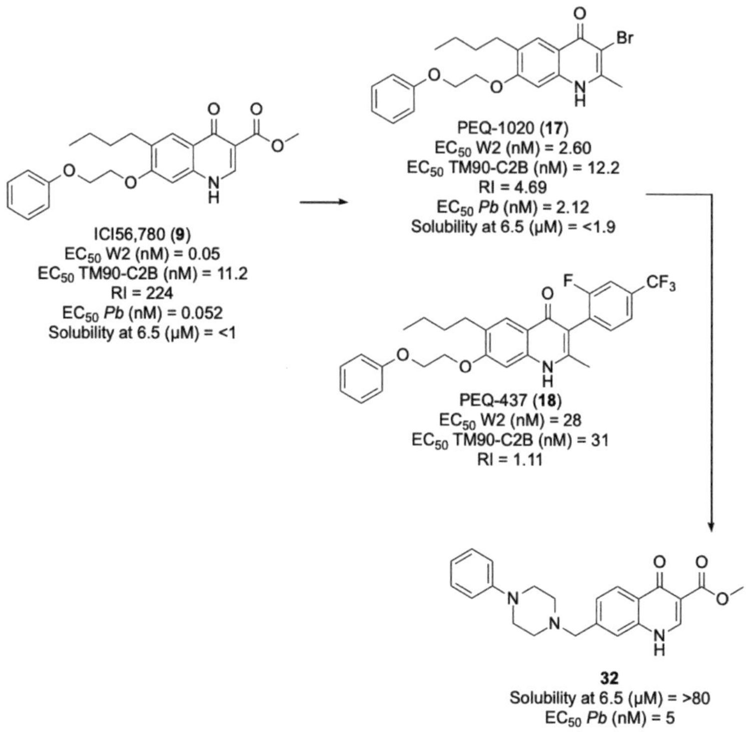

Figure 10.
Optimization of ICI56,780.

Given the necessity to improve aqueous solubility, ionizable piperazinyl-substituted analogues were developed. The linker length between the piperazine moiety and the benzenoid ring was investigated, along with the various piperazinyl-substituent. Ethylene linker analogues were found to diminish blood stage activity, while methylene linker analogues were most active. Amongst the *N*-phenylpiperazinyl, *N*-benzylpiperazinyl, and *p*-methoxybenzylpiperazinyl substituents, *N*-phenylpiperazinyl was most potent. When the piperazinyl-substituent was placed on the 6-position rather than the 7-position, the analogues were void of activity. Based on previously developed analogues, 3-position was investigated. Similarly, 3-halo substituted analogs improved RI; however, diminished activity compared to that of the methyl ester at the 3-position. This led to the discovery of **32** and due to its high potency against *in vitro* liver stage activity, **32** was further evaluated in an *in vivo* assay against liver stage. Compound **32** was able to generate cures at oral doses of 25 mg/kg or higher [44].

2.2.3 Optimization of endochin

Endochin (7) was discovered during World War II by Hans Andersag, a German chemist from Bayer [45, 46]. This compound had been identified to be a causal prophylactic and potent erythrocytic stage agent in avian models [47]. However, it was deemed ineffective against human malaria due to its physicochemical properties and its inactive metabolite that formed in the presence of cytochrome P450 (CYP450) enzymes [45]. This had inspired research teams, like the one of Manetsch and Kyle or Riscoe, to diversify such molecule.

The two groups worked together to synthesize a series of compounds, termed ELQ for endochin-like quinolones and P4Q for phenyl/aryl substituted in the 4-position of 4(1*H*)-quinolones, to undertake SAR and SPR studies. By removing either substituent on the 3- or 7-position, it was determined that the 3-position is essential to the activity of endochin. Because the alkyl chain on the 3-position was metabolically labile, they modified the 3-position. By diversifying the 3-position, it suggested that the active site was hydrophobic with a reasonably sized pocket. The substituents on the benzenoid ring was also investigated, where installing a chlorine at the 6-position and a methoxy- group on the 7-position increased potency through the nature of electronics. The chlorine increases the binding affinity by increasing the acidity of N-H. The methoxy-group increases the potential of the carbonyl to accept hydrogen bonds with the active site. Substitutions at the 5- and 8-positions were not tolerated well. To optimize variably in the SAR study, further studies utilized 3-alkylphenyl-4(1*H*)-quinolones. It was revealed that *para* position observed higher activity, *para* and *ortho* position had acceptable RI, and *ortho* position exhibited the higher aqueous solubility. Of this series, P4Q-146 (**19**) and P4Q-158 (**20**) were the compounds with the best characteristics – single-digit nanomolar activity with acceptable RI and lack of toxicity. To further optimize the aryl-substituent, moieties with two aromatic rings were investigated, where some were inspired by the GSK pyridones. This led to P4Q-390 (**21**). P4Q-391 (**22**), and ELQ-300 (**23**), where they exhibited low single-digit nanomolar activity with acceptable RI (**Figure 11**). P4Q–391 (**22**) and ELQ-300 (**23**) are especially unique because of its activity against exo-erythrocytic stage, which includes liver schizonts, gametocytes, and ookinetes and oocytes. Antimalarials that are capable of preventing the transmission of malaria is extremely important. For this reason, ELQ-300 (**23**) was selected by Medicines for Malaria Venture (MMV) to undergo preclinical development, where it resulted in causal prophylaxis in mice malarial models and complete inhibition of oocyst formation. Unlike the structurally similar GSK 4(1*H*)-pyridone, **23** was a species–specific inhibitor. However, due to the poor solubility of this compound, a proper safety margin could not be established and was, therefore, abandoned for future tests [48–54].

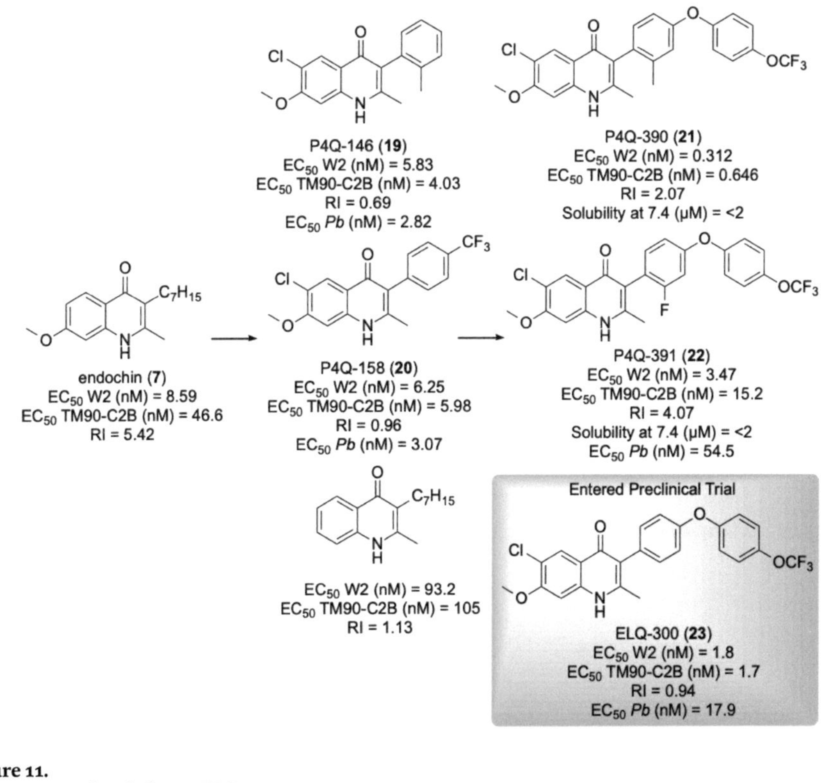

Figure 11.
Optimization of endochin to ELQ-300.

2.2.4 Optimization of TDR molecules

The Guy laboratory is also one of the various groups that are working to optimize quinolones to develop a potent antimalarial; however, their approach was slightly different. Rather than utilizing the older antimalarials, this group utilized two compounds that had confirmed antimalarial activity through the WHO's Special Programme for Tropical Disease Research (TDR). TDR42098 (**24**) and TDR17516 (**25**), differing in the position of the methoxy group on the benzenoid ring, was identified and confirmed to have antimalarial activity from a screening campaign by TDR at Tibotec using 17,472 non-proprietary compounds sourced from SPECS (**Figure 12**) [55].

Utilizing **24** and **25** as the reference compound, the Guy laboratory modified the 2-, 3-, 5-, and 7-position to see its effect on the activity, solubility, and permeability. In the first series of compounds, the 3-position was investigated. Removal of the carboxyl ester resulted in the total loss of activity and solubility for both analogues of **24** and **25**. Replacing the carboxylate with either an acid or amide also resulted in the total loss of activity and due to its hydrophilic nature, loss of permeability was observed. In the next series, quinoline analogues were investigated, where any alterations to the 4-oxo observed total loss of activity. It is possible that the ability for the quinolones to undergo tautomerization is a necessary characteristic to have antimalarial activity. Finally, they investigated the 2-position by installing varying aryl groups. Alterations of analogue **25** at the 2-position diminished antimalarial activity; however, analogues of **24** observed different results. Installing an unsubstituted phenyl group decreased activity by approximately two-fold, while maintaining solubility and increasing permeability. *Ortho* substituted phenyl rings diminished any activity. *Para* substituted phenyl rings either decreased activity by four-fold or completely, in addition to significant decrease in aqueous solubility. *Meta* substituted rings observed the best potency with acceptable aqueous solubility and increased permeability (**Figure 13**) [56].

Findings from the initial SAR study prompted the Guy laboratory to further investigate 3-carboxy-4(1*H*)-quinolones. Various *meta* substituted phenyl rings were installed to the 2-position. Introduction of hydrophobic groups, such as methyl, vinyl, and phenyl, retained similar potency to **24**. Installation of alkoxy groups on the *meta* position displayed great improvement to the potency. Strong electron withdrawing groups, such as nitro, acetyl, and methyl sulfonyl, and H-bond donors

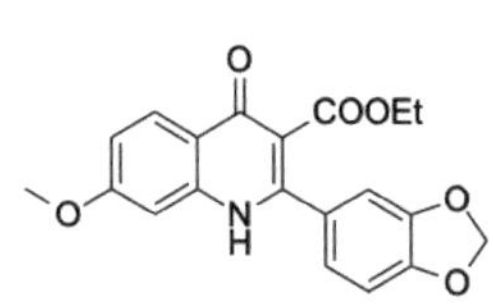

TDR42098 (**24**)
EC_{50} K1 (μM) = 0.25
EC_{50} 3D7 (μM) = 0.24
Solubility at 7.4 (μM) = >100

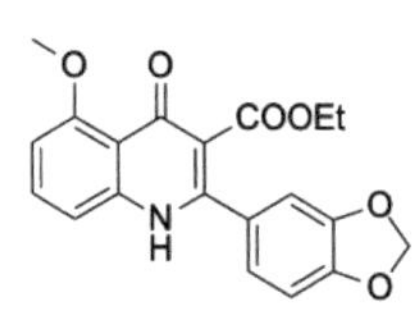

TDR17516 (**25**)
EC_{50} K1 (μM) = 3.01
EC_{50} 3D7 (μM) = 2.81
Solubility at 7.4 (μM) = >100

Figure 12.
TDR molecules identified as compounds with antimalarial activity.

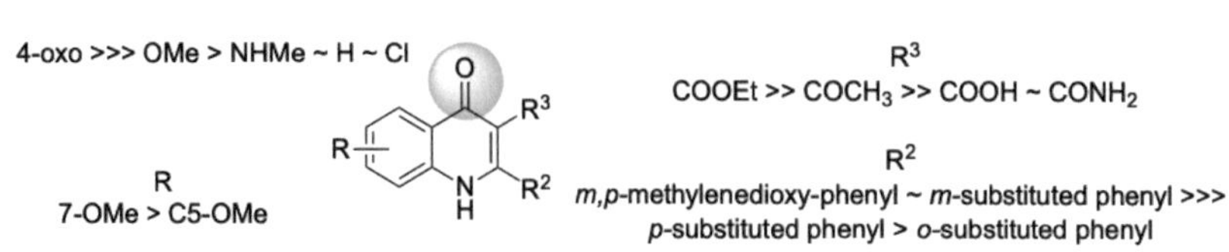

Figure 13.
Initial optimization of TDR molecules.

resulted in loss of activity. This suggests that hydrophobic electron-donating group on the *meta*-position of the phenyl group is most ideal; however, like other quinolones, increasing activity with hydrophobic substituents tends to decrease aqueous solubility and permeability – essential characteristics for oral bioavailability [57].

7-position was also investigated, where findings also displayed that small hydrophobic electron-donating group improves potency, while an electron withdrawing group diminishes the potency [57].

Multi-substituted benzenoid ring was investigated to observe if there are any synergistic effect of varying substituents. 5,7- and 6,7- dihalogenated compounds were inactive towards multidrug-resistant (MDR) strains. Similar results were observed from 6,7-dimethoxy analogues. Simultaneous incorporation of a methoxy and halo group was investigated, where it exhibited sub-micromolar to nanomolar activity when the halogen was on the 6 position and the methoxy was on the 7 position. When installing a methoxy group on the 6 position and the halogen on the 7 position, antimalarial activity against all strains were lost [57].

Finally, the carbonyl substituent on the 3-position was investigated. Varying chain lengths and incorporation of morpholinyl, pyrrolidinyl, and *N,N*-dimethyl amino functionalities were installed; however, these changes reduced potency without any increase in solubility of the compounds (**Figure 14**) [57].

13 compounds that had an appropriate balance amongst activity, solubility and permeability were selected by the Guy laboratory to test for microsomal activity. Compounds **26** and **27** displayed the most promising liver microsomal activity ($CL_{int,in\ vitro}$ < 4 uL/min/mg in human and mouse microsomes). These two compounds also displayed highest C_{max} and AUC, which is indicative of extensive systemic exposure after oral administration. This was observed in *in vivo* antimalarial activity assay, where these two compounds were the only compounds that suppressed parasite growth (**Figure 15**) [57].

2.2.5 Optimization of HDQ

Similar to the Guy laboratory, the O'Neill and Ward utilized a unique approach that led them to study quinolones to treat malaria. Originally, hydroxy-2-dodecyl-4(1*H*)-quinolone (HDQ, **28**) was known to be active against alternative NADH

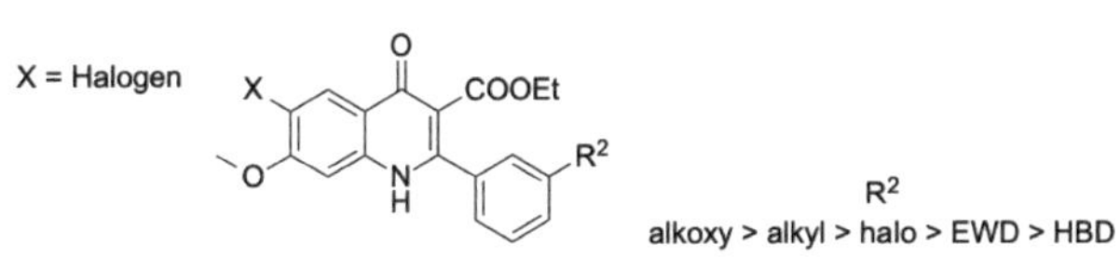

Figure 14.
Recent optimization of TDR molecule by the guy lab.

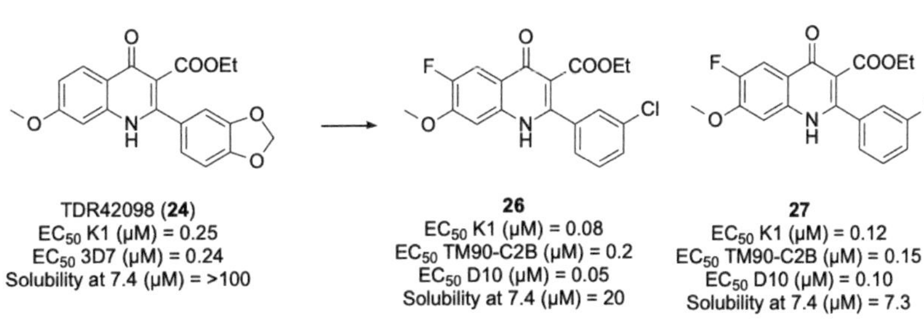

Figure 15.
Overall optimization of TDR molecule to frontrunner compounds.

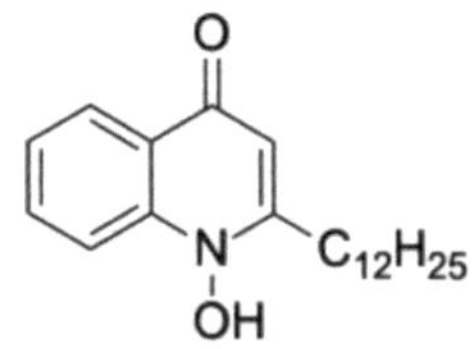

HDQ (**28**)

Figure 16.
Hydroxy-2-dodecyl-4(1H)-quinolone (HDQ).

dehydrogenase from the fungus *Yarrowia lipolytica* (**Figure 16**). In 2007, HDQ (**28**) exhibited nanomolar activity against *P. falciparum* and *T. gondii* [58]. This led O'Neill and Ward to perform various chemoinformatic methods (molecular fingerprinting, turbo similarity, principal component analysis, Bayesian modeling, and bioisosteric replacements) to select compounds for high-throughput screening. 17,000 compounds were selected from a commercial library of approximately 750,000 compounds from Biofocus DPI. Afterwards, these molecules were subjected to a sequential high-throughput screening method utilizing an *in vitro* assay against recombinant PfNDH2. This led to the selection of quinolone core as the main target chemotype for their SAR study [59–61].

Quinolones with 2-substituted monoaryl were selected as the template, as it contained a lipophilic side chain that was not metabolically labile like the aliphatic chain on HDQ (**28**) [59–61].

Initially, the quinolone core was modified. Installing a 8-aza-4(1*H*)-quinolone core reduced antimalarial activity. Similar to the previous optimization of various quinolones, chlorine and fluorine is well-tolerated, methoxy on the 7-position is well-tolerated, and large substituents on the benzenoid ring is not well tolerated. Interestingly, unsubstituted 3-position provides a slight increase in activity; however, this small advantage is outweighed by the decrease in solubility. Given that there is a large hydrophobic pocket at the active site, these researchers investigated 2-substituted biaryl quinolones. It became clear to the researchers that a monoaryl group could not obtain an IC_{50} of below 500 nM. Investigation of the biaryl began with modification of the linkers. Variations on linkers (*p*-CH_2, *m*-CH_2, and *p*-O) did not affect the activity of the compound, as they were all well-tolerated. The terminal substituent on the distal phenyl group is also dependent on the other substituents on the molecule. In general, OCF_3 is the optimal terminal group, while a large EWG was less tolerated. This led to the discovery of CK-2-68 (**29**). Due to poor solubility, the use of prodrug moiety and altering formulations provided a proof of concept that CK-2-68 (**29**) clears the parasites *in vivo* [59–62].

To improve solubility properties, heterocyclic substituents were introduced to the quinolone core. It was observed that the distal ring is most favorable as a phenyl ring; however, a pyridine ring for the replacement of the proximal aromatic ring demonstrates great potency, reduced ClogP, and improved solubility. However, even with the improved solubility, the *in vivo* testing had to utilize a prodrug moiety to establish a proof of concept that **30** does clear the parasites *in vivo* [60].

The most recent attempt to improve solubility was to utilize a bioisostere of benzene rings. Pyrazoles have been well-documented to improve solubility by reducing ClogP. The optimization of the other substituents follows their previous findings (**Figure 17**) [62].

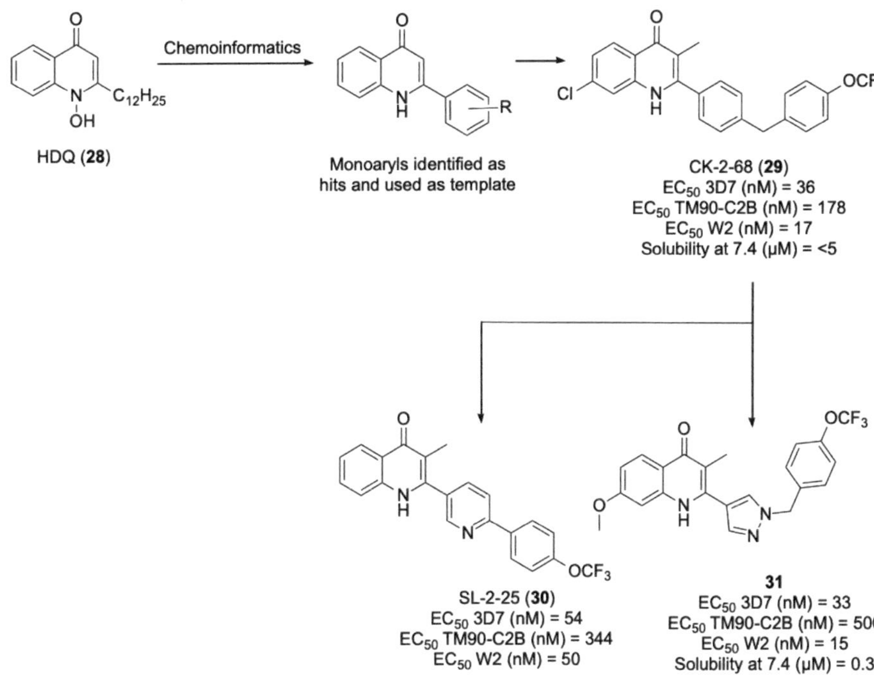

Figure 17.
Optimization of HDQ.

3. Conclusion

While malaria remains to be a global health threat, developing a novel class of drugs has become essential to treat and prevent the spread of this disease. 4(1*H*)-quinolones and 4(1*H*)-pyridones both display potential of developing into potent antimalarial agents due to recent re-evaluation of old 4(1*H*)-quinolones and 4(1*H*)-pyridones possessing antimalarial activity. These historical quinolones display promising activity against both erythrocytic and exo-erythrocytic stages of the parasite. Various research groups invested their efforts and resources to optimize these 4(1*H*)-pyridones or 4(1*H*)-quinolones since it is perfect for the malaria eradication initiative.

The frontrunner compound for 4(1*H*)-pyridone is **13**, which displayed single-digit nanomolar activity against the erythrocytic stage with excellent solubility. However, after entering first-time in human study, **13** displayed toxicity, which terminated the study.

Unlike 4(1*H*)-pyridones, 4(1*H*)-quinolones (P4Qs, ELQs, THAs, TDR analogues, and HDQ analogues) lack cytotoxicity. This is essential to develop a species-specific inhibitor. The frontrunner compounds for ELQ/P4Q are **22** and **23**, which displayed low nanomolar activity for both the erythrocytic and exo-erythrocytic stages. In addition to this, **22** and **23** displayed activity against the transmitting stages, making these molecules especially important. The frontrunner compounds for PEQ are **17**, **18**, and **32**, which displayed low nanomolar activity for both the erythrocytic and liver stages. Another molecule that is promising. The frontrunner compounds for THA are **15** and **16**, which displayed nanomolar activity for the erythrocytic stage. The frontrunner compound for TDR analogues are **26** and **27**, which displayed nanomolar activity for the erythrocytic stage. The frontrunner compound for HDQ analogues are **30** and **31**, which displayed nanomolar activity for the erythrocytic stage.

Since many research teams focus solely on the activity against the blood stage, compounds **22**, **23**, **17**, **18**, and **32** are especially promising, as these display exo-erythrocytic activity, along with the erythrocytic activity.

Nevertheless, one major downfall with the development of 4(1*H*)-quinolones and 4(1*H*)-pyridones is the poor aqueous solubility. This prevents proper development of pharmacokinetic profiles for drug candidacy; therefore, failed clinical development and development was halted in the early 80s.

Thankfully, by early 2000s, the field of medicinal chemistry advanced, where researchers could optimize historical quinolones to develop them into drug-like molecules. Even with the variety of chemotypes, the approach towards optimization is quite similar amongst the various research teams.

Despite these obstacles, 4(1*H*)-quinolones have a great potential of becoming the next class of antimalarials. These molecules lack toxicity and have acceptable physicochemical properties, aside from solubility. With increased understanding to improve aqueous solubility, it is recommended to continue research on antimalarial quinolones, as they have great potential of becoming orally bioavailable antimalarials.

Acknowledgements

We would like to thank Medicines for Malaria Venture and the National Institutes of Health for supporting our efforts in developing 4(1H)-quinolones with antimalarial activity. In particular, we are grateful for MMV awards 08/0068, 11/0022 and 16/00421 and NIH awards GM097118 and AI144464.

Conflict of interest

The authors declare no conflict of interest.

Author details

Ami H. Asakawa and Roman Manetsch*
Department of Pharmaceutical Sciences, Northeastern University, Boston, MA, USA

*Address all correspondence to: r.manetsch@northeastern.edu

References

[1] *World Malaria Report 2020*. World Health Organization.

[2] *World Malaria Report 2009*. World Health Organization.

[3] Phillips MA, Burrows JN, Manyando C, et al. Malaria. *Nature Reviews Disease Primers* 2017; 3: 17050.

[4] Cowman AF, Healer J, Marapana D, et al. Malaria: Biology and Disease. *Cell* 2016; 167: 610-624.

[5] Frevert U. Sneaking in through the back entrance: the biology of malaria liver stages. *Trends in Parasitology* 2004; 20: 417-424.

[6] Siciliano G, Alano P. Enlightening the malaria parasite life cycle: bioluminescent Plasmodium in fundamental and applied research. *Front Microbiol*; 6. Epub ahead of print 2015. DOI: 10.3389/fmicb.2015.00391.

[7] Mueller I, Galinski MR, Baird JK, et al. Key gaps in the knowledge of *Plasmodium vivax*, a neglected human malaria parasite. *The Lancet Infectious Diseases* 2009; 9: 555-566.

[8] *World Malaria Report 2019*. World Health Organization.

[9] Sevene E, González R, Menéndez C. Current knowledge and challenges of antimalarial drugs for treatment and prevention in pregnancy. *Expert Opinion on Pharmacotherapy* 2010; 11: 1277-1293.

[10] Kumar S, Bhardwaj TR, Prasad DN, et al. Drug targets for resistant malaria: Historic to future perspectives. *Biomedicine & Pharmacotherapy* 2018; 104: 8-27.

[11] Teixeira C, Vale N, Pérez B, et al. "Recycling" Classical Drugs for Malaria. *Chem Rev* 2014; 114: 11164-11220.

[12] Achan J, Talisuna AO, Erhart A, et al. Quinine, an old anti-malarial drug in a modern world: role in the treatment of malaria. *Malaria Journal* 2011; 10: 144.

[13] Parhizgar AR, Tahghighi A. Introducing New Antimalarial Analogues of Chloroquine and Amodiaquine: A Narrative Review. *Iran J Med Sci* 2016; 42: 115-128.

[14] Schlagenhauf P, Adamcova M, Regep L, et al. The position of mefloquine as a 21st century malaria chemoprophylaxis. *Malaria Journal* 2010; 9: 357.

[15] Schlitzer M. Malaria Chemotherapeutics Part I: History of Antimalarial Drug Development, Currently Used Therapeutics, and Drugs in Clinical Development. *ChemMedChem* 2007; 2: 944-986.

[16] Jensen M, Mehlhorn H. Seventy-five years of Resochin® in the fight against malaria. *Parasitology Research* 2009; 105: 609.

[17] Ashley EA, Recht J, White NJ. Primaquine: the risks and the benefits. *Malaria Journal* 2014; 13: 418.

[18] White NJ. Antimalarial drug resistance. *J Clin Invest* 2004; 113: 1084-1092.

[19] Anderson RM, White N. Antimalarial drug resistance and combination chemotherapy. *Philosophical Transactions of the Royal Society of London Series B: Biological Sciences* 1999; 354: 739-749.

[20] Phyo AP, Nkhoma S, Stepniewska K, et al. Emergence of artemisinin-resistant malaria on the western border of Thailand: a longitudinal study. *The Lancet* 2012; 379: 1960-1966.

[21] White NJ. Qinghaosu (Artemisinin): The Price of Success. *Science* 2008; 320: 330.

[22] Baird JK. Effectiveness of Antimalarial Drugs. *N Engl J Med* 2005; 352: 1565-1577.

[23] Burrows JN, Hooft van Huijsduijnen R, Möhrle JJ, et al. Designing the next generation of medicines for malaria control and eradication. *Malaria Journal* 2013; 12: 187.

[24] Burrows JN, Duparc S, Gutteridge WE, et al. New developments in anti-malarial target candidate and product profiles. *Malaria Journal* 2017; 16: 26.

[25] Bueno JM, Herreros E, Angulo-Barturen I, et al. Exploration of 4(1H)-pyridones as a novel family of potent antimalarial inhibitors of the plasmodial cytochrome bc1. *Future Medicinal Chemistry* 2012; 4: 2311-2323.

[26] Monastyrskyi A, Dennis K, Manetsch R. 4(1H)-Pyridone and 4(1H)-Quinolone Derivatives as Antimalarials with Erythrocytic, Exoerythrocytic, and Transmission Blocking Activities. *Current Topics in Medicinal Chemistry* 2014; 14: 1693-1705.

[27] Lipinski CA, Lombardo F, Dominy BW, et al. Experimental and computational approaches to estimate solubility and permeability in drug discovery and development settings1PII of original article: S0169-409X(96)00423-1. The article was originally published in Advanced Drug Delivery Reviews 23 (1997) 3-25.1. *Advanced Drug Delivery Reviews* 2001; 46: 3-26.

[28] Veber DF, Johnson SR, Cheng H-Y, et al. Molecular Properties That Influence the Oral Bioavailability of Drug Candidates. *J Med Chem* 2002; 45: 2615-2623.

[29] Lovering F, Bikker J, Humblet C. Escape from Flatland: Increasing Saturation as an Approach to Improving Clinical Success. *J Med Chem* 2009; 52: 6752-6756.

[30] Markley LD, Van Heertum JC, Doorenbos HE. Antimalarial activity of clopidol, 3,5-dichloro-2,6-dimethyl-4-pyridinol, and its esters, carbonates, and sulfonates. *J Med Chem* 1972; 15: 1188-1189.

[31] Fry M, Williams RB. Effects of decoquinate and clopidol on electron transport in mitochondria of Eimeria tenella (Apicomplexa: coccidia). *Biochemical Pharmacology* 1984; 33: 229-240.

[32] Yeates CL, Batchelor JF, Capon EC, et al. Synthesis and Structure–Activity Relationships of 4-Pyridones as Potential Antimalarials. *J Med Chem* 2008; 51: 2845-2852.

[33] Bueno JM, Manzano P, García MC, et al. Potent antimalarial 4-pyridones with improved physico-chemical properties. *Bioorganic & Medicinal Chemistry Letters* 2011; 21: 5214-5218.

[34] Bueno JM, Calderon F, Chicharro J, et al. Synthesis and Structure–Activity Relationships of the Novel Antimalarials 5-Pyridinyl-4(1H)-Pyridones. *J Med Chem* 2018; 61: 3422-3435.

[35] Corey VC, Lukens AK, Istvan ES, et al. A broad analysis of resistance development in the malaria parasite. *Nat Commun* 2016; 7: 11901-11901.

[36] Schmidt LH. Antimalarial Properties of Floxacrine, a Dihydroacridinedione Derivative. *Antimicrob Agents Chemother* 1979; 16: 475.

[37] Dorn A, Scovill JP, Ellis WY, et al. Short report: floxacrine analog WR 243251 inhibits hematin polymerization.

The American Journal of Tropical Medicine and Hygiene 2001; 65: 19-20.

[38] Suswam E, Kyle D, Lang-Unnasch N. Plasmodium falciparum: The Effects of Atovaquone Resistance on Respiration. *Experimental Parasitology* 2001; 98: 180-187.

[39] Cross RM, Maignan JR, Mutka TS, et al. Optimization of 1,2,3,4-Tetrahydroacridin-9(10H)-ones as Antimalarials Utilizing Structure–Activity and Structure–Property Relationships. *J Med Chem* 2011; 54: 4399-4426.

[40] Puri SK, Dutta GP. Quinoline esters as potential antimalarial drugs: effect on relapses of *Plasmodium cynomolgi* infections in monkeys. *Transactions of The Royal Society of Tropical Medicine and Hygiene* 1990; 84: 759-760.

[41] Ryley JF, Peters W. The antimalarial activity of some quinolone esters. *Annals of Tropical Medicine & Parasitology* 1970; 64: 209-222.

[42] Cross RM, Namelikonda NK, Mutka TS, et al. Synthesis, Antimalarial Activity, and Structure–Activity Relationship of 7-(2-Phenoxyethoxy)-4(1H)-quinolones. *J Med Chem* 2011; 54: 8321-8327.

[43] Maignan JR, Lichorowic CL, Giarrusso J, et al. ICI 56,780 Optimization: Structure–Activity Relationship Studies of 7-(2-Phenoxyethoxy)-4(1H)-quinolones with Antimalarial Activity. *J Med Chem* 2016; 59: 6943-6960.

[44] Neelarapu R, Maignan JR, Lichorowic CL, et al. Design and Synthesis of Orally Bioavailable Piperazine Substituted 4(1H)-Quinolones with Potent Antimalarial Activity: Structure–Activity and Structure–Property Relationship Studies. *J Med Chem* 2018; 61: 1450-1473.

[45] Winter R, Kelly JX, Smilkstein MJ, et al. Optimization of endochin-like quinolones for antimalarial activity. *Experimental Parasitology* 2011; 127: 545-551.

[46] Kikuth W, Mudrow-Reichenow L. Über kausalprophylaktisch bei Vogelmalaria wirksame Substanzen. *Zeitschrift für Hygiene und Infektionskrankheiten* 1947; 127: 151-165.

[47] Cross RM, Monastyrskyi A, Mutka TS, et al. Endochin Optimization: Structure−Activity and Structure−Property Relationship Studies of 3-Substituted 2-Methyl-4(1H)-quinolones with Antimalarial Activity. *J Med Chem* 2010; 53: 7076-7094.

[48] LaCrue AN, Sáenz FE, Cross RM, et al. 4(1H)-Quinolones with Liver Stage Activity against Plasmodium berghei. *Antimicrob Agents Chemother* 2013; 57: 417.

[49] Winter R, Kelly JX, Smilkstein MJ, et al. Optimization of endochin-like quinolones for antimalarial activity. *Experimental Parasitology* 2011; 127: 545-551.

[50] Cross RM, Monastyrskyi A, Mutka TS, et al. Endochin Optimization: Structure−Activity and Structure−Property Relationship Studies of 3-Substituted 2-Methyl-4(1H)-quinolones with Antimalarial Activity. *J Med Chem* 2010; 53: 7076-7094.

[51] Cross RM, Flanigan DL, Monastyrskyi A, et al. Orally Bioavailable 6-Chloro-7-methoxy-4(1H)-quinolones Efficacious against Multiple Stages of Plasmodium. *J Med Chem* 2014; 57: 8860-8879.

[52] Nilsen A, LaCrue AN, White KL, et al. Quinolone-3-Diarylethers: A New Class of Antimalarial Drug. *Science Translational Medicine* 2013; 5: 177ra37.

[53] Nilsen A, Miley GP, Forquer IP, et al. Discovery, Synthesis, and Optimization of Antimalarial 4(1H)-Quinolone-3-Diarylethers. *J Med Chem* 2014; 57: 3818-3834.

[54] Miley GP, Pou S, Winter R, et al. ELQ-300 Prodrugs for Enhanced Delivery and Single-Dose Cure of Malaria. *Antimicrob Agents Chemother* 2015; 59: 5555.

[55] Nwaka S, Ramirez B, Brun R, et al. Advancing Drug Innovation for Neglected Diseases—Criteria for Lead Progression. *PLOS Neglected Tropical Diseases* 2009; 3: e440.

[56] Zhang Y, Guiguemde WA, Sigal M, et al. Synthesis and structure–activity relationships of antimalarial 4-oxo-3-carboxyl quinolones. *Bioorganic & Medicinal Chemistry* 2010; 18: 2756-2766.

[57] Zhang Y, Clark JA, Connelly MC, et al. Lead Optimization of 3-Carboxyl-4(1H)-Quinolones to Deliver Orally Bioavailable Antimalarials. *J Med Chem* 2012; 55: 4205-4219.

[58] Saleh A, Friesen J, Baumeister S, et al. Growth Inhibition of Toxoplasma gondii and *Plasmodium falciparum* by Nanomolar Concentrations of 1-Hydroxy-2-Dodecyl-4(1H)Quinolone, a High-Affinity Inhibitor of Alternative (Type II) NADH Dehydrogenases. *Antimicrob Agents Chemother* 2007; 51: 1217.

[59] Pidathala C, Amewu R, Pacorel B, et al. Identification, Design and Biological Evaluation of Bisaryl Quinolones Targeting *Plasmodium falciparum* Type II NADH:Quinone Oxidoreductase (PfNDH2). *J Med Chem* 2012; 55: 1831-1843.

[60] Leung SC, Gibbons P, Amewu R, et al. Identification, Design and Biological Evaluation of Heterocyclic Quinolones Targeting *Plasmodium falciparum* Type II NADH:Quinone Oxidoreductase (PfNDH2). *J Med Chem* 2012; 55: 1844-1857.

[61] Nixon GL, Pidathala C, Shone AE, et al. Targeting the mitochondrial electron transport chain of *Plasmodium falciparum*: new strategies towards the development of improved antimalarials for the elimination era. *Future Medicinal Chemistry* 2013; 5: 1573-1591.

[62] David Hong W, Leung SC, Amporndanai K, et al. Potent Antimalarial 2-Pyrazolyl Quinolone bc1 (Qi) Inhibitors with Improved Drug-like Properties. *ACS Med Chem Lett* 2018; 9: 1205-1210.

Chapter 11

Stable Artesunate Resistance in A Humanized Mouse Model of *Plasmodium falciparum*

Sheetal Saini, Rajinder Kumar and Rajeev K. Tyagi

Abstract

Plasmodium falciparum, the most devastating human malaria parasite, confers higher morbidity and mortality. Although efforts have been made to develop an effective malaria vaccine, stage- and species-specific short-lived immunity crippled these efforts. Hence, antimalarial drug treatment becomes a mainstay for the treatment of malaria infection in the wake of the unavailability of an effective vaccine. Further, there has been a wide array of antimalarial drugs effective against various developmental stages of *P. falciparum* due to their different structures, modes of action, and pharmacodynamics as well as pharmacokinetics. The development of resistance against almost all frontline drugs by *P. falciparum* indicates the need for combination therapy (artemisinin-based combination therapy; ACT) to treat patients with *P. falciparum*. A higher pool of parasitemia under discontinuous *in vivo* artemisinin drug pressure in a developed humanized mouse allows the selection of artesunate resistant (ART-R) *P. falciparum*. Intravenously administered artesunate, using either single flash doses or a 2-day regimen, to the *P. falciparum*-infected human blood chimeric NOD/SCID.IL-2R$\gamma^{-/-}$ immunocompromised (NSG) mice, with progressive dose increments upon parasite recovery, was the strategy deployed to select resistant parasites. Parasite susceptibility to artemisinins and other antimalarial compounds was characterized *in vitro* and *in vivo*. *P. falciparum* has shown to evolve extreme artemisinin resistance as well as co-resistance to antimalarial drugs. Overall, the present information shall be very useful in devising newer therapeutic strategies to treat human malaria infection.

Keywords: artemisinin, artesunate resistance, co-resistance, *Plasmodium falciparum*, humanized mouse model

1. Introduction

1.1 Malaria biology

Malaria is a leading parasitic disease caused by protozoans belonging to the genus *Plasmodium* (*P.*) when injected by the female mosquito (*Anopheles*) in humans during a blood meal. Out of 172 species of *Plasmodium* parasite, only five species are reportedly known to cause malaria infection: *Plasmodium falciparum*, *Plasmodium malariae*, *Plasmodium vivex*, *Plasmodium ovale*, and *Plasmodium knowlesi*. The parasite completes its sexual and asexual cycles in a very complicated manner [1]. *Plasmodium* gametocytes are taken up during the blood meal from the human host and travel through salivary glands to the gut of *Anopheles* and continue the sexual multiplication. The haploid male and female gametes fertilize and give rise to zygote in the gut, which further grows and elongates into the ookinetes. Ookinetes following several replication processes become oocyst that transforms into sporozoites [2]. These sporozoites move from the gut to salivary glands and are released by the mosquitoes into the human bloodstream during a blood meal.

Once sporozoites are released in the bloodstream, the asexual development stage gets started [3]. Sporozoites traverse to their first incubation site, that is, hepatocytes (pre-erythrocytic stage), and later continues the asexual blood-stage infection inside red blood cells (RBCs). The asexual blood-stage infection results in clinical manifestations of the disease. Some sporozoites reach the liver within a few hours and penetrate the hepatocyte and undergo asexual replication known as exo-erythrocytic schizogony. Each sporozoite develops into a schizont containing 18–26 merozoites. The entire pre-erythrocytic phase lasts about 5–16 days depending upon the parasite species. RBCs are "center stage" and host the asexual development of *Plasmodium*. The merozoites (infective form) released from the liver recognize, attach, and enter the RBCs quickly. Merozoite passes through a developmental transformation beginning with a characteristic ring stage and leading to the formation of a multinucleated schizont within RBCs. Mature schizont ruptures to release the merozoites and continues the multiplication in RBCs. Each mature schizont contains around 18–26 merozoites, and these are released following the lysis of RBC to invade fresh RBCs. It is the lysis of RBCs that induces the bouts of fever and anemia in the infected individual, whereas, in *P. vivax* and *P. ovale* infection, a few merozoites remain in dormant stages for four months or year causing malaria relapse [4].

1.2 Malaria vaccine

Globally, malaria is one of the leading causes of mortality (0.3–2.3%), and Africa and Asia are highly endemic regions among the other continents [5]. According to World Health Organization, approximately 299 million cases of malaria and 400,000 deaths have been reported worldwide in 2019 [6]. A variety of antimalarial drugs are available but the emergence of resistance has been a major setback in containing malaria infection. Currently, Mosquirix (RTS,S/AS01) developed by GlaxoSmithKline is the only vaccine available in the market against malaria. RTS,S/AS01 is an engineered vaccine comprising of the genes from the outer protein of *P. falciparum* circumsporozoites and a portion of a hepatitis B surface antigen with chemical adjuvant to boost the immune responses. Mosquirix reduced malaria cases in children to nearly half [7] and has had 40% efficacy in children receiving four vaccine doses [8]. However, the efficacy dropped to 26% in children receiving only three vaccine doses and 33% efficacy was observed during the first year in infants (up to 3 months old). Further, the effectiveness of Mosquirix is only for one year and failed to provide long-term protection but could be combined with chemotherapy to prevent the transmission of malaria in low-endemic regions [9].

A variety of vaccines focusing on irradiated sporozoites is under trial, which may give exposure to the array of antigens and help induce protective immunity against malaria [1].

1.3 Drug-based therapy

Antimalarial drugs are the most commonly used treatment option for malaria in tropical regions. Three types of antimalarial drugs are currently available *viz.* aryl amino alcohol compounds (quinine, lumefantrine, chloroquine, amodiaquine, mefloquine, etc.), antifolate compounds (pyrimethamine and sulfadoxine), and artemisinin and derivatives [10]. *Plasmodium* parasites have a complex life cycle that involves a mammalian and an invertebrate host. All the symptoms are caused by the repeated rupture and penetration of erythrocytes by the asexual blood-stage parasites (merozoites). Hence, most of the antimalarial drugs target the asexual erythrocytic stage of the parasite. As per WHO's Model List of Essential Medicines (MLEM), currently, there are 14 curative drugs for the treatment of malaria (treatment postinfection) and 6 prophylactic medicines (treatment before infection), either single or in combination [11]. Curative drugs for *P. falciparum* are mostly artemisinin-based combinations with artemisinin derivative (short half-life) in combination with partner drug(s) with a different mechanism of action (longer half-life). Out of 14 curative drugs, chloroquine is used for *P. vivax*, primaquine is used for *P. vivax* and *P. ovale* both, and the rest 12 are used for treating *P. falciparum* malaria.

1.3.1 Quinine

First isolated from the bark of the cinchona tree in 1820, and it remained one of the most effective malaria treatment options till the early 2000s [12]. Even today, quinine is obtained entirely from its natural source due to its difficult synthesis of the active molecule. Resistance for quinine was first reported in the 1980s, and since 2006, not being used as a frontline antimalarial drug [12]. However, the drug is still present on the WHO's list of essential medicines and is used wherever artemisinins are not available [11]. Quinine has blood schizonticidal and gametocytocidal activity against *P. vivax* and *P. malariae*. Quinine also inhibits heme polymerase activity (required to convert toxic heme into nontoxic hemazoin) and, hence, leads to the accumulation of heme (cytotoxic substrate) in parasites.

1.3.2 Chloroquine

It was used to treat all forms of malaria infections with fewer side effects in the 1940s [13]. Blood stage of *P. vivax*, *P. ovale,* and *P. malariae*, sensitive strains of *P. falciparum*, and gametocytes of *P. vivax* are sensitive to chloroquine. It is highly effective in controlling acute malaria infection as compared to quinine. Moreover, it has been efficient and safer to use to treat sensitive cases. The first resistance case was reported in the 1950s and by the time, many malaria parasites have developed resistance against chloroquine. As per MLEM, chloroquine is used as a curative and prophylactic drug against *P. vivax* in the regions where resistance is not known to evolve (Central American regions) [11].

1.3.3 Amodiaquine

It was first synthesized in 1948 [14] and used in combination with artesunate for treating uncomplicated *P. falciparum* malaria (Camoquine® or Coarsucam™) [15]. The mechanism of action of amodiaquine is similar to that of chloroquine involving inhibition of hemozoin formation [16].

1.3.4 Pyrimethamine and sulfadoxine

In the early 1950s, Elion G and Hitchings G developed pyrimethamine [17] and Elion, Hitchings, and Black won the joint Nobel Prize in Physiology or Medicine (1988) for "their discoveries of important principles for drug treatment." Sulfadoxine was developed in the early 1960s [18] and in 1981, the pyrimethamine and sulfadoxine combination was approved for the treatment of malaria. The emergence of high levels of resistance against the combination of pyrimethamine and sulfadoxine led to its discontinuation as a prophylactic drug since both drugs inhibit the parasite's folate biosynthesis pathway (dihydrofolate reductase, DHFR and dihydropteroate synthetase, respectively) [19].

1.3.5 Primaquine

Primaquine, an 8-aminoquinoline, was first used in early 1950s. 8-aminoquinolines eliminates mature *P. falciparum* gametocytes, exo-erythrocytic (hepatic) stage of all *Plasmodium* species, and prevents the relapse cases of *P. vivax* and *P. ovale* showing suboptimal blood-stage activity. Despite its remarkable antimalarial properties, primaquine is reportedly known to confer severe side effects [20].

1.3.6 Piperaquine

It was developed as a part of the Chinese National Malaria Elimination Programme in the 1960s [21]. Although China used this drug as a replacement for chloroquine, the emergence of resistance against piperaquine prohibited its use as monotherapy. Currently, this is used with a partner drug with DHA (Eurartesim®) as a combination therapy [22]. It binds to heme-containing species by blocking heme detoxification and acts through getting accumulated in the digestive vacuole [14].

1.3.7 Doxycycline

In the early 1960s, Pfizer Inc. (USA) invented doxycyclin, a synthetically derived broad-spectrum bacteriostatic agent from *Streptomyces* sp. Doxycyclin is an efficacious prophylactic drug and, in combination with a partner drug, is highly effective as a curative drug for *Plasmodium* infection. Doxycycline is particularly used as a preventive drug in the regions with chloroquine and multidrug-resistant (MDR) *P. falciparum* malaria. It is not recommended for pregnant women and children below 8 years of age, but adverse effects were scarcely reported [23].

1.3.8 Mefloquine

American Army developed mefloquine in the 1970s [24] and is still part of the MLEM. Initially introduced for the treatment of chloroquine-resistant malaria, mefloquine has been used as a curative (in combination with artesunate) and prophylactic drug. In the late 1980s, resistance cases were reported for mefloquine [25]. Further, antimalarial action is mediated by disrupting the hemoglobin digestion in the asexual erythrocytic stage of the parasite [14]. The rendered adverse effects on the central nervous system prohibited its use as an antimalarial drug [26].

1.3.9 Artemisinin and its derivatives

Tu Youyou first isolated artemisinin in 1971, from a traditional Chinese medicine plant *Artemisia annua* [27], and was conferred Nobel Prize (2015) in Physiology or Medicine for "her discoveries concerning a novel therapy against malaria." Artemisinin and its derivatives (artemether, artesunate, and arteether) are metabolized to its active compound DHA and are effective against all MDR forms of *P. falciparum*. Artemisinins acts in multiple ways including the generation of free radicals after being activated by heme, which, in turn, destroys proteins essentially required for the parasite growth and development [28]. Additionally, its action is associated with upregulation of unfolded protein response (UPR) pathways [29] and downregulation of *P. falciparum* phosphatidylinositol-3-kinase (PfPI3K) [30] and Ca2+ transporter (PfATP6) [31]. Artemisinins are crucial to fight the battle against malaria with artemisinin combination therapy (ACT) accounting for the majority of current antimalarial treatments [22], and in the late 2000s, emerging artemisinin resistance was noticed in Southeast (SE) Asia [5, 32].

1.3.10 Lumefantrine

Chinese antimalarial research effort "Project 523" that led to the discovery of artemisinin also synthesized lumefantrine in 1976 [33]. Currently, lumefantrine is used in combination with artemether. Lumefantrine is known to inhibit the transcriptional and translational pathway of malaria parasites [16].

2. Artemisinin resistance

One of the greatest challenges in achieving malaria control is antimalarial drug resistance (**Figure 1**). It has been associated with the malaria dissemination to new areas and resurgence in areas where the disease had been eliminated from. The situation is worsened by the incomplete treatments as it puts massive drug selection pressure on *P. falciparum* parasites, and hence, it helps evolve resistance against all frontline drugs. Chloroquine resistance leads to the resurgence and spread of malaria for decades in most countries in the 1960s [34]. Pyrimethamine, amodiaquine (chloroquine analog), arylaminoalcohols mefloquine, and halofantrine too suffered reduced efficacy in the 1980s, spreading resistant parasites. WHO recommended the combined use of two or more compounds with different modes of action to provide necessary cure rates and delay the development and spread of resistance. With low mixed-strain transmission rates, Southeast (SE) Asia was historically the first region to show resistance to frontline drugs [32]. Resistance to chloroquine, mefloquine, and sulfadoxine-pyrimethamine was initially seen in SE Asia [35, 36]. Artemisinin-based combination therapies (ACTs) have been seen as effective in controlling malaria. ACTs were a first-line treatment option for malaria since the early 2000s and were quickly adopted worldwide [34].

The mechanism of action of most antimalarials depends on targeting a single pathway/molecule, for example, DHFR-mediated folate synthesis (sulfadoxine-pyrimethamine), cytochrome bc1 (atovaquone), and heme detoxification (chloroquine). The artemisinin(s) binds to an array of parasite proteins and influences multiple cellular processes including glycolysis, translational pathway, and cell cycle regulation [37–40]. Some studies also suggest that artemisinin may target and depolarize the mitochondrial membrane potential [41, 42]. Due to these functional

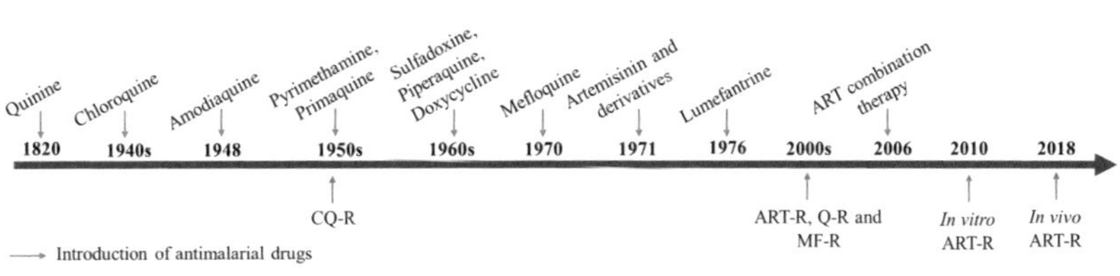

Figure 1.
Timeline for the introduction of antimalarial drugs and emergence of resistance. Image illustrates the approximate timeline for the discovery of antimalarial drugs and evolution of resistance. In vitro and in vivo (huRBCs-reconstituted human blood chimeric/humanized mice) induction of artsunare resistance in laboratory strains of P. falciparum *to confirm the emergence of resistance. CQ-R, chloroquine resistance; ART-R, artemisinin resistance; Q-R, quinine resistance; MF-R, mefloquine resistance.*

attributes, artemisinin eliminates the asexual blood stage and early sexual gametocyte forms of *P. falciparum* parasites at low concentrations (nM) regardless of its short half-life (<1 h). To overcome the half-life issue, artemisinin and its derivatives (artemether, artesunate, and dihydroartemisinin; DHA) are used in combination with a drug of longer half-life. In Southeast Asia (SE), primary artemisinin derivative combinations used are artesunate with mefloquine and DHA with piperaquine, whereas in Africa artemether with lumefantrine and artesunate and amodiaquine. In the late 2000s, emerging artemisinin resistance was noticed in SE Asia [5, 32] and the most problematic situation currently is the rapid increase in failure rates of DHA used in combination with piperaquine. Later have been the first-line treatment and the preferred ACT in most of the SE Asia [43, 44]. Artemisinin resistance enchants potential pressure on partner drugs to work quickly and effectively in case of efficacy failure of artemisinin. *P. falciparum* Kelch 13 (Pf-Kelch13) (located on chromosome 13) is shown to be primarily responsible for artemisinin resistance. Kelch13 protein is involved in intraerythrocytic parasite development and many other cellular processes including hemoglobin endocytosis responsible for parasite growth and antimalarial activity of artemisinin. K13 mutations in parasites mediate artemisinin resistance through the reduced killing potential of artemisinin drugs. Moreover, mutations in K13 drive the enhanced removal of damaged proteins by the parasite [45].

Triple artemisinin-based combination therapies (TACTs) and mass drug administration (MDA) are proposed to combat artemisinin resistance [46, 47]. Combining more than two drugs with different modes of action prevents the chances of multidrug resistance and its spread. MDA targets the asymptomatic malaria receptacles that may serve as hotbeds for the transmission and perseverance of resistant parasites. TACT efficacy is currently in the second phase; with underway Tracking Resistance to Artemisinin Collaboration II (TRAC II) multiple-site study. DHA, piperaquine and mefloquine, and artemether and lumefantrine along with amodiaquine combinations have shown promising results and might help to defer the evolution of artemisinin resistance. Moreover, TACTs might reinstate the artemisinin sensitivity in the areas prevalent for artemisinin resistance [48].

2.1 Experimental induction of artesunate resistance *in vitro* and *in vivo* (human RBCs-reconstituted NSG mice [humanized mice])

Various studies have been performed to understand artemisinin (ACT) resistance being evolved in laboratory strains of *P. falciparum in vitro* and in human blood chimeric mice. Human studies suggest single-dose artemisinin-induced dormant parasites in *P. falciparum* 3D7 or K13-infected strains of *P. falciparum*-infected patients. These parasites are most likely a reservoir for recrudescent infection following artemisinin mono- and combination therapy (ACT). Artemisinin-resistant *P. falciparum* may be experimentally selected following different regimens *in vitro*. The selected resistant parasites could employ different mechanism(s) of action to escape drug pressure for extended survival. Witkowski et al. [49] submitted laboratory *P. falciparum* (F32-Tanzania) to artemisinin pressure for over 3 years/100 cycles to select artemisinin-resistant parasites. These artemisinin-resistant parasite could survive up to 7000× of the initial IC50 of artemisinin (~10 nM) with unaltered chemosensitivity. Further, under high artemisinin pressure, parasites were arrested at the ring stage and re-gained their sensitive phenotype when drug pressure was removed. This unstable resistance phenotype questions the experimental generation of resistant phenotype [49]. Chavchich et al. [50] findings directly associated the development of resistance against artemisinin derivatives in *P. falciparum* strains (W2 and TM91C235) with the pfmdr1 gene and protein expression. However, there were no changes seen in these markers when D6 parasites were submitted to a similar drug pressure [50]. These findings were attested by Tucker et al. [51]. After continuous exposure of DHA for 1–2 months (320 nM maximum), Cui et al. were able to generate DHA-resistant *P. falciparum* strains 7G8, Dd2, HB3, and D10 but 3D7. DHA resistance was not seen limited to the ring stage but also occurred in trophozoites and schizonts like artemisinin [52]. Rocamora et al. [53] generated artemisinin-resistant *P. falciparum* parasite lines from 6A and 11C clones of the 3D7 strain of *P. falciparum*. Resistant clones displayed a significant decrease in artemisinin sensitivity within 1.5 months of selection and showed the enhanced cellular response against oxidative stress (antioxidant defense) and protein damage (unfolded protein response; UPR) [53]. Major pathways associated with UPR against artemisinin resistance are reported to be *Plasmodium* reactive oxidative stress complex (PROSC) and TCP-1 ring complex (TRiC) [29].

Rodrigues et al. [54] generated artesunate- and mefloquine-resistant *P. chabaudi* parasite in Balb/c mice and confirmed that resistance could be generated against combination drugs even when both drugs are administered simultaneously [54]. Maslachah et al. used *P. berghei* ANKA-infected Swiss mice and observed repeated passages of artemisinin-treated parasites in mice increased the effective dose of artemisinin from 50% to 90% with the reduced parasite clearance time and recrudescence time. Additionally, repeatedly artemisinin exposed parasites showed dormancy and vacuole formation [55]. Humans share >85% similarity with murines, but for the complexity of the cellular system and specificity of the human immune system, *in vivo* mouse models are far close to an ideal model for studying human malaria parasites. Rodent parasites are used as surrogates for human parasites, but the genetic differences between rodent and human parasites make it difficult to correlate with human studies. Human pathogens, which do not infect other animal species, require an animal model that could reconstitute or replicate the human immune system [56]. Fortunately, the mouse-human chimeric animals present a viable preclinical *in vivo* model to study the interaction of the human immune system with infectious agents. Immunodeficient mice engrafted with human RBCs (humanized mice) support the development of asexual blood-stage infection of *P. falciparum* [57, 58]. Artesunate-resistant (ART-R) *P. falciparum* (Uganada, Palo Alto Marburg) was experimentally selected by submitting discontinuous artesunate pressure on *P. falciparum*-infected humanized NOD/SCID IL-2R$\gamma^{-/-}$ immunocompromised mice reconstituted with human erythrocytes (huRBC). This humanized animal model supported the incremental increase in artesunate dosage to select 100 times ART-R parasites (240 mg/kg) to that of clinical dose (2.4 mg/kg). ART-R phenotype exhibited two patterns of IC50 in the selected parasites *in vivo*. Further, the first-stage phenotype showed substantial resistance to artemisinin *in vivo* (400×) without a shift seen in IC50, and the second-stage resistance phenotype showed an absence of response to a very high artemisinin dose (3200×) with a shift in IC50 and co-resistance to quinine, halofantrine, and amodiaquine. This phenotype was further demonstrated as having high-grade and stable artemisinin resistance phenotype. This is the first report of its kind [59], wherein a humanized mouse model was developed and a stable ART-R phenotype was achieved. Moreover, mimicking the clinical double doe regime (for consecutive two days and 24 h apart), 41% survival was observed with the highest dose of artemisinin (80 mg/kg) in contrast to 80% survival in the single-dose protocol (240 mg/kg) (**Figure 2**) [59]. There have been humanized mouse models to study asexual blood and liver stage infection of *P. falciparum* [57, 58, 60–62] and *P. vivax* [63, 64].

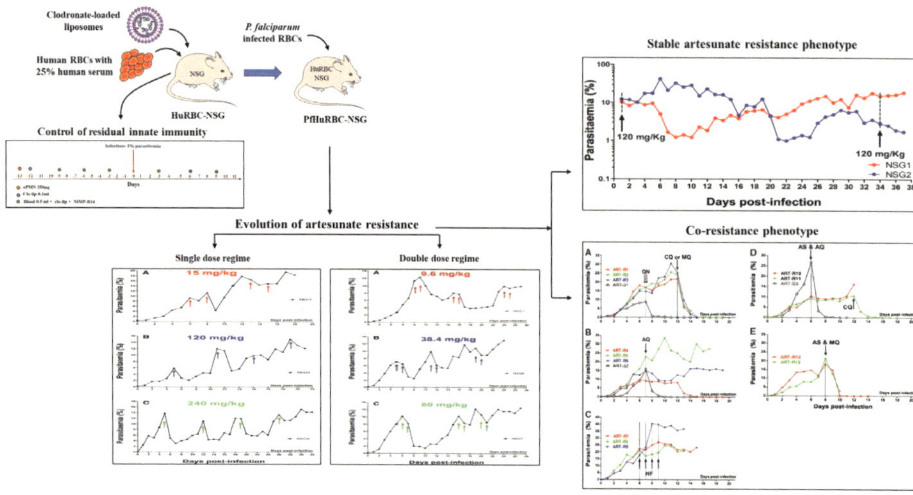

Figure 2.
Experimental selection of artesunate-resistant P. falciparum in a huRBCs-reconstituted NSG mice (PfhuRBC-NSG). NOD.PrkdcscidIl2rg$^{-/-}$ (NSG) mice non-adaptively controlled residual immune responses and reconstituted with human RBCs (HuRBCs) were used to study of asexual blood-stage infection of P. falciparum. *The artesunate resistance (ART-R) was developed by the stepwise selection in experimental humanized mice using single/flash dose (the highest dose: 240 mg/kg) and double-dose (the highest dose: 80 mg/kg) regimens. The stability of the resistance (ART-R) phenotype was attested in vivo by removing ART pressure for one month and then submitting the parasite to ART pressure. ART-R parasites exhibited co-resistance to quinine (QN), amodiaquine (AQ), and halofantrine (HF), and a combination of artesunate (AS) and AQ. These ART-R parasites showing cross-resistance were susceptible to chloroquine (CQ) and mefloquine (MQ).*

3. Conclusion and future perspectives

Human malaria infection remains a biggest challenge to humanity and extensive research is *en route* to find newer therapeutic options to treat this systemic infectious disease, *P. falciparum.* Basic research has been focused to decipher the mechanisms of infection of *Plasmodium* species and biochemical, genomics, proteomics, and metabolomics pathways. This information is used to advance the applied research wherein incessant efforts are being made to design vaccines and drugs against this menace. An effective vaccine development against *P. falciparum* has been a cumbersome process as it takes longer durations than drug therapies. A variety of drugs are developed acting against all developmental stages of different species. The development of drug resistance is affected by various genetic factors (mutations in genes involved in drug transport and metabolism) as well as environmental factors (drug pressure, the geographical distribution of the parasite, etc.). Currently, artemisinin and its derivatives are the cornerstones of effective malaria therapy regimens. These drugs are used in "artemisinin-based combination therapy" for treating malarial infections where artemisinin or its derivatives are given in combination with another unrelated partner drug. Despite ACTs, a parasite is gaining resistance against almost all drugs at a frightening pace suggesting an urgent need to devise novel antimalarial drug(s). Advanced techniques in genomics and proteomics help in developing novel drugs and drug targets. Since single-drug therapy may lead to problems such as ineffective parasite clearance and development of resistance, newer drug combinations are also being developed to clear parasites at even lower doses.

In the end, we developed humanized mice (huRBCs-reconstituted NSG mice) and selected stable ART-resistant *P. falciparum* that showed co-resistance to amodiaquine, quinine, and halofantrine. If resistance to artesunate and artemisinins evolves at such a speed along with co-resistance to quinine and other antimalarials, we would be left with no satisfactory option for treating severe malaria and a compromised choice of treatments for uncomplicated malaria. Indeed, the current dependence on ARTs for both uncomplicated and severe malaria, together with a lack of viable therapeutic alternatives, is a compromising situation. We believe this may have dire consequences and would cripple efforts to achieve malaria control globally. Therefore, novel approaches are needed to devise newer drug and their targets to address this drug resistance issue.

Acknowledgements

Rajeev Tyagi would like to offer his sincere thanks to DBT, New Delhi, Govt. of India, for financially supporting this study in the form Ramalingaswami Re-entry Fellowship-2019 (D.O. NO. BT/HRD/35/02/2006) Sanction order (BT/RLF/Re-entry/27/2018).

Author's contribution

RKT, SS, and RK contributed to conceptualization and writing; SS, RK, and RKT contributed to writing—review and editing. All authors have read and agreed to the final version of the manuscript.

Conflict of interests

Authors declare no conflict of interests exists. The funders had no role in the design of the study; in the collection, analyses, or interpretation of data; in the writing of the manuscript; or in the decision to publish the results.

Author details

Sheetal Saini, Rajinder Kumar and Rajeev K. Tyagi*
Division of Cell Biology and Immunology, Biomedical Parasitology and Nano-immunology Lab, CSIR-Institute of Microbial Technology (IMTECH), Chandigarh, India

*Address all correspondence to: rajeevtyagi@imtech.res.in; rajeev.gru@gmail.com

References

[1] Phillips M, Burrows J, Manyando C, et al. Malaria. Nature Reviews. Disease Primers. 2017;**3**:17050. DOI: 10.1038/nrdp.2017.50

[2] Baker DA. Malaria gametocytogenesis. Molecular and Biochemical Parasitology. 2010;**172**:57-65

[3] Cowman AF, Healer J, Marapana D, Marsh K. Malaria: Biology and disease. Cell. 2016;**167**:610-624

[4] White NJ. Determinants of relapse periodicity in *Plasmodium vivax* malaria. Malaria Journal. 2011; **10**:297

[5] White NJ, Pukrittayakamee S, Hien TT, et al. Malaria. Lancet. 2014;**383**:723-735

[6] WHO/Malaria Key facts. 2021 Available from: https://www.who.int/news-room/fact-sheets/detail/malaria [Accessed: 07 July 2021]

[7] RTS,S Clinical Trials Partnership (CTP). Efficacy and safety of RTS,S/AS01 malaria vaccine with or without a booster dose in infants and children in Africa: Final results of a phase 3, individually randomised, controlled trial. Lancet. 2015;**386**:31-45

[8] Penny MA, Verity R, Bever CA, et al. Public health impact and cost-effectiveness of the RTS,S/AS01 malaria vaccine: A systematic comparison of predictions from four mathematical models. Lancet. 2015;**387**:367-375

[9] Gosling R, von Seidlein L. The future of the RTS,S/AS01 malaria vaccine: An alternative development plan. PLoS Medicine. 2016;**13**:e1001994

[10] Golenser J, Waknine JH, Krugliak M, et al. Current perspectives on the mechanism of action of artemisinins. International Journal for Parasitology. 2006;**36**(14):1427-1441

[11] WHO Model List of Essential Medicines. 2019. Available from: https://www.who.int/groups/expert-committee-on-selection-and-use-of-essential-medicines/essential-medicines-lists. [Accessed: 07 July 2021]

[12] Achan J, Talisuna AO, Erhart A, et al. Quinine, an old anti-malarial drug in a modern world: Role in the treatment of malaria. Malaria Journal. 2011;**10**:144

[13] Loeb F. Activity of a new antimalarial agent, chloroquine (SN 7618). Journal of the American Medical Association. 1946;**130**:1069-1070

[14] Tse EG, Korsik M, Todd MH. The past, present and future of anti-malarial medicines. Malaria Journal. 2019;**18**:93

[15] Bompart F, Kiechel JR, Sebbag R, Pecoul B. Innovative public-private partnerships to maximize the delivery of anti-malarial medicines: Lessons learned from the ASAQ Winthrop experience. Malaria Journal. 2011;**10**:143

[16] Combrinck JM, Mabotha TE, Ncokazi KK, et al. Insights into the role of heme in the mechanism of action of antimalarials. ACS Chemical Biology. 2012;**8**:133-137

[17] Russell PB, Hitchings GH. 2,4-Diaminopyrimidines as antimalarials. III. 5-Aryl derivatives. Journal of the American Chemical Society. 1951;**73**:3763-3770

[18] Laing AB. Treatment of acute falciparum malaria with sulphorthodimethoxine (Fansil). British Medical Journal. 1965;**1**:905-907

[19] Lumb V, Das MK, Singh N, et al. Multiple origins of *Plasmodium falciparum* dihydropteroate synthetase

mutant alleles associated with sulfadoxine resistance in India. Antimicrobial Agents and Chemotherapy. 2011;**55**:2813-2817

[20] Ashley EA, Recht J, White NJ. Primaquine: The risks and the benefits. Malaria Journal. 2014;**13**:418

[21] Chen L, Qu FY, Zhou YC. Field observations on the antimalarial iperaquine. Chinese Medical Journal. 1982;**95**:281-286

[22] Eastman RT, Fidock DA. Artemisinin-based combination therapies: A vital tool in efforts to eliminate malaria. Nature Reviews. Microbiology. 2009;**7**:864-874

[23] Tan KR, Magill AJ, Parise M, Arguin PM. Centers for Disease Control and Prevention. Doxycycline for malaria chemoprophylaxis and treatment: Report from the CDC expert meeting on malaria chemoprophylaxis. The American Journal of Tropical Medicine and Hygiene. 2011;**84**(4):517-531

[24] Trenholme C, Williams R, Desjardins R, et al. Mefloquine (WR 142,490) in the treatment of human malaria. Science. 1975;**190**:792-794

[25] Brasseur P, Druilhe P, Kouamouo J, et al. High level of sensitivity to chloroquine of 72 *Plasmodium falciparum* isolates from Southern Cameroon in January 1985. The American Journal of Tropical Medicine and Hygiene. 1986;**35**:711-716

[26] Nevin RL, Croft AM. Psychiatric effects of malaria and anti-malarial drugs: Historical and modern perspectives. Malaria Journal. 2016;**15**:332

[27] Qinghaosu Antimalaria Coordinating Research Group (QACRG). Antimalarial studies on Qinghaosu. Chinese Medical Journal. 1979;**92**:811-816

[28] Tilley L, Straimer J, Gnädig NF, et al. Artemisinin action and resistance in *Plasmodium falciparum*. Trends in Parasitology. 2016;**32**:682-696

[29] Mok S, Ashley EA, Ferreira PE, et al. Drug resistance. Population transcriptomics of human malaria parasites reveals the mechanism of artemisinin resistance. Science. 2015;**347**(6220):431-435

[30] Mbengue A, Bhattacharjee S, Pandharkar T, et al. A molecular mechanism of artemisinin resistance in *Plasmodium falciparum* malaria. Nature. 2015;**520**:683-687

[31] Shandilya A, Chacko S, Jayaram B, Ghosh I. A plausible mechanism for the antimalarial activity of artemisinin: A computational approach. Scientific Reports. 2013;**3**:2513

[32] Menard D, Dondorp A. Antimalarial drug resistance: A threat to malaria elimination. Cold Spring Harbor Perspectives in Medicine. 2017;**7**: a025619

[33] Cui L, zhuan Su X. Discovery, mechanisms of action and combination therapy of artemisinin. Expert Review of Anti-Infective Therapy. 2009;**7**:999-1013

[34] White NJ. Antimalarial drug resistance. Journal of Clinical Investigation. 2004;**113**:1084-1092

[35] Roper C, Pearce R, Nair S, et al. Intercontinental spread of pyrimethamine-resistant malaria. Science. 2004;**305**:1124

[36] Blasco B, Leroy D, Fidock DA. Antimalarial drug resistance: Linking *Plasmodium falciparum* parasite biology to the clinic. Nature Medicine. 2017;**23**:917-928

[37] Shaw PJ, Chaotheing S, Kaewprommal P, et al. *Plasmodium*

parasites mount an arrest response to dihydroartemisinin, as revealed by whole transcriptome shotgun sequencing (RNA-seq) and microarray study. BMC Genomics. 2015;**16**:830

[38] Wang J, Zhang CJ, Chia WN, et al. Haem-activated promiscuous targeting of artemisinin in *Plasmodium falciparum*. Nature Communications. 2015;**6**:10111

[39] Ismail HM, Barton V, Phanchana M, et al. Artemisinin activity-based probes identify multiple molecular targets within the asexual stage of the malaria parasites *Plasmodium falciparum* 3D7. PNAS. 2016;**113**:2080-2085

[40] Bridgford JL, Xie SC, Cobbold SA, et al. Artemisinin kills malaria parasites by damaging proteins and inhibiting the proteasome. Nature Communications. 2018;**9**:3801

[41] Li W, Mo W, Shen D, et al. Yeast model uncovers dual roles of mitochondria in action of artemisinin. PLoS Genetics. 2005;**1**:e36

[42] Wang J, Huang L, Li J, et al. Artemisinin directly targets malarial mitochondria through its specific mitochondrial activation. PLoS One. 2010;**5**:e9582

[43] Phuc BQ, Rasmussen C, Duong TT, et al. Treatment failure of dihydroartemisinin/piperaquine for *Plasmodium falciparum* malaria, Vietnam. Emerging Infectious Diseases. 2017;**23**:715-717

[44] van der Pluijm RW, Imwong M, Chau NH, et al. Determinants of dihydroartemisinin-piperaquine treatment failure in *Plasmodium falciparum* malaria in Cambodia, Thailand, and Vietnam: A prospective clinical, pharmacological, and genetic study. The Lancet Infectious Diseases. 2019;**19**:952-961

[45] Kathryn JW, Mok S, Fidock DA. Molecular mechanisms of drug resistance in *Plasmodium falciparum* Malaria. Annual Review of Microbiology. 2020;**74**:431-454

[46] Dini S, Zaloumis S, Cao P, et al. Investigating the efficacy of triple artemisinin-based combination therapies for treating *Plasmodium falciparum* malaria patients using mathematical modeling. Antimicrobial Agents and Chemotherapy. 2018;**62**:e01068-e01018

[47] von Seidlein L, Peto TJ, Landier J, et al. The impact of targeted malaria elimination with mass drug administrations on falciparum malaria in Southeast Asia: A cluster randomised trial. PLoS Medicine. 2019;**16**: e1002745

[48] van der Pluijm RW, Tripura R, Hoglund RM, et al. Triple artemisinin-based combination therapies versus artemisinin-based combination therapies for uncomplicated *Plasmodium falciparum* malaria: A multicentre, open-label, randomised clinical trial. Lancet. 2020;**395**:1345-1360

[49] Witkowski B, Lelièvre J, Barragán MJ, et al. Increased tolerance to artemisinin in *Plasmodium falciparum* is mediated by a quiescence mechanism. Antimicrobial Agents and Chemotherapy. 2010;**54**(5):1872-1877

[50] Chavchich M, Gerena L, Peters J, et al. Role of pfmdr1 amplification and expression in induction of resistance to artemisinin derivatives in *Plasmodium falciparum*. Antimicrobial Agents and Chemotherapy. 2010;**54**(6):2455-2464

[51] Tucker MS, Mutka T, Sparks K, et al. Phenotypic and genotypic analysis of in vitro-selected artemisinin-resistant progeny of *Plasmodium falciparum*. Antimicrobial Agents and Chemotherapy. 2012;**56**(1):302-314. 21

[52] Cui L, Wang Z, Miao J, et al. Mechanisms of in vitro resistance to dihydroartemisinin in *Plasmodium falciparum*. Molecular Microbiology. 2012;**86**(1):111-128

[53] Rocamora F, Zhu L, Liong KY, et al. Oxidative stress and protein damage responses mediate artemisinin resistance in malaria parasites. PLoS Pathogens. 2018;**14**(3):e1006930

[54] Rodrigues LA, Henriques G, Borges ST, et al. Experimental evolution of resistance to artemisinin combination therapy results in amplification of the mdr1 gene in a rodent malaria parasite. PLoS One. 2010;**5**(7):e11593

[55] Maslachah L, Widiyatno TV, Yustinasari LR, Plumeriastuti H. Phenotypic approach artemisinin resistance in malaria rodent as in vivo model. Veterinary World. 2017;**10**(7):790-797

[56] Rämer PC, Chijioke O, Meixlsperger S, et al. Mice with human immune system components as in vivo models for infections with human pathogens. Immunology and Cell Biology. 2011;**89**:408-416

[57] Tyagi RK, Tandel N, Deshpande R, et al. Humanized mice are instrumental to the study of *Plasmodium falciparum* infection. Frontiers in Immunology. 2018;**9**:2550

[58] Tyagi RK. Plasmodium falciparum infected humanized mice: A viable preclinical tool. Immunotherapy. 2021; DOI: 10.2217/imt-2021-0102

[59] Tyagi RK, Gleeson PJ, Arnold L, et al. High-level artemisinin-resistance with quinine co-resistance emerges in *P. falciparum* malaria under in vivo artesunate pressure. BMC Medicine. 2018;**16**:181

[60] Arnold L, Tyagi RK, Mejia P, et al. Analysis of innate defences against *Plasmodium falciparum* in immunodeficient mice. Malaria Journal. 2010;**9**:197

[61] Arnold L, Tyagi RK, Meija P, et al. Further improvements of the *P. falciparum* humanized mouse model. PLoS ONE. 2011;**6**(3):e18045

[62] Duffier Y, Lorthiois A, Cisteró P, et al. A humanized mouse model for sequestration of *Plasmodium falciparum* sexual stages and in vivo evaluation of gametocytidal drugs. Scientific Reports. 2016;**6**:35025

[63] Minkah NK, Schafer C, Kappe SHI. Humanized mouse models for the study of human malaria parasite biology, pathogenesis, and immunity. Frontiers in Immunology. 2018;**9**:807

[64] Schafer C, Roobsoong W, Kangwanrangsan N, et al. A humanized mouse Model for *Plasmodium vivax* to test interventions that block liver stage to blood stage transition and blood stage infection. IScience. 2020;**23**:101381

Chapter 12

Drug Design for Malaria with Artificial Intelligence (AI)

Bhaswar Ghosh and Soham Choudhuri

Abstract

Malaria is a deadly disease caused by the plasmodium parasites. Approximately 210 million people get affected by malaria every year resulting in half a million deaths. Among several species of the parasite, *Plasmodium falciparum* is the primary cause of severe infection and death. Several drugs are available for malaria treatment in the market but plasmodium parasites have successfully developed resistance against many drugs over the years. This poses a serious threat to efficacy of the treatments and continuing discovery of new drug is necessary to tackle the situation, especially due to failure in designing an effective vaccine. People are now trying to design new drugs for malaria using AI technologies which can substantially reduce the time and cost required in classical drug discovery programs. In this chapter, we provide a comprehensive overview of a road map for several AI based computational techniques which can be implemented in a malaria drugs discovery program. Classical computers has limiting computing power. So, researchers are also trying to harness quantum machine learning to speed up the drug discovery processes.

Keywords: Malaria, *Plasmodium falciparum*, machine learning, drug design, Quantum machine learning, Topological data analysis

1. Introduction

Malaria is an infectious and dreadful disease caused by the plasmodium parasites. The parasite is transmitted to humans through the bites of infected mosquitoes. Around 210 million people get infected by malaria every year resulting in 440,000 deaths, especially children under the age of five [1]. The *Plasmodium falciparum* is the primary cause of severe infection and death in most cases. So far, numerous drugs are available in the market such as Quinine, Mepacrine, Chloroquine, Mefloquine, Halofantrine, Artemisinin and their derivatives. Unfortunately, malaria parasites, especially the falciparum species, developed resistance against many of these drugs if not all after some time posing a serious threat to the medication's efficacy [2]. As a result, the continued discovery of new drugs against malaria becomes essential to mitigate this threat. During the last decade, various drug design programs focusing on malaria are initiated all over the world. Drug discovery is a time-consuming and complex process that can be broadly divided into four main phases: (i) the target selection and validation, (ii) screening and optimization of lead compounds, (iii) preclinical studies, and (iv) clinical trials. First, the targets associated with specific diseases need to be identified. This requires an evaluation of cellular and genetic targets, genomics and proteomics analysis, and prediction bioinformatics. The next step was to hit identification. The compound is identified from the library Molec-snake using combinatorial chemistry, high-throughput screening, and virtual screening. Furthermore, in vivo pharmacokinetic studies are performed to conduct toxicity tests on animals. After, the preclinical tests are conducted successfully, clinical trials are performed on the infected patients. Clinical trial is conducted in three phases. The Phase I constitutes drug safety test with few people; In Phase II, the dose amount of the drug necessary to eliminate the infection is determined on few patients and finally Phase III comprises of precisely quantifying the efficacy of the drug on large number of patients. After the drug candidates' safety and efficacy are confirmed in the clinical phases, agencies such as the FDA review this compound for approval and commercialization. The total cost of a conventional drug development pipeline is projected to be USD 2.6 billion, and it can take more than 12 years for a complete traditional workflow.

2. Malaria disease overview

Malaria has a wide effect in the subtropical and tropical continents. Sub-Saharan Africa has the most malaria cases as well as significant cases in India, Brazil, Afghanistan, Sri Lanka, Thailand, Indonesia, Vietnam, Cambodia, and China [3, 4]. In many medium climate areas, such as Western Europe and the United States, public health measures and economic development have succeeded in achieving elimination of malaria, apart from occasionally imported cases through international travels. Female Anopheles mosquitoes transmit malaria. There are approximately 400 species of Anopheles in the world. Among them, 30 species are responsible for malaria. Plasmodium species can also infect animals, birds, etc. The four species of malaria parasites namely *Plasmodium falciparum*, *Plasmodium vivax*, Plasmodium ovale and Plasmodium malariae, can infect humans under natural conditions. *Plasmodium falciparum* is the major killer among these species. In August 1897, Ronald Ross for first time reported that the parasites can infect female mosquitoes and further showed that the parasite completed it's development cycle in the female mosquitoes which is the primary source of the spread of infection from one infected patient to another healthy individual.

2.1 Life cycle

Malaria infection begins when the anopheles mosquito bites someone and injects plasmodium parasitse into the bloodstream in the form of sporozoites. Sporozoites are then passed to the human liver and multiply asexually in liver cells for the next 7 to 10 days, but do not cause any symptom. In animals, parasites are released from liver cells to the vesicles in the form of merozoites which then enter into the heart and in the lungs and finally stays in the lung capillary.

The vesicles eventually disintegrate, enabling the merozoites to progress to the blood stage of development. Merozoites enter red blood cells (erythrocytes) in the bloodstream and multiply until the cells burst [5] resulting in released merozoites which further penetrate more erythrocytes. Each time parasites invade the blood cells, this cycle is repeated, causing fever. Some parasites inside the infected blood cells leave the asexual multiplication cycle [6]. Instead of replicating, these parasites in those blood cells develop into sexual forms of parasites, called gametocytes flowing through the bloodstream. When an anopheles mosquito bites an infected human, it swallows the gametocytes, which develop further into mature sex cells

DOI: http://dx.doi.org/10.5772/intechopen.98695

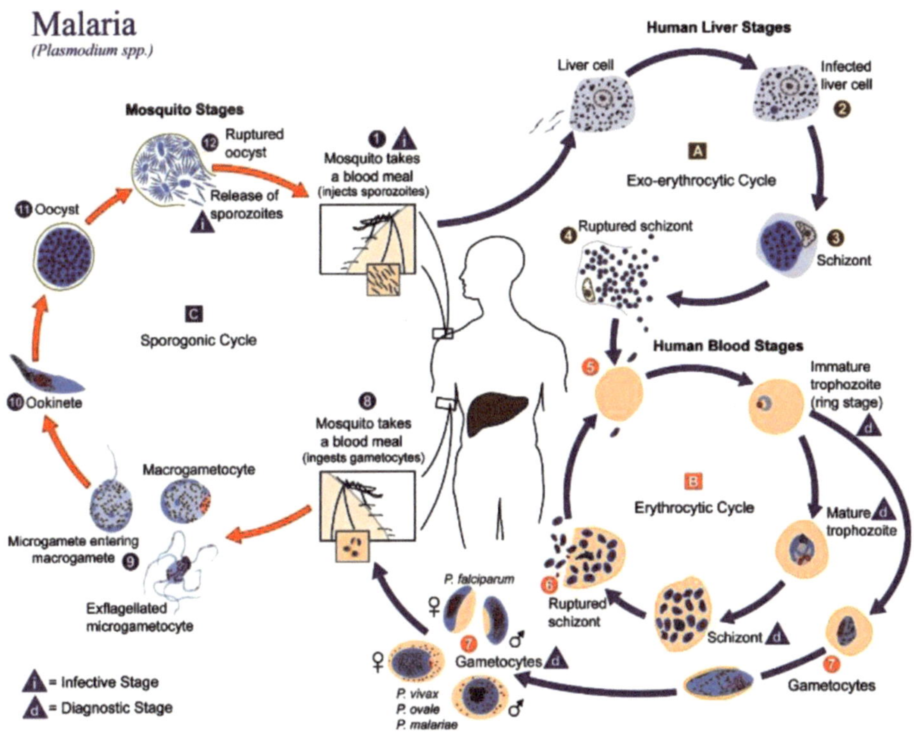

Figure 1.
Malaria parasite life cycle. This pictute is downloaded from (https://www.ncbi.nlm.nih.gov/books/NBK5951/figure/malaria_LifeCycle/).

called gametes [7]. The female gametes that have been fertilized grow into actively moving ookinetes which form oocysts outside the surface. Thousands of active sporozoites develop within the oocyst and eventually, the oocyst bursts, releasing sporozoites into the body's cavity that fly to the salivary glands of the mosquito [8]. As the mosquito bites another person injecting the sporozoites the cycle of human infection begins again (**Figure 1**).

2.2 Drug design for malaria using deep learning and others in silico techniques

For the last few years, several reports have been published on drug design for malaria using machine learning or others computational methods. Arash et al. [9] devised a deep learning based technique (DeepMalaria) using a graph based model and SMILE to predict the anti-malarial inhibitory compounds. There are few studies which delineate In Silico approaches of analysing anti-plasmodium compounds. Monika Samant et al. [10] has developed a protein–protein interaction network of *Plasmodium falciparum* and human host by integrating experimental data and computational prediction of interactions using the interolog method. Manila et al. [11] has also studied inhibitor against the plasmepsin II. This is an aspartic protease encoded by the malarial parasite that is essential for host haemoglobin degradation. They have studied target protein structure and searched a suitable molecule that has a high binding affinity towards the target protein. Although there are few studies on In silico drug target identification or drug design for malaria but real-life implementation of these drugs which have been designed by computational methods is not successfully achieved yet. One of the main reasons for this is that these

Description	References
DeepMalaria (a graph based model using SMILE)	[9]
Analysis of malaria inhibitors	[10]
Prediction of antimalarial drug target	[12]
inhibitor designing against malarial parasite	[11]

Note: These are the most significant paper for in-silico malaria research and DeepMalaria is the only paper where authors has used deep neural network for malaria drug design.

Table 1.
Different approaches for in silico antimalarial drug discovery.

computation methods are only optimizing physical or chemical properties but these methods are not able to predict whether the designed drug is biologically relevant for malaria. In the next sections, we will provide a road map to harness recent developments in several genomics and AI technique which can be used in drug design programs (**Table 1**).

3. Drug target selection using genomics data

The first step in the drug discovery project is to identify a potential target. Transcriptomics data can be effectively utilized for target identification. Differential gene expression analysis provides information about differences in gene expression between normal and diseased states. For malaria parasites, plasmoDB database [13] provides a large variety of trarencriptomics datasets at different stages of the life cycle or at different times after it infects the RBC's. However, bulk RNA-sequencing data does not have the ability to recognize cell to cell variability within a population as a result of which some essential feature may remain undetected. For example, recent single cell RNA-seq experiment was able to differentiate between sexually and asexually committed scizont from a population of parasites [14]. With the launch of such single cell RNA sequencing (RNA-seq), it is now possible to measure RNA levels on the entire genome scale to gain insights into cellular processes and illuminate the specifics of many important molecular events such as alternative splicing, gene fusion, variation of single nucleotide, and differential genes expression. ScRNA-seq enables analysis of individual cell transcriptomes. ScRNA-seq is generally used to examine transcriptional similarities and variations within the cell population. RNA sequencing technologies continue to advance and provide new ideas for understanding biological processes. Early findings revealed previously unrecognised levels of heterogeneity in embryonic and immune cell population [15, 16]. Thus, the analysis of heterogeneity remains a core reason to embark on scRNA-seq studies. Similarly, assessments of transcriptional variations between individual cells have been used to distinguish unusual cell populations that would otherwise go undetected in pooled cell analysis [17], such as malignant tumor cells within a tumor mass [18], or hyper-responsive immune cells within an otherwise homogeneous group [19]. The scRNA-seq technique is also ideal for the examination of individual cells where each cell is essentially unique, such as individual T lymphocytes expressing highly diverse T-cell receptors [20], brain neurons [21], or early-stage embryo cells [22]. In scenarios such as embryonic development, cancer, myoblast, and lung epithelium differentiation and lymphocyte fate diversification, scRNA-seq is also increasingly used to trace the lineage and developmental relationships between heterogeneous yet related cellular states [22–27].

In addition to solving cellular heterogeneity, scRNA-seq can also provide important information on essential gene expression characteristics which include studying the expression of monoallelic genes [15, 28, 29], splicing patterns [30], as well as noise during transcriptional responses [30–32]. Importantly, the study of gene co-expression patterns at the single-cell level could enable the identification of co-regulated gene modules and even inference of gene-regulatory networks underlying functional heterogeneity and cell-type specifications [32, 33]. Additionally, we can extract many more information such as how many genes can be detected and whether a particular gene of interest is being expressed, or whether there has been differential splicing, depending on the procedure of generating the mRNA data. Several single cell RNA-seq experiments have been performed in the last couple of years for plasmodium parasites which paved a much more sophisticated way to characterise gene expression at different stages of the life cycle [14, 34–36]. Both supervised and unsupervised learning methods can be used to identify deferentially expressed genes at different life cycle stages [37, 38]. These information can be harnessed in a gene ontology analysis or a genome-scale metabolic model to identify function of the genes and subsequently potential target for a drug.

4. Drug discovery with AI

Classical approach of drug discovery is a time consuming and complex process. It takes almost 12 years to discover a drug with the cost soaring to billions of dollars. Several pharma-companies are working on drug discovery but 90 percent of all drug discovery programs are failing due to limitations both at the computational as well as clinical phases. We can divide drug discovery into four major steps (1) target selection and validation; (2) compound screening and lad optimization; (3) pre-clinical studies; (4) clinical trials. Bio-pharmaceutical industries are focusing on computational approaches in order to enhance the drug discovery processes as well as to reduce research and development expenses by diminishing failure rates in clinical trials and ultimately generate superior medicines. Different machine learning approaches help to identify drug targets, find suitable molecules from data libraries, suggest chemical modifications, etc. There are several steps for drug discovery and we will discuss how computational approaches help in each step of drug discovery process.

4.1 Primary drug screening with AI

4.1.1 Image processing and usage of AI to sort and classify cells

AI technology performs well at classifying images that contained various objects or features [39, 40]. Various dimension reduction techniques like principal component analysis(PCA) can be utilized to reduce the features of the images and then we can use AI-based techniques to classify the cells [41]. Least square support vector machine (LS-SVM), which use classification and regression techniques shows the highest accuracy (95.34) during classification. Modern devices like activated cell sorting images (IACS) are used to measure the optical, electrical, and mechanical properties of cells for highly versatile and scalable cell sorting automation. This instrument use neural network algorithms to do decision-making and high-speed digital image processing. AI is recently used to interpret computerized electrocardiography (ECG). This process plays an significant role in the diagnosis/clinical treatment of the workflow.

4.2 Secondary drug screening with AI

4.2.1 Physical properties predictions

For drug design, features like bioavailability, bioactivity and toxicity are very important defining characteristics of a compound. The Partition coefficient (logP) and melting point affect a drug molecule's bioavailability. The melting point of a drug indicates how easily it dissolves in water, whereas logP quantifies relative solubility between oil and water. logP is used to calculate cellular drug absorption. A molecular fingerprint, SMILE(simplified molecular input line-entry system) string, potential energy measurements (e.g., from ab initio calculations), molecular graphs with varying weights for atoms or bonds, Coulomb matrices, molecular fragments or bonds, and atomic coordinates in 3D are examples of molecular representations used in an AI drug design algorithm that takes these properties into account [42]. These inputs can be utilized in the DNN training phase and can be processed by various DNNs in different stages, including generative and predictive stages. We can also use reinforcement learning (RL). The generative stage of a DNN is trained to generate chemically feasible SMILES strings using SMILES inputs in a typical sample, while the predictive stage is trained to predict molecule properties. Although the two stages are initially trained separately using supervised learning algorithms, different kinds of biases may be introduced by rewarding or penalising specific properties when the two stages are trained simultaneously.

4.2.2 Predictions of bioactivity and toxicity

The toxicity and bioactivity profiles are significant properties of a compound. Matched molecular pair (MMP) analysis can be used to explore the local changes of the drug molecule and its significance on the molecular properties as well as bioactivity [43]. MMP is used to study the quantitative structure–activity relationship (QSAR) [43]. Random forest(RF), gradient boosting machine (GBMs), and DNNs, the machine learning techniques previously applied without MMP, are used to gather new transformations, fragments as well as modifications of the core static. When it comes to predicting compound activity, DNN outperforms RF and GBM. MMP with ML has been used to predict many properties of bioactivity such as oral exposure, the distribution coefficient (log D) [44, 45], the intrinsic clearance, the absorption, distribution, metabolism, and excretion (ADME), and mode of action owing to the rapid increase of public databases (such as ChEMBL and PubChem) containing a significant amount of structure–activity relationships (SAR). A few methods for predicting the bioactivity of a drug candidate have recently been created. For example, few researcher used a network coding convolution graph with discrete chemicals to extract the drug target sites' signature into a sustainable space latent vectors (LVS). LVS enables optimization based on molecule gradients in space, allowing predictions to be made based on the model's differential affinity and other binding properties. The DeepTox algorithm is important for toxicity prediction [46].

4.3 AI in drug design

4.3.1 Prediction of target proteins 3D structure

The 3D structure of a target protein's ligand-binding site is usually used to design new drug molecules [47, 48]. As a result, researchers have used homology modelling and de novo protein design in the past [49–51]. With the development of AI-based approaches, prediction of the 3D structure of a target protein can be performed more accurately. The AI tool AlphaFold is successfully implemented to predict the 3D structure of a drug target protein in the recent Crucial Assessment of Protein Structure Prediction contest and performed amazingly well. AlphaFold correctly predicted 25 of 43 structures using only primary protein sequences. These results outperformed the second-place finisher, who correctly predicted just three of the 43 test sequences. AlphaFold is based on deep neural networks (DNNs) trained to predict proteins' properties based on their primary sequences. It measures the angles between peptide bonds in close proximity as well as the distances between pairs of amino acids. These two features are then combined to generate a score that can be used to predict the accuracy of a proposed 3D protein structure model. These scoring functions are used by AlphaFold to examine the protein structure landscape and find structures that match predictions.

4.3.2 Predicting drug-protein interactions

Quantum mechanics (QM) is a very effective tool for predicting protein–ligand (drug) interactions [52, 53]. These methods takes the help of quantum effects for the simulated system at the atomic resolution, resulting in substantially higher precision than conventional MM methods. The time–cost of QM-based methods is far higher than that of MM methods since MM methods only use basic energy functions based on atomic coordinates [54, 55]. As a result, applying AI methods to QM calculations necessitates a tradeoff between QM accuracy and molecular mechanics(MM) models' favorable time–cost [56]. AI models have been trained to replicate QM energies from atomic coordinates, and they can outperform MM methods in terms of calculation speed. Deep learning can be used to predict the potential energies of small molecules, thus replacing computationally challenging quantum chemistry calculations with a fast ML method [56]. AI is mainly utilized for atomic simulations and predictions of electrical properties, while DL has been utilized to predict the potential energies of small molecules, thus replacing computationally demanding quantum chemistry calculations with a fast ML method. DFT (density functional theory) potential energies derived from quantum chemistry have been measured and used to train DNNs for large data sets. For example, the accuracy of an ML model improved with increasing sample size in a study of two million elpasolite crystals, reaching 0.1 eV/atom for DFT formation energies trained on 10,000 structures. The model was then used to test different compositional choices for different properties (**Table 2**) [57].

4.4 Possibility of drug design using topological data analysis

If we have a dataset containing information about compounds with respect to their structural features, toxicity, binding affinity to the target then we can use TDA, a mathematical technique to create a similarity network of the compounds by studying shapes preserving high-dimensionality. TDA will enable us to visualize our compound library as a two-dimensional network, with compounds (located in nodes) linked by a series of edges indicating their degree of mutual similarity. As a result, two compounds with identical properties will appear closer together in the network, whereas two compounds with vastly different properties will appear farther apart. This network would make it simple to create subgroups or families of related compounds, which could then be used to choose the best compound.

Tools name	Description	Reference
AlphaFold	Protein 3D structure prediction	
Chemputer	A more structured format for documenting a procedure for chemical synthesis	[58]
DeepChem	A python-based AI platform for different predictions of drug discovery tasks	[59]
DeepNeuralNet-QSAR	Molecular activity predictions	[60]
DeepTox	Toxicity predictions	[46]
DeltaVina	A scoring feature for protein-ligand binding affinity rescoring	[61]
Hit Dexter	ML models for molecule prediction that could react to biochemical assays	[62]
Neural Graph Fingerprints	Prediction of properties for novel molecules	[63]
NNScore	For protein-ligand interactions, neural network-based scoring mechanism	[64]
ODDT	A robust chemoinformatics and molecular modelling toolkit for use	[65]
ORGANIC	An powerful method for molecular generation to build molecules with desired characteristics	[66]
PotentialNet	Ligand-binding prediction of affinity on the basis of a convolution Neural Network (CNN)	[67]
PPB2	Polypharmacology prediction	[68]
QML	A Python toolkit for quantum ML	
REINVENT	Using RNN (recurrent neural network) and RL (reinforcement learning), molecular de novo architecture	[69]
SCScore	A scoring feature for the assessment of a molecule's synthesis complexity	[70]
SIEVE-Score	An improved method of virtual screening based on structure via interaction-energy-based learning	[71]

Table 2.
List of AI-Based Computational Tools for Drug Discovery.

4.5 Possibility drug design using Quantum machine learning

The Quantum Computer Algorithm (QC) was introduced as a way to speed up classical machine learning algorithm. However, modern computers are not enough to analyze the behavior of the atoms in a molecule. Even the most powerful super-computers at this time can only simulate relatively simple molecules by significantly limiting their ability to predict the interaction of complex molecules and atoms. Classical computing (CC) and big data analysis methods can screen desired properties of molecules. Researchers use Molecular simulator to simulate interactions between electrons of each atom to test how they react with each other in the real world. However, due to CC's relatively limited processing capacity, the computationally designed drug fails to deliver the desired results in 90 percent cases during the first phase of the clinical trial causing loss of billions of dollars every year. When Google announced a successful quantum computing experiment (QC) that has achieved what is called "quantum supremacy" (calculations that are too complex to do using CC), it was praised by many peoplearound the world as a key moment for QC.

It is also an important development for drug discovery. Indeed, QC can change the drug discovery game entirely by packing enough computational muscles to enable molecular analysis at an unprecedented scale which was completely unimaginable with a CC. Additionally, quantum machine learning (QML) which uses quantum algorithms to perform complex algorithms of learning assignments [72] can augment the computational tools of drug discovery programs even further. Classical machine learning has already shown a significant promise in drug discovery. QML allows scientists to translate classical ML algorithms into quantum circuits to run an ultra-strong quantum computer efficiently. This quantum computer will become more efficient in future as the quantum technologies become less prone to mistakes. Scientists from the University of Warwick, the University of Luxembourg, and the University of Berlin recently created a deep ML algorithm that could predict the molecule's quantum state faster than before. "Solve the fundamental equation of quantum mechanics in conventional ways requires high-performance computing resources and computational months," explained the laboratory news. The team said that "the new AI algorithm developed can provide accurate predictions in seconds on a laptop or cellphone." Researchers from Pfizer have made similar progress, using modeling techniques called predictions of the crystal structure (CSP) to map molecular 3D structures - calculations that usually take months to solve. However, there is a long path to travel before we can say that we have achieved a practical quantum advantage. However, QC and QML hold extraordinary promises for the pharmaceutical business - which, when refined, will pave the way towards the development of new drugs as well as safer and cheaper health products for patients in the future.

5. Conclusions

Many pharmaceutical companies are using AI tools in drug discovery process. Costs and time remain big challenges in drug discovery programs. There are usually about 1 million compounds in a standard high-throughput screening library, where designing each compound typically costs 50–100 USD. As a result, an initial screening phase would cost several million dollars and take months to complete. AI or ML techniques help to do optimization of lead compound. It takes only few days to find the lead compounds by AI, when classical approach takes several years. AI helps to predict bio-activity, toxicity, physical properties, structure prediction of potential drug. There are few companies like Merck, Novartis etc. who are using AI technologies to design drug. Classical computer has some limiting computing power. So, Researcher are trying to make quantum computer or using quantum machine learning algorithm in Classical computer to do computation in a faster way. Since, malaria is one of the major health burdens in the developing world, AI based drug design programs will be immensely helpful in aiding WHO's goal to reduce cases of malaria by 90 percent by 2030. The inefficacy of vaccination strategies further impose all the burdens on continuous discovery of new drugs. We strongly suggest through this review that AI based drug program would substantially benefit in tackling this debilitating disease with respect to saving human life at lower amount of time and cost.

Acknowledgements

Authors thank Department of Biotechnology (No. BT/RLF/Re-entry/32/2017), Government of India for funding this project.

The authorship criteria are listed in our Authorship Policy:
https://www.intechopen.com/page/authorship-policy.
This section of your manuscript may also include funding information.

Author details

Bhaswar Ghosh† and Soham Choudhuri*†
Center for Computational Natural Sciences and Bioinformatics, International Institute of Information Technology, Hyderabad, India

*Address all correspondence to: choudhurisoham@gmail.com

† These authors contributed equally.

References

[1] World Malaria Report 2020. https://www.who.int/news-room/fact-sheets/detail/malaria (2020)

[2] White, Nicholas J. "Antimalarial drug resistance." The Journal of clinical investigation vol. 113,8 (2004): 1084–92. doi:10.1172/JCI21682

[3] Snow RW, Craig M, Deichmann U Marsh K: Estimating mortality, morbidity and disability due to malaria among Africa's non-pregnant population. 1999, Bull WHO 77, 624–640. https://pubmed.ncbi.nlm.nih.gov/10516785/ [Accessed: 21 January 2021]

[4] Breman JG, Egan A Keusch GT, The intolerable burden of malaria: a new look at the numbers. 2001, J Trop Med Hyg 64, (Suppl. 1–2), iv–vii https://core.ac.uk/reader/13114159?utm_source=linkout [Accessed: 21 January 2021]

[5] Yamauchi LM, Coppi A, Snounou G Sinnis P (2007)*Plasmodium sporozoites* trickle out of the injection site. Cell Microbiol [Epub ahead of print].

[6] Mota MM, Pradel G, Vanderberg JP, Hafalla JC, Frevert U, Nussenzweig RS, Nussenzweig V Rodriguez A (2001) Migration of *Plasmodium sporozoites* through cells before infection. Science 291, 141–144.

[7] Frevert U, Sinnis P, Cerami C, Shreffler W, Takacs B Nussenzweig V (1993) Malaria circumsporozoite protein binds to heparan sulfate proteoglycans associated with the surface membrane of hepatocytes. J Exp Med 177, 1287–1298.

[8] Sturm A, Amino R, van de Sand C, Regen T, Retzlaff S, Rennenberg A, Krueger A, Pollok JM, Menard R Heussler VT (2006) Manipulation of host hepatocytes by the malaria parasite for delivery into liver sinusoids. Science 313, 1287–1290.

[9] Arash Keshavarzi Arshadi, Milad Salem, Jennifer Collins, Jiann Shiun Yuan and Debopam Chakrabarti : DeepMalaria: Artificial Intelligence Driven Discovery of Potent Antiplasmodials. Frontiers in pharmacology. 15th January 2020;doi: 10.3389/fphar.2019.01526. https://www.frontiersin.org/articles/10.3389/fphar.2019.01526/full [Accessed: 26th February 2021]

[10] Monika Samant, Nidhi Chadha, Anjani K. Tiwari, and Yasha Hasija: In Silico Designing and Analysis of Inhibitors against Target Protein Identified through Host-Pathogen Protein Interactions in Malaria. 17 November 2015. International Journal of Medicinal Chemistry Volume 2016, Article ID 2741038, 13 pages http://dx.doi.org/10.1155/2016/2741038 https://www.hindawi.com/journals/ijmc/2016/2741038/ [Accessed: 27th February 2021]

[11] Manila Kashyap, Vipan Kumar Sohpal and Parul Mahajan: In silico approaches for inhibitor designing against Plasmepsin-II of malarial parasite, Plasmodium malariae. Biotechnological Communication. Biosci. Biotech. Res. Comm. 9(1): 25–31 (2016) https://www.researchgate.net/publication/333822594_In_silico_approaches_for_inhibitor_designing_against_Plasmepsin-II_of_malarial_parasite_Plasmodium_malariae [Accessed: 27th February 2021]

[12] Philipp Ludin, Ben Woodcroft, Stuart A Ralph, Pascal Mäser: In silico prediction of antimalarial drug target candidates. 2012 Jul , Int J Parasitol Drugs Drug Resist17;2:191–9. doi: 10.1016/j.ijpddr.2012.07.002 https://pubmed.ncbi.nlm.nih.gov/24533280/ [Accessed: 27th February 2021]

[13] Bahl, A., Brunk, B., Crabtree, J., Fraunholz, M. J., Gajria, B., Grant, G. R.,

Ginsburg, H., Gupta, D., Kissinger, J. C., Labo, P., Li, L., Mailman, M. D., Milgram, A. J., Pearson, D. S., Roos, D. S., Schug, J., Stoeckert, C. J., Jr, Whetzel, P. (2003). PlasmoDB: the Plasmodium genome resource. A database integrating experimental and computational data. Nucleic acids research, 31(1), 212–215. https://doi.org/10.1093/nar/gkg081.

[14] Ruberto, A.A., Bourke, C., Merienne, N. et al. Single-cell RNA sequencing reveals developmental heterogeneity among Plasmodium berghei sporozoites. Sci Rep 11, 4127 (2021). https://doi.org/10.1038/s41598-021-82914-w

[15] Deng Q, Ramskold D, Reinius B, Sandberg R. *Single-cell RNA-seq reveals dynamic, random monoallelic gene expression in mammalian cells.* Science. 2014;343:193–6.

[16] Jaitin DA, Kenigsberg E, Keren-Shaul H, Elefant N, Paul F, Zaretsky I, et al. *Massively parallel single-cell RNAseq for marker-free decomposition of tissues into cell types. Science.* 2014;343:776–9.

[17] Miyamoto DT, Zheng Y, Wittner BS, Lee RJ, Zhu H, Broderick KT, et al. *RNA-Seq of single prostate CTCs implicates noncanonical Wnt signaling in antiandrogen resistance.* Science. 2015; 349:1351–6.

[18] Tirosh I, Izar B, Prakadan SM, Wadsworth MH, Treacy D, Trombetta JJ, et al. *Dissecting the multicellular ecosystem of metastatic melanoma by single-cell RNA-seq. Science.* 2016;352: 189–96.

[19] Shalek AK, Satija R, Shuga J, Trombetta JJ, Gennert D, Lu D, et al. *Single-cell RNA-seq reveals dynamic paracrine control of cellular variation.* Nature. 2014;510:363–9.

[20] Stubbington MJ, Lonnberg T, Proserpio V, Clare S, Speak AO, Dougan G, et al. *T cell fate and clonality inference from single-cell transcriptomes.* Nat Methods.2016;13:329–32.

[21] Zeisel A, Munoz-Manchado AB, Codeluppi S, ~Lonnerberg P, La Manno G, Jurëus A, et al. *Brain structure. Cell types in the mouse cortex and hippocampus revealed by single-cell RNA-seq.* Science. 2015;347:1138–42.

[22] Blakeley P, Fogarty NM, Del Valle I, Wamaitha SE, Hu TX, Elder K, et al. *Defining the three cell lineages of the human blastocyst by single-cell RNA-seq.* Development. 2015; 142:3613.

[23] Treutlein B, Brownfield DG, Wu AR, Neff NF, Mantalas GL, Espinoza FH, et al. *Reconstructing lineage hierarchies of the distal lung epithelium using single-cell RNA-seq.* Nature. 2014; 509:371–5.

[24] Trapnell C, Cacchiarelli D, Grimsby J, Pokharel P, Li S, Morse M, et al. *The dynamics and regulators of cell fate decisions are revealed by pseudotemporal ordering of single cells.* Nat Biotechnol. 2014;32:381–6.

[25] Petropoulos S, Edsgard D, Reinius B, Deng Q, Panulä SP, Codeluppi S, et al. *Single-cell RNA-seq reveals lineage and X chromosome dynamics in human preimplantation embryos Cell.* 2016;167: 285.

[26] Lonnberg T, Svensson V, James KR, Fernandez-Ruiz D, Sebina I, Montandon R, et al. *Single-cell RNA-seq and computational analysis using temporal mixture modelling resolves Th1/Tfh fate bifurcation in malaria.* Sci Immunol.2017;2:eaal2192.

[27] Venteicher AS, Tirosh I, Hebert C, Yizhak K, Neftel C, Filbin MG, et al. *Decoupling genetics, lineages, and microenvironment in IDH-mutant gliomas by single-cell RNAseq.* Science. 2017;355: eaai8478.

[28] Tang F, Barbacioru C, Nordman E, Bao S, Lee C, Wang X, et al. *Deterministic and stochastic allele specific gene expression in single mouse blastomeres.* PLoS One.2011;6:e21208.

[29] Reinius B, Mold JE, Ramskold D, Deng Q, Johnssön P, Michaelsson J, et al. *Analysis of allelic expression patterns in clonal somatic cells by single-cell RNA-seq. Nat Genet.* 2016;48:1430–5.

[30] Shalek AK, Satija R, Adiconis X, Gertner RS, Gaublomme JT, Raychowdhury R, et al. *Single-cell transcriptomics reveals bimodality in expression and splicing in immune cells.* Nature. 2013;498:236–40.

[31] Kim JK, Kolodziejczyk AA, Ilicic T, Illicic T, Teichmann SA, Marioni JC. *Characterizing noise structure in singlecell RNA-seq distinguishes genuine from technical stochastic allelic expression.* Nat Commun. 2015;6:8687.

[32] Kar G, Kim JK, Kolodziejczyk AA, Natarajan KN, Torlai Triglia E, Mifsud B, et al. *Flipping between Polycomb repressed and active transcriptional states introduces noise in gene expression.* Nat Commun. 2017;8:36.

[33] Liu S, Trapnell C. *Single-cell transcriptome sequencing: recent advances and remaining challenges.* F1000Res. 2016;5:182.

[34] Katelyn A. Walzer,Hélène Fradin, Liane Y. Emerson,David L. Corcoran,Jen-Tsan Chi. Latent transcriptional variations of individual *Plasmodium falciparum* uncovered by single-cell RNA-seq and fluorescence imaging. December 19, 2019, https://doi.org/10.1371/journal.pgen.1008506.

[35] Virginia M. Howick, Andrew J. C. Russell, Tallulah Andrews, Haynes Heaton, Adam J. Reid, Kedar, The Malaria Cell Atlas: Single parasite transcriptomes across the complete Plasmodium life cycle, Science 23 Aug 2019: Vol. 365, Issue 6455, eaaw2619, DOI: 10.1126/science.aaw2619.

[36] Reid AJ, Talman AM, Bennett HM, et al. Single-cell RNA-seq reveals hidden transcriptional variation in malaria parasites. Elife. 2018;7:e33105. Published 2018 Mar 27. doi:10.7554/eLife.33105.

[37] Xishuang Dong, Shanta Chowdhury, Uboho Victor, Xiangfang Li, Lijun Qian, Cell Type Identification from Single-Cell Transcriptomic Data via Semi-supervised Learning, 6 May 2020 in arXiv. url: https://arxiv.org/abs/2005.03994.

[38] Jian Hu, Xiangjie Li, Gang Hu, Yafei Lyu, Katalin Susztak, Mingyao Li, Iterative transfer learning with neural network for clustering and cell type classification in single-cell RNA-seq analysis,February 03, 2020. doi: https://doi.org/10.1101/2020.02.02.931139 Nature Machine Intelligence doi: 10.1038/s42256-020-00233-7

[39] Zhou, L.Q. et al. (2019) *Artificial intelligence in medical imaging of the liver.* World J. Gastroenterol. 25, 672–682

[40] Ho, C.W.L. et al. (2019) *Governance of automated image anal-ysis and artificial intelligence analytics in healthcare.* Clin. Radiol. 74, 329–337

[41] Samui, P. and Kothari, D.P. (2011) Utilization of a least square support vector machine (LSSVM) for slope stability analysis. Sci. Iran. 18, 53–58

[42] Sanchez-Lengeling, B. and Aspuru-Guzik, A. (2018) Inverse molecular design using machine learning: generative models for matter engineering. Science 361, 360–365

[43] Tyrchan, C. and Evertsson, E. (2017) Matched molecular pair analysis in short: algorithms, applications and limitations. Comput. Struct. Biotechnol. J. 15, 86–90

[44] Warner, D.J. et al. (2010) WizePairZ: a novel algorithm to identify, encode, and exploit matched molecular pairs with unspec-ified cores in medicinal chemistry. J. Chem. Inf. Model. 50, 1350–1357

[45] Lapins, M. et al. (2018) A confidence predictor for logD using conformal regression and a support-vector machine.J. Cheminform. 10, 17.

[46] Mayr, A. et al. (2016) DeepTox: toxicity prediction using deep learning. Front. Environ. Sci. 3, 80.

[47] Chan, H.C.S. et al. (2019) New binding sites, new opportunities for GPCR drug discovery. Trends Biochem. Sci. 44, 312–330.

[48] Chan, H.C.S. et al. (2018) Exploring a new ligand binding site of G protein-coupled receptors. Chem. Sci. 9, 6480–6489.

[49] Kufareva, I. et al. (2014) Advances in GPCR modeling evalu-ated by the GPCR Dock 2013 assessment: meeting new chal-lenges. Structure 22, 1120–1139.

[50] Yang, Z. et al. (2012) UCSF Chimera, MODELLER, and IMP: an integrated modeling system. J. Struct. Biol. 179, 269–278.

[51] Cavasotto, C.N. and Phatak, S.S. (2009) Homology modeling in drug discovery: current trends and applications. Drug Discov. Today 14, 676–683.

[52] Wang, M. et al. (2018) Predicting relative binding affinity using nonequilibrium QM/MM simulations. J. Chem. Theory Comput. 14, 6613–6622

[53] Hayik, S.A. et al. (2010) A mixed QM/MM scoring function to predict protein–ligand binding affinity. J. Chem. Theory Comput. 6, 3079–3091

[54] Ryde, U. (2016) QM/MM calculations on proteins. Methods Enzymol. 577, 119–158

[55] Smith, J.S. et al. (2017) ANI-1: an extensible neural network potential with DFT accuracy at force field computational cost. Chem. Sci. 8, 3192–3203

[56] Zhang, Y.J. et al. (2018) The potential for machine learning in hybrid QM/MM calculations. J. Chem. Phys. 148, 241740.

[57] Faber, F.A. et al. (2016) Machine learning energies of 2 million elpasolite (ABC2D6) crystals. Phys. Rev. Lett. 117, 135502.

[58] Steiner, S. et al.: Organic synthesis in a modular robotic system driven by a chemical programming language.2019, Science 363, eaav2211 https://science.sciencemag.org/content/363/6423/eaav2211#:~:text=CONCLUSION,robotic%20platform%20for%20organic%20synthesis. [Accessed: 21th February 2021]

[59] Ramsundar, B. et al.: Deep Learning for the Life Sciences, 2019, O'Reilly Media. https://www.oreilly.com/library/view/deep-learning-for/9781492039822/ [Accessed: 16 November 2016] [Accessed: 15th February 2021]

[60] Xu, Y. et al.: Demystifying multitask deep neural networks for quantitative structure–activity relationships.2017, J. Chem. Inf. Model. 57, 2490–2504. https://pubs.acs.org/doi/10.1021/acs.jcim.7b00087 [Accessed: 15th February 2021]

[61] Wang, C. and Zhang, Y.: Improving scoring-docking-screening powers of protein–ligand scoring functions using random forest., 2017, J. Comput. Chem. 38, 169–177 https://pubmed.ncbi.nlm.nih.gov/27859414/ [Accessed: 15th February 2021].

[62] Stork, C. et al., Hit Dexter 2.0: machine-learning models for the prediction of frequent hitters.,2019, J. Chem. Inf. Model. 59, 1030–1043. https://pubs.acs.org/doi/10.1021/acs.jcim.8b00677 [Accessed: 15th February 2021].

[63] Duvenaud, D.K. et al.: Convolutional networks on graphs for learning molecular fingerprints., 2015, In Advances in Neural Information Processing Systems (Vol. 28) (Cortes, C., et al., eds), pp. 2224–2232, NIPS Foundation. https://arxiv.org/abs/1509.09292 [Accessed: 10th February 2021].

[64] Durrant, J.D. and McCammon, J.A.: NNScore 2.0: a neural-network receptor–ligand scoring function., 2011, J. Chem. Inf. Model. 51, 2897–2903.

[65] Wojcikowski, M. et al. (2015) Open Drug Discovery Toolkit (ODDT): a new open-source player in the drug discovery field. J. Cheminform. 7, 26.

[66] Benjamin, S-L. et al. (2017) Optimizing distributions over molecular space. An objective-reinforced generative adversarial network for inverse-design chemistry (ORGANIC). ChemRxiv Published online August, 17, 2017. https://chemrxiv.org/articles/ORGANIC$_{1p}$*df*/5309668.

[67] Feinberg, E.N. et al. (2018) PotentialNet for molecular property prediction. ACS Cent. Sci. 4, 1520–1530

[68] Awale, M. and Reymond, J.L. (2019) Polypharmacology browser PPB2: target prediction combining nearest neighbors with machine learning. J. Chem. Inf. Model. 59, 10–17

[69] Olivecrona, M. et al. (2017) Molecular de-novo design through deep reinforcement learning. J. Cheminform. 9, 48

[70] Coley, C.W. et al. (2018) SCScore: synthetic complexity learned from a reaction corpus. J. Chem. Inf. Model. 58, 252–261

[71] Yasuo, N. and Sekijima, M. (2019) Improved method of structure-based virtual screening via interaction-energy-based learning. J. Chem. Inf. Model. 59, 1050–1061

[72] Batra, Kushal; Zorn, Kimberley M.; Foil, Daniel H.; Minerali, Eni; Gawriljuk, Victor O.; Lane, Thomas R.; et al. (2020): Quantum Machine Learning for Drug Discovery. ChemRxiv. Preprint. https://doi.org/10.26434/chemrxiv.12781232.v1.

Chapter 13

Plasmodium vivax and Drug Resistance

Puji Budi Setia Asih and Din Syafruddin

Abstract

Resistance to antimalarial drugs is a threat to global efforts to eliminate malaria by 2030. Currently, treatment for vivax malaria uses chloroquine or ACT for uncomplicated *P. vivax* whereas primaquine is given to eliminate latent liver stage infections (a method known as radical cure). Studies on *P. vivax* resistance to antimalarials and the molecular basis of resistance lags far behind the *P. falciparum* as *in vitro* cultivation of the *P. vivax* has not yet been established. Therefore, data on the *P. vivax* resistance to any antimalarial drugs are generated through *in vivo* studies or through monitoring of antimalarial treatments in mixed species infection. Indirect evidence through drug selective pressure on the parasites genome, as evidenced by the presence of the molecular marker(s) for drug resistance in areas where *P. falciparum* and *P. vivax* are distributed in sympatry may reflect, although require validation, the status of *P. vivax* resistance. This review focuses on the currently available data that may represent the *state-of-the art* of the *P. vivax* resistance status to antimalarial to anticipate the challenge for malaria elimination by 2030.

Keywords: *Plasmodium vivax*, antimalarials, resistance status, genetic marker(s)

1. Introduction

Plasmodium vivax presents a major challenge to achieving the global effort to eliminate malaria by 2030. The global distribution and factors that are associated with *P. vivax* occurrence in wider geographic regions in tropical, subtropical and temperate zones have extensively been reviewed recently [1, 2]. The ability of this species to undergo dormancy in the form of single-celled hypnozoites in the human liver, a safe haven from immune attack during the long mosquito-free cold seasons contributed to this phenomenon (**Figure 1**) [3]. Currently, *P. vivax* is present in 51 countries across Central and South America, the horn of Africa, Asia and the Pacific islands. Global malaria control and elimination programme successfully brought down the malaria incidence from 238 million cases in 2000 to 229 millions in 2019. The proportion of *P. vivax* cases declined from 7% in 2000 to 3% in 2019 [4]. Between 2000 and 2015, global malaria case incidence declined by 27%, and between 2015 and 2019 it declined by less than 2%, indicating a slowing of the rate of decline since 2015. Different from other human malaria, *P. vivax* uses Duffy antigen as its receptor in human to invade exclusively the young red blood cell (reticulocytes). Therefore, individuals who do not express the Duffy antigen are considered to be genetically resistant to *P. vivax* infection and this is particularly true in the majority of African sub-saharan population [5]. However, evidence for

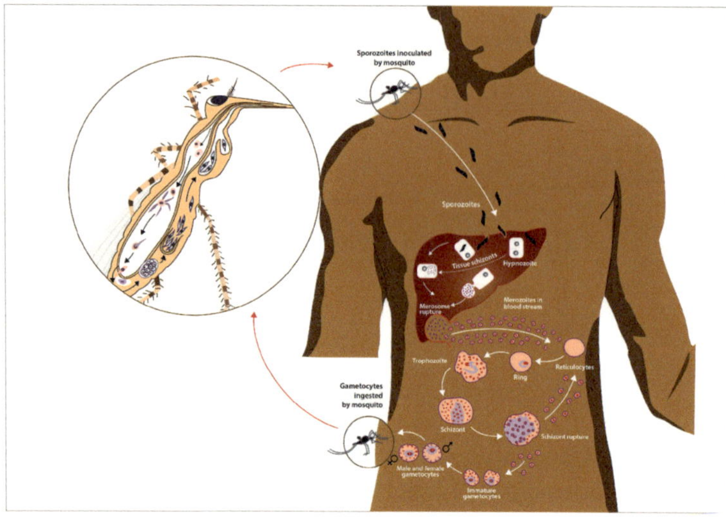

Figure 1.
Plasmodium vivax *life cycle [3].*

P. vivax infections in Duffy negative patients raise the possibility of an alternative invasion mechanism to Duffy [6, 7].

Plasmodium vivax in most geographic regions is distributed in sympatry with *P. falciparum*. This situation requires special attention during diagnosis and before prescription of drugs to the infected people. The biological characteristic of the *P. vivax* exhibit multiple exoerythrocytic cycle (relapses) from a single mosquito inoculation, and coupled with the very early emergence of gametocytes in the course of blood-stage infection, perhaps enables parasite survival and transmit to mosquito vector silently despite relatively low probability of propagation in blood. This propensity presents a unique challenge to the chemotherapeutic intervention against vivax malaria cases in which radical cure to block the reactivation of hypnozoites should be given in addition to blood schizontocide. Although *P. vivax* has been known to be less severe than *P. falciparum*, a growing body of evidence indicates that severe and fatal outcome also occurred in many *P. vivax* cases and necessitate the importance of reversing the historic neglect of this infection [8–10].

Treatment of *P. vivax* currently relies on either chloroquine or ACTs, supplemented both with 14 days primaquine as anti-hypnozoites. The only available drug for radical cure is primaquine but its use in vivax endemic region is limited by its potential serious complication among the people who inherit glucose-6-phosphate dehydrogenase (G6PD) enzyme deficiency.

The present review focuses on the recent progress that has been achieved to try to circumvent the problem of drug resistance in *P. vivax*. The global spread of chloroquine-resistant *P. vivax* has forced some countries to adopt artemisinin-based combination therapy (ACTs) to replace chloroquine as the first line drug to treat uncomplicated *P. vivax* and this policy change also impact the use of primaquine, the sole agent for anti-relapse. Many studies and reviews have been exclusively focused to elucidate the basic mechanism(s) of drug resistance in the malarial parasite using *P. falciparum* or other rodent and avian plasmodia as model while *P. vivax*, as usual, is consistently neglected. In discussing the topic, we will review all antimalarial drugs that used to be used or have been used to treat vivax malaria since the early development of quinine to date. Rapid development of resistance to the antimalarial drug mainstays from the early days to date will also be discussed to provide better perspectives for circumventing the problem of antimalarial drug resistance. The global extent of the drug-resistant *P. vivax* will also be reviewed to determine the appropriate measures based on drug policies that have been adopted by World Health Organisation (WHO) and implemented on local setting by member countries.

2. Challenges in the validation of drug resistance in *Plasmodium vivax*

2.1 Detection of hypnozoites

Historically, until to date, very few, if any, progress that has been achieved with regard to the biology of hypnozoites. Owing to its relatively "benign" clinical manifestation, the need for developing a more effective and less side effect radical cure have been hindered by our inability to detect the presence of hypnozoites in the liver cells. The occurrence of relapses in *P. vivax* after primaquine therapy would be assumed to be the most reliable indication of resistance. Nevertheless, recurrent parasite following primary attack may originate from failed therapy against asexual blood stages (recrudescence), biting infectious anopheline mosquitoes (reinfection), and reactivation of hypnozoites (relapse).

Since parasite arising from relapse may be genetically heterologous [11–13], distinguishing these events using molecular technologies is not yet possible, and this imposes limitations in estimating primaquine efficacy against relapse or resistance. Our inability to detect the presence of hypnozoite lead us to the assumption that every acute attack of *P. vivax* shall also harbour hypnozoites in the liver cell and this is supported by the fact that without prescription of anti-relapse, almost all acute attack will experience relapse within a year [14, 15]. Recent studies have tried to identify any protein (s) that are released by hypnozoites during its dormancy and some progress have been achieved in this endeavour. Although the finding is still a proof-of-principle, the presence of human arginase-I and an uncharacterized *P. vivax* protein in plasma-derived exosomes deserves further exploration on the potential to identify biomarkers of hypnozoite infection [16].

2.2 *In vitro* cultivation of *Plasmodium vivax*

Studies on *P. vivax* resistance to drugs used either as blood schizontocide or radical cure lags far behind *P. falciparum*. The absence of *in vitro* culture system for propagating the blood stage of *P. vivax* has made the *in vivo* test is the only way to determine the *P. vivax* drug response to any antimalarial drugs [17]. Advance in molecular and cellular biology within the last few decades have contributed significantly to the progress in the establishment and refinement of ex vivo drug test and repeatable *in vitro* cultivation in *P vivax* [18–20]. It has long been known that *P. vivax* invade exclusively young erythrocyte (reticulocytes) of Duffy antigen positive vertebrate host for asexual development in human and non human primate [21]. Recent progress have identified more specifically that *Plasmodium vivax* preferentially invade stage I reticulocytes $CD71^{high}TO^{high}$) [22]. Other progress also showed the success for long term cultivation, including cryopreservation and re-cultivation of *P. vivax* using blood of certain non-human primate [23]. With the aforementioned evidence, *ex vivo* and *in vitro* drug testing platform of *P. vivax* for novel drug development is now workable.

3. History of antimalarial drug use in vivax malaria

3.1 Quinine

Originally extracted from a Peruvian tree bark in South America, quinine was initially named cinchona in 1742 by Linnaeus. In 1820, two French chemists isolated quinine from the cinchona bark and this compound became a treatment of reference for intermittent fever throughout the world [24, 25] until the resistance of *P. falciparum* was first reported in Brazil in 1910 [26]. Quinine is also used for malaria prophylaxis. It was not clear as to whether the resistance rendered complete inefficacy of quinine to cure the falciparum malaria nor that it also occurred in other species, including *P. vivax* but it was evident that quinine was still widely used as the antimalarial mainstay until the second world war when the new antimalarial, chloroquine was introduced. As the advance in parasite biology provide more insight into parasite species diversity in human and other primates, the resistance phenomenon has attracted attention to investigate in animal model but the results were not conclusive [27]. At the end of 1930s, pamaquine, a new compound targeted at *P. vivax* liver stage was introduced, but 20 years later it was replaced by primaquine, a new 8-aminoquinoline compound. Primaquine is also still used until now as anti-hypnozoites for *P. vivax* [28] and malaria prophylactic [29] and anti-gametocyte drug for *P. falciparum* [30].

In response to the resistance to quinine in 1910 [26], scientists across the globe explore to find alternative treatment. Mepacrine was first synthesised in 1931 at Bayer, Germany. The product was one of the first synthetic substitutes for quinine although later superseded by chloroquine. Mepacrine (Atabrine) was used extensively during the second World War by Allied forces fighting in North Africa and the Far East to prevent malaria. This compound is also used for the treatment of giardiasis (an intestinal parasite) and has been researched as an inhibitor of phospholipase A2. Establishment of mepacrine-resistant strain in rodent plasmodia model indicated that the drug interfere with the haemozoin formation as that of quinine-resistant and primaquine-resistant strain [31]. The major breakthrough achieved during this period is the establishment of testing platform to raise drug-resistant malarial parasites in rodent model [32].

3.2 Primaquine (8-aminoquinoline)

Primaquine has long been used for radical cure to prevent relapse of malaria due to *P. vivax* and *P. ovale*. Primaquine kills hypnozoites, the dormant liver stage of the parasite. However, primaquine is known to cause severe haemolysis in patients with G6PD deficiency, a genetic disorder present in approximately 8% of the population in malaria endemic countries [33]. To prevent relapses, the World Health Organisation recommends the co-administration of CQ and standard- (total, 3.5 mg/kg) or high-dose PQ (total, 7.0 mg/kg) distributed over 14 days to patients aged >6 months with normal G6PD activity who are neither pregnant nor breast-feeding [34]. Nevertheless, adherence to such prolonged course in malaria endemic areas is poor and coupled with the fear of G6PD deficiency, prescription of this drug is mostly inadequate. Following reports of primaquine resistance in *P. vivax* in several geographic areas [35–40]. Collins and Jeffrey in1996 conducted a review and concluded that the data on the efficacy of primaquine as an anti relapse remains few and inconclusive. Therefore, the need for a standardised tool to determine primaquine resistance status should be developed [41, 42]. Primaquine is also known to possess blood schizontocidal activity as well as gametocytocidal activity in *P. falciparum*. In the context of anti-relapse activity in *P. vivax*, it is important to distinguish as to whether the observed recurrent parasite following a radical cure indeed originates from reactivated hypnozoites or recrudescence. Attempts to prescribe safer and shorter dose of primaquine rendered several improvements but dependence on G6PD screening could not be excluded [34]. Review on primaquine use in *P. vivax* concluded that the currently suggested indications in relation to vivax malaria, namely; causal prophylaxis, terminal prophylaxis, and radical cure is still highly effective [43, 44]. With regard to primaquine treatment failure in some areas, the presence of host genetic factors, such as single nucleotide polymorphisms (SNPs) in the gene encoding enzyme involved in primaquine metabolism, CYP2D6, may also be considered before claiming primaquine resistance [45, 46].

A new compound of 8-aminoquinoline class, tafenoquine was introduced following clinical trials in several countries [47, 48]. Despite single dose prescription, tafenoquine did not show any superiority to primaquine [49]. Therefore, development of a novel compound for anti-hypnozoites that does not depend on G6PD status still has to be prioritised.

3.3 Aminoquinoline antimalarials

Chloroquine was discovered in 1934, by Hans Andersag and co-workers at the Bayer laboratories. Research by German scientists to discover a substitute for quinine led to the synthesis in 1934 of Resochin (chloroquine) and Sontochin (3-methyl-chloroquine). After the war, chloroquine have for decades been the mainstays for malaria treatment and prevention during the global malaria eradication campaign by WHO in 1950s. This safe and inexpensive 4-aminoquinoline compound is believed to exert its antimalarial property through accumulation in the food vacuole [50]. The mechanisms by which chloroquine selectively accumulates may include protonation and ion trapping of the chloroquine due to the low pH of the food vacuole, active uptake of chloroquine by a parasite transporter(s), and/or binding of chloroquine to a specific receptor in the food vacuole [51–55].

After a decade of its use, chloroquine resistant *P. falciparum* arose in four separate locations, starting with the Thai-Cambodian border around 1957; in Venezuela and parts of Colombia around 1960; in Papua New Guinea in the mid-1970s and in Africa in 1978 in Kenya and Tanzania [56]. Resistance of *P. falciparum* to chloroquine changed the treatment policy to use several drugs such as halofantrine, lumefantrine, pyronaridine, mefloquine, and sulfadoxine-pyrimethamine (SP), while chloroquine and primaquine remain effective to treat *P. vivax* until few decades.

Resistance by *P. vivax* to chloroquine was unknown until 1989, when Australians repatriated from Papua New Guinea failed routine treatment [57]. Subsequent reports affirmed that finding and CQ-resistant *P. vivax* (CRPV) was reported from Indonesia [58] and Guyana [59]. A review and meta-analytic study evaluating chloroquine clinical trials performed during the period of 1960 to 2014 found out a contrasting evidence, indicating chloroquine sensitivity as shown by elimination of the asexual parasite by day 3 [60]. Although in some studies, a high degree of resistance was confirmed, the trials exhibited heterogeneity in study design and the presence of confounding factors such as interpretation of a recurrent parasites to distinguish relapse or recrudescence. In addition, technical issues on the quality and the dose of chloroquine used may also play role as the chloroquine possesses a wide therapeutic windows that enable to increase the dose. A therapeutic efficacy study to determine the efficacy of chloroquine in uncomplicated vivax malaria was conducted in Papua, Indonesia in 2007 isolated few recurrent parasites that survive chloroquine at blood concentration ranged from 100 ng/ml to 516 ng/ml [61]. Other study performed *in vitro* chloroquine sensitivity assay on either freshly collected or cryopreserved *P. vivax* isolates collected from Papua and Thailand [62]. The global spread of chlroquine-resistant *P. vivax* was later summarised in 2016 [63], as shown in **Figure 2**.

The absence of reliable, robust, sensitive methods for detection and monitoring of antimalarial drug efficacy in *P. vivax* has almost certainly contributed to the delayed recognition of this emerging problem [57]. Other factors include the relatively small parasite biomass in *P. vivax* infections, concomitant medication, such as primaquine to kill hypnozoites, early transmission due to the early presence of gametocytes, and high genetic diversity in natural population of *P. vivax* [64]. This delay has had important public health implications in areas where high-grade chloroquine-resistant *P. vivax* is prevalent (such as Indonesia and Oceania), partly effective drug treatments and consequent recurrent infections are an important contributing factor to severe anaemia from *P. vivax* malaria [65].

3.4 Resistance to antifolate and sulpha drugs

Proguanil, also known as chlorguanide and chloroguanide, is the first antifolate used to treat malaria. Proguanil is converted by the liver to its active metabolite, cycloguanil. The success of proguanil in treating human malaria led to further study of its chemical class and to the development of pyrimethamine in 1952. Resistance to the monotherapies of proguanil or pyrimethamine developed rapidly (within one year in the case of proguanil). A clear cut resistance to antifolate was proven in *P. falciparum, P. vivax* and *P. malariae* [66–68]. Sulfones and sulfonamides were then combined with proguanil or pyrimethamine in hopes of increasing efficacy and preventing or delaying resistance. By 1953, *P. falciparum* resistance had already been noted in Tanzania. When Sulfadoxine-pyrimethamine (SP) was introduced in Thailand in 1967, resistance appeared in the same year and spread quickly throughout South-East Asia. Resistance to SP in Africa remained low until the late 1990s but since then it has spread rapidly [69]. The SP has never been recommended for *P. vivax* treatment but evidence suggest that this compound is also effective to treat uncomplicated *P. vivax* [70, 71]. In response to resistance to SP and chloroquine, a combination of proguanil with a new class antimalarial compound, atovaquone, was introduced in 1999 by Glaxo-Smith Kline [72]. Nevertheless, prior

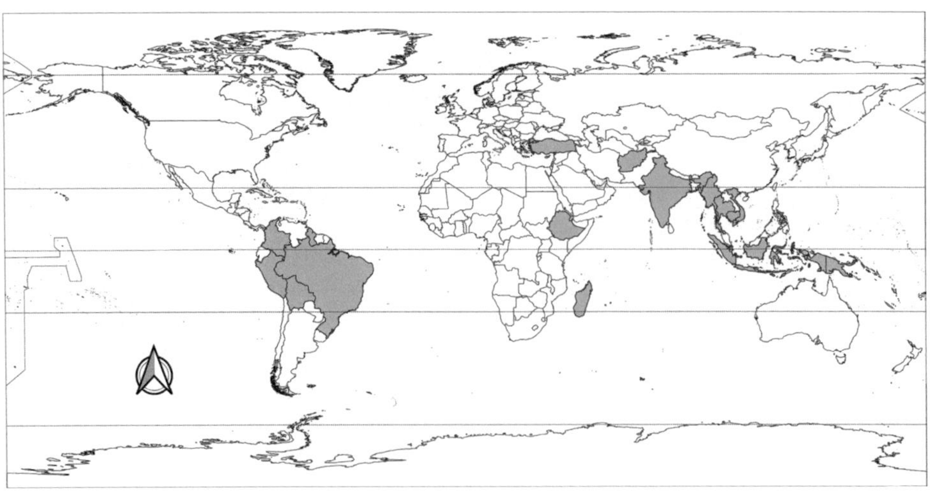

Figure 2.
Chloroquine -resistant P. vivax *infections. Source: World Wide Antimalarial Resistance Network (WWARN), available at: http://www.wwarn.org/vivax/surveyor/#0 and [64].*

to its introduction, resistance to atovaquone has been rapidly selected up in rodent plasmodia and *P. falciparum* [73, 74]. Since 2011, atovaquone-proguanil is available as a generic drug.

3.5 Artemisinin-based combination therapy (ACTs)

Artemisinin is a sesquiterpene lactone, containing the peroxide group, extracted and isolated from the leaves of *Artemisia annua.* by Chinese scientists in 1972 [75]. The drug and its derivatives play a role in killing *Plasmodium falciparum* by inhibiting the activity of phosphatidylinositol-3-kinase (PfPI3K) [76]. Initially, it was used as monotherapy to treat uncomplicated malaria but due to high recrudescence rate, a combination therapy was advised. Artemisinin-based Combination Therapy (ACTs), particularly artesunate-mefloquine, was introduced in Thailand during the early 1990s [77]. Since 2001, artemisinin (ART) combination therapy (ACT) has been recommended as the first-line treatment in the national treatment guidelines of most malaria endemic countries and have played an important role in reducing global malaria-associated mortality and morbidity [78].

Resistance to artemisinin was first detected in the Greater Mekong Subregion (GMS) region in 2008 [79]. Since then, ART resistance has spread and/or emerged in other areas of the GMS [80–83]. Exposure of the parasite population to artemisinin monotherapies in subtherapeutic doses for over 30 years, and the availability of substandard artemisinin, have probably been the main driving force in the selection of the resistant phenotype in the region. ART resistance is defined as the parasite clearance half-life of >5 h or presence of parasites in patients 3 days after treatment but has been more challenging to define, mostly because artemisinin act potently and rapidly clear parasites from the bloodstream by a unique mechanism involving the spleen [84, 85].

Currently, several drugs have been recommended (**Table 1**) for the treatment of severe and uncomplicated vivax malaria [34, 63, 86–90] and WHO is considering

	Drugs
Severe	
1	Artesunate
2	Artemether
3	Quinine
Uncomplicated	
1	Artesunate - Amodiaquine
2	Artemether - Lumefantrine
3	Artesunate - Mefloquine
4	Artesunate - Pyronaridine
5	Artesunate – Sulfadoxine/Pyrimethamine
6	Dihydroartemisinin - Piperaquine
7	Chloroquine
Antirelapse	
1	Primaquine
2	Tafenoquine

Table 1.
Antimalarial drugs for the treatment of Plasmodium vivax *malaria.*

the use of artesunate-pyronaridine, in areas where other ACTs are failing. In the absence of resistance, all six partner drugs would be highly efficacious as monotherapies at the dose used in the ACTs. Two injectable treatments, artesunate and artemether, are recommended for the treatment of severe malaria and should be followed by an ACTs once the patient can tolerate oral therapy [34].

Studies to monitor the efficacy of the ACTs on both *P. falciparum* and *P. vivax* have been conducted since the introduction of this drug in 2001. Evidence to date revealed that resistance of *P. falciparum* to artemisinin so far is not only confined to the Greater Mekong Subregion (GMS). Recent evidence indicated that *P. falciparum* isolates carrying the kelch13 C580Y mutation has been found in Papua New Guinea [91]. The finding is quite worrying as both PNG and Indonesia shared terrestrial border and the mutations may have spread to Indonesia. Therapeutic efficacy studies (TES) conducted during the period of 2009–2018 in various sites in Indonesia, including the Indonesia-PNG border documented no cases of either *P. falciparum and P. vivax* resistance nor treatment failure associated with artemisinin in Indonesia [92–96]. Nevertheless, recurrent parasite at late observation day was reported and this recurrence certainly nothing to do with artemisinin but rather with partner drug.

4. Molecular basis of *P. vivax* resistance to antimalarial drugs

The advent of molecular and cellular parasitology within the last 4 decades have brought along a lot of substantial innovations in the antimalarial drug testing platforms, molecular assays to phenotype as well as genotype the malarial parasite, although it mainly attributed to *P. falciparum*. In *P. vivax*, attempts to develop a repeatable *in vitro* drug resistance test continue to elude us, although certain progress has been achieved [23]. As a consequence, progress on the studies to elucidate the molecular basis of the *P. vivax* resistance to antimalarial drugs, particularly chloroquine and artemisinin is lagged far behind *P. falciparum*. While studies on molecular basis of resistance to chloroquine and artemisinin successfully identified candidate gene (s) through a clear phenotypic and genotypic assay, similar progress in *P. vivax* could not be achieved. The molecular basis of *Plasmodium* resistance to antifolates and sulpha drugs had been well described [97–99]. This evidence also applies to *P. vivax*, and the underlying genetic polymorphisms in dhfr and dhps genes, conferring resistance to antifolates and sulpha drugs, respectively. Likewise, resistance to atovaquone, a partner drug of proguanil has been associated genetic polymorphisms in the *cytb* gene of the malarial parasite [73, 74].

Resistance to chloroquine, has long been subject for research in many laboratories around the globe. A yet unclear mechanism of action of this compound making it more attractive for elucidation using molecular tool. Initially the role of *Plasmodium falciparum* multidrug resistance 1 (pfmdr1), homologous to the mammalian multiple drug resistance (MDR) gene were incriminated [100–102]. The product of thePfmdr1gene, P-glycoprotein homolog 1 *(Pgh1)* has been localized to the membrane of the digestive vacuole of mature blood stage parasites. This model predicted that thePfmdr1gene would be amplified and/or over expressed in CQ-resistant isolates. Further study, however identified different mechanism for chloroquine resistance but support for the role of this pfmdr1 in other antimalarials such as mefloquine, halofantrine and quinine [103–106]. Chloroquine-resistant parasites pump chloroquine out at 40 times the rate of chloroquine-sensitive parasites; the pump is coded by the *P. falciparum* chloroquine resistance transporter (*PfCRT*) gene [107, 108]. The natural function of the chloroquine pump is to transport peptides: mutations to the pump that allow it to pump chloroquine out impairs its function as a peptide pump and comes at a cost to the parasite, making it less fit.

Several genetic polymorphisms at the PfCRT gene have been associated with resistance to chloroquine in a wide geographic regions of malaria endemic areas [108]. Nevertheless, attempts to prove this finding in CRPV still fail, primarily because the technical difficulties in proving the resistant phenotype in *P. vivax*. Molecular analysis of the *P. vivax* isolates that have been phenotypically determined to be resistant in a rigorous *in vivo* and limited in vitro tests did not reveal any polymorphisms in the PvCRT gene as that of PfCRT. Instead, amplification of Pvmdr1 and several SNPs in the pvmdr1 was found to associate with CRPV [62]. Recent evidence found out that increases in PvCRT copy number associated with the *P. vivax* resistance to chloroquine [109–113].

The molecular basis for artemisinin resistance in the malarial parasite have also been described recently. Since mammalian kelch proteins can detect oxidants and other stressors, mutations in K13-propeller were reasonably implicated in mediating resistance to artemisinin and have been proposed as molecular marker [114–117]. Subsequent studies provided a more detail biochemical impact of the *PfKelch13* mutations on the decreased abundance of PfKelch13 protein, decreased haemoglobin digestion, and enhanced glutathione production [118]. However, the finding on the interaction of dihydroartemisinin with phosphatidylinositol-3-phosphate kinase, and that elevated phosphatidyl-inositol-3 phosphate can be associated with resistance in the absence of PfK13 mutations suggested for other mechanism [119]. In line with this evidence, Tyagi *et al* [120] raised a clear-cut artemisinin resistant isolates of *P. falciparum* following artesunate drug pressure in humanised mouse and the molecular analyses of the ART-resistant isolates revealed no mutations in PfK13 gene. Instead, an obvious selective pressure on RAD5 gene. Interestingly, the ART-resistant isolates also exhibited concomitant resistance to quinine, a second line drug used for treating severe malaria cases. The association between mutations in RAD5 gene and the resistance to artemisinin require further confirmation through either reverse genetics or genetic gross in mosquito.

Resistance of *P. vivax* to artemisinin so far has never been reported in areas where ACTs have long been used as first line drug for *P. vivax* malaria in South and Southeast Asia and the Pacific islands to replace chloroquine. This evidence, however, has to be carefully considered as *P. vivax* perhaps has long experienced with artemisinin pressure as that of *P. falciparum*, particularly in the GMS region where both species are distributed in sympatry and undetectable mixed species infection are common [121]. In support of this assumption, molecular analysis of *P. vivax* isolate from the GMS region revealed a high diversity and *ex vivo* analysis indicate reduced sensitivity to chloroquine, mefloquine, pyronaridine, piperaquine, quinine, artesunate and dihydroartemisinin [122, 123]. In this context, regular monitoring of the antimalarial treatment as well as genomic surveillance of the PvK12 gene, orthologues of the PfK13, in *P. vivax* and other relevant gene (s) should be conducted to monitor the emergence of artemisinin-resistant *P. vivax* and to contain the spread of the resistance to other regions [124, 125].

5. Conclusion

Reports of *P. vivax* resistance to primaquine and chloroquine have been well documented. Nevertheless, attempts to validate the resistance status of primaquine rendered an equivocal results. With the current limitation in testing platform both *in vivo* and *in vitro*, the use of primaquine as anti-relaps compound is still recommended. Therefore, factors that may limit its use in *P. vivax* endemic setting such as G5PD deficiency should be excluded by deploying a cheap, easy to use Point-of-Care (PoC) G6PD test.

Plasmodium vivax resistance to chloroquine present different burden to each geographic areas. Therefore, the use of alternative drug ACTs should be tailored following the degree of resistance to chloroquine, as well as therapeutic response to any available ACTs.

Plasmodium vivax resistance to artemisinin has never been found in any of the *P. vivax* isolates examined from different geographic regions but resistance to partner drug such as amodiaquine, piperaquine, lumefantrine, mefloquine and pyronaridine should be regularly monitored to safeguard our arsenal for achieving malaria elimination by 2030.

6. Future perspectives

Resistance of *P. vivax* to the antimalarial drug mainstays, chloroquine and primaquine poses a serious challenge to achieving the global malaria elimination that has been set up in 2030. Despite ambiguous evidence on both of this drug, chloroquine and primaquine deserve further exploration on its efficacy in different geographic setting before being side lined. To ensure the safe provision of primaquine treatment in *P. vivax,* local capacity to determine the existence host genetic factors such as G6PD deficiency as well as CYP2D6 allelic frequency should be established to mitigate the treatment failure that potentially increasing the risk of severe and fatal outcome.

Recent progress on the *in vitro* cultivation of *P. vivax* renew our interest to carefully validate the clinical phenotype of *P. vivax* isolates to the antimalarial drug mainstays, chloroquine, ACT and primaquine as well as the association with the genotype through genome-wide association study. In this context, progress achieved in *P. falciparum* certainly provide guidance to circumvent the limitations in *P. vivax*.

The proven efficacy of ACTs to vivax malaria in general and CRPV in particular, also support for our readiness to circumvent the problem of *P. vivax* resistance toward the remaining years ahead. Although the ACT is hastily paired with primaquine, evidence to date is still supportive.

Apart from our readiness to cope in turn the chemotherapeutic issue in combating *P. vivax,* efforts to mitigate the transmission through vector control should also be encouraged. A regular vector surveillance and control around the dwelling areas should be promoted to prevent the silent transmission of the parasite to Anopheles vector.

Acknowledgements

We gratefully acknowledge Prof. Amin Soebandrio MD, Ph.D, Clin. Microbiol, Chairman of the Eijkman Institute for Molecular Biology for his encouragement and advice and Prof. dr. Budu, Ph.D., Sp.M (K), M.Med.Ed, Dean of the Faculty of Medicine, Hasanuddin University for the support to DS. Therapeutics efficacy studies (TES) for period 2012–2021 in Eijkman Institute are supported by Government of Indonesia (Ministry of Research and Technology/National Research and Innovation Agency and Ministry of Health) and World Health Organisation.

List of acronyms

ACT	Artemisinin-based combination therapy
ART	Artemisinin

CQ	Chloroquine
CRPV	Chloroquine Resistant *Plasmodium vivax*
Cyp2D6	Cytochrome P450 2D6
G6PD	Glucose-6-phospate dehydrogenase
PfCRT	*P. falciparum* chloroquine resistance transporter
PfMDR	*P. falciparum* multidrug resistance
Pfdhfr	*Plasmodium falciparum* dihydrofolate reductase
Pfdhps	*Plasmodium falciparum* dihydropteroate synthetase
SNPs	Single nucleotide polymorphisms
SP	Sulfadoxine/Pyrimethamine
TES	Therapeutic efficacy studies

Author details

Puji Budi Setia Asih[1] and Din Syafruddin[1,2,3]*

1 Eijkman Institute for Molecular Biology, Jakarta, Indonesia

2 Hasanuddin University Medical Research Centre, Makassar, Indonesia

3 Department of Parasitology, Faculty of Medicine, Hasanuddin University, Makassar, Indonesia

*Address all correspondence to: din@eijkman.go.id

References

[1] Howes RE, Battle KE, Mendis KN, Smith DL, Cibulskis RE, Baird JK, Hay SI. Global Epidemiology of *Plasmodium vivax*. The American Journal Tropical Medicine and Hygiene. 2016; 95(6). DOI: 10.4269/ajtmh.16-0141

[2] Battle KE, Lucas TCD, Nguyen M, Howes RE, Nandi AK, Twohig KA, Pfeffer DA, Cameron E, Rao PC, Casey D, Gibson HS, Rozier JA, Dalrymple U, Keddie SH, Collins EL, Harris JR, Guerra CA, Thorn MP, Bisanzio D, Fullman N, Huynh CK, Kulikoff X, Kutz MJ, Lopez AD, Mokdad AH, Naghavi M, Nguyen G, Shackelford KA, Vos T, Wang H, Lim SS, Murray CLJ, Price RN, Baird JK, Smith DL, Bhatt S, Weiss DJ, Hay SI, Gething PW. Mapping the global endemicity and clinical burden of P*lasmodium vivax*, 2000-17: a spatial and temporal modelling study. Lancet. 2019;394(10195):332-343. DOI: 10.1016/S0140-6736(19)31096-7

[3] Mueller I, Galinski MR, Baird JK, Carlton JM, Kochar DK, Alonso PL, del Portillo HA. Key gaps in the knowledge of *Plasmodium vivax*, a neglected human malaria parasite. Lancet Infectious Diseases. 2009;(9):555-566. DOI: 10.1016/S1473-3099(09)70177-X

[4] World Health Organization. World Malaria Report. 2020. ISBN 978-92-4-001579-1

[5] Howes RE, Patil AP, Piel FB, Nyangiri OA, Kabaria CW, Gething PW, Zimmerman PA, Barnadas C, Beall CM, Gebremedhin A, Menard D, Williams TN, Weatherall DJ, Hay SI. 2011. The global distribution of the Duffy blood group. Nature Communication. 2011;2:266. DOI: 10.1038/ncomms1265

[6] Ménard D, Barnadas C, Bouchier C, Henry-Halldin C, Gray LR, Ratsimbasoa A, Thonier V, Carod JF, Domarle O, Colin Y, Bertrand O, Picot J, King CL, Grimberg BT, Mercereau-Puijalon O, Zimmerman PA. *Plasmodium vivax* clinical malaria is commonly observed in Duffy-negative Malagasy people. Proceedings of the National Academy of Sciences of the United States of America. 2010; 107(13):5967-5971. DOI: 10.1073/pnas.0912496107

[7] Zimmerman PA, Ferreira MU, Howes RE, Mercereau-Puijalon O. Red blood cell polymorphism and susceptibility to *Plasmodium vivax*. Advances in Parasitology. 2013;81:27-76. DOI: 10.1016/B978-0-12-407826-0.00002-3

[8] Rahimi BA, Thakkinstian A, White NJ, Sirivichayakul C, Dondorp AM, Chokejindachai W. Severe vivax malaria: A systematic review and meta-analysis of clinical studies since 1900. Malaria Journal. 2014;13: 481. DOI: 10.1186/1475-2875-13-481

[9] Baird JK, 2013. Evidence and implications of mortality associated with acute *Plasmodium vivax* malaria. Clinical Microbiology Review. 2013;26(1):36-57. DOI: 10.1128/CMR.00074-12

[10] Nicholas M Anstey, Nicholas M Douglas, Jeanne R Poespoprodjo, Ric N Price *Plasmodium vivax*: Clinical spectrum, risk factors and pathogenesis. Advance Parasitology. 2012; 80:151-201. DOI: 10.1016/B978-0-12-397900-1.00003-7

[11] Chen N, Auliff A, Rieckmann K, Gatton M, Cheng Q. Relapses of *Plasmodium vivax* infection result from clonal hypnozoites activated at predetermined intervals. The Journal Infectious Diseases. 2007; 195(7):934-941. DOI: 10.1086/512242

[12] Imwong M, Snounou G, Pukrittayakamee S, Tanomsing N, Kim JR, Nandy A, Guthmann JP, Nosten F, Carlton J, Looareesuwan S, Nair S, Sudimack D, Day NP, Anderson TJC, White NJ. Relapses of *Plasmodium vivax* infection usually result from activation of heterologous hypnozoites. The Journal Infectious Diseases. 2007;195(7):927-933. DOI: 10.1086/512241

[13] Imwong M, Boel M, Pagornrat W, Pimanpanarak M, McGready R, Day NPJ, Nosten F, White NJ. The first *Plasmodium vivax* relapses of life are usually genetically homologous. The Journal Infectious Diseases. 2012;205(4):680-683. DOI: 10.1093/infdis/jir806

[14] Baird JK, Hoffman SL. Primaquine therapy for malaria. Clinical Infectious Diseases. 2004; ;39(9):1336-45. DOI: 10.1086/424663

[15] Thomas D, Tazerouni H, Sundararaj KGS, Cooper JC. Therapeutic failure of primaquine and need for new medicines in radical cure of plasmodium vivax. Acta Tropica. 2016;160:35-38. DOI: 10.1016/j.actatropica.2016.04.009

[16] Gualdrón-López M, Flannery EL, Kangwanrangsan N, Chuenchob V, Fernandez-Orth D, Segui-Barber J, Royo F, Falcón-Pérez JM, Fernandez-Becerra C, Lacerda MVG, Kappe SHI, Sattabongkot J, Gonzalez JR, Mikolajczak SA, Del-Portillo HA. Characterization of plasmodium vivax proteins in plasma-derived exosomes from malaria-infected liver-chimeric humanized mice. Front Microbiology. 2018;9:1271. DOI: 10.3389/fmicb.2018.01271

[17] Udomsangpetch R, Kaneko O, Chotivanich K, Sattabongkot J. Cultivation of *Plasmodium vivax*. Trends Parasitology. 2008;24(2):85-88. DOI: 10.1016/j.pt.2007.09.010

[18] Shaw-Saliba K, Clarke D, Santos JM, Menezes MJ, Lim C, Mascarenhas A, Chery L, Gomes E, March S, Bhatia SN, Rathod PK, Ferreira MU, Catteruccia F, Duraisingh MT. Infection of laboratory colonies of anopheles mosquitoes with plasmodium vivax from cryopreserved clinical isolates. International Journal Parasitololy. 2016;46(11):679-683. DOI: 10.1016/j.ijpara.2016.06.003.

[19] Rangel GW. Empowering the Experimental Biology of Plasmodium Vivax Through Elucidating Requirements for Ex Vivo Culture. 2019. Doctoral Disertation, Harvard university, Graduare School of Arts and Sciences.

[20] Rangel GW, Clark MA, Kanjee U, Lim C, Shaw-Saliba K, Menezes MJ, Mascarenhas A, Chery L, Gomes E, Rathod PK, Ferreira MU, Duraisingh MT. Enhanced ex vivo plasmodium vivax Intraerythrocytic enrichment and maturation for rapid and sensitive parasite growth assays. Antimicrobial Agents Chemotherapy. 2018;62(4):e02519-e02517. DOI: 10.1128/AAC.02519-17. Print 2018 Apr.

[21] King CL, Adams JH, Xianli J, Grimberg BT, McHenry AM, Greenberg LJ, Siddiqui A, Howes RE, da Silva-Nunes M, Ferreira MU, Zimmerman PA. Fy(a)/Fy(b) antigen polymorphism in human erythrocyte Duffyantigen affects susceptibility to *Plasmodium vivax* malaria. Proceedings of the National Academy of Sciences of the United States of America. 2011;108(50):20113-20118. DOI: 10.1073/pnas.1109621108

[22] Bermúdez M, Moreno-Pérez DA, Arévalo-Pinzón G, Curtidor H, Patarroyo MA. *Plasmodium vivax in vitro* continuous culture: The spoke in the wheel. Malaria Journal. 2018; 17:301. DOI: https://doi.org/10.1186/s12936-018-2456-5

[23] Mehlotra RK, Blankenship D, Howes RE, Rakotomanga TA,

Ramiranirina B, Ramboarina S, Franchard T, Linger MH, Zikursh-Blood M, Ratsimbasoa AC, Zimmerman PA, Grimberg BT. Long term in vitro culture of plasmodium vivax isolates from Madagascar maintained in *Saimiri boliviensis* blood. Malaria Journal. 2017;16:442. DOI: 10.1186/s12936-017-2090-7

[24] Achan J, Talisuna AO, Erhart A, Yeka A, Tibenderana JK, Baliraine FN, Rosenthal PJ, D'Alessandro U. Quinine, an old anti-malarial drug in a modern world: Role in the treatment of malaria. Malaria journal. 2011;10:144. DOI: https://doi.org/10.1186/1475-2875-10-144

[25] Bunnag D, Karbwang J, Na-Bangchang K, Thanavibul A, Chittamas S, Harinasuta T. Quinine-tetracycline for multidrug resistant falciparum malaria. The Southeast Asian Journal of Tropical Medicine and Public Health. 1996;27:15-18. PMID: 9031393

[26] Da Silva AF, Benchimol F. Malaria and quinine resistance: A medical and scientific issue between Brazil and Germany, (1907-1919). Medical history. 2014:58(1):1-26. DOI: 10.1017/mdh.2013.69

[27] Peters W. Plasmodium: Resistance To Antimalarial Drugs. Annales de Parasitologie Humaine et Comparee. 1990; 65:603-606

[28] John GK, Douglas NM, von Seidlein L, Nosten F, Baird JK, White NJ, Price RN. Primaquine radical cure of *Plasmodium vivax*: A critical review of the literature. Malaria Journal. 2012; 11:280. DOI: 10.1186/1475-2875-11-280

[29] Hill DR, Baird JK, Parise ME, Lewis LS, Ryan ET, Magill AJ. Primaquine: Report from CDC expert meeting on malaria chemoprophylaxis I. The American Journal Tropical Medicine and Hygiene. 2006;75:402-415. PMID: 16968913

[30] World Health Organization: Single dose primaquine as a gametocytocide in Plasmodium falciparum malaria. Geneva, Switzerland: October 2012. Archived from the original on 2 January 2014

[31] Peters W. Mepacrine- and Primaquine-resistant strains of plasmodium berghei, Vincke and lips, 1948, 1964. Nature. 208:1290. DOI: https://doi.org/10.1038/208693a0

[32] Peters W. Chemotherapy and Drug Resistance in Malaria. 2nd ed. *Academic Press,* London, 1987.

[33] Howes RE, Piel FB, Patil AP, Nyangiri OA, Gething PW, Dewi M, Hogg MM, Battle KE, Padilla CD, Baird JK, Hay SI. G6PD deficiency prevalence and estimates of affected populations in malaria endemic countries: A geostatistical model-based map. PLoS Medicine. 2012;9: e1001339. DOI: doi: 10.1371/journal.pmed.1001339

[34] World Health Organization: Guidelines for the treatment of malaria. 3rd ed. Geneva. 2015 (http://apps.who.int/iris/bitstream/10665/162441/1/9789241549127_eng.pdf. opens in new tab)

[35] Krotoski WA, 1980. Frequency of relapse and primaquine resistance in southeast Asian vivax malaria. The New England journal of medicine. 303: 587. DOI: 10.1056/NEJM198009043031022

[36] Rombo L, Edwards G, Ward SA, Eriksson G, Lindquist L, Lindberg A, Runehagen A, Bjorkman A, Hylander NO. Seven patients with relapses of *Plasmodium vivax* or *P. ovale* despite primaquine treatment. Tropical Medicine and Parasitology. 1987;38(1):49-50. PMID: 3299660

[37] Cabezos J, Duran E, Tomas D, Bada JL. Resistencia de *Plasmodium vivax* a la primaquina. Medicina Clinica. 1994; 103. PMID: 8072336

[38] Luzzi GA, Warrell DA, Barnes AJ, Dunbar EM. Treatment of primaquine-resistant plasmodium vivax malaria. Lancet. 1992; 340: 310. DOI: 10.1016/0140-6736(92)92404-4

[39] Charoenlarp P. Harinasuta T, 1973. Relapses of vivax malaria after a conventional course of primaquine and chloroquine: Report of 2 cases. The Southeast Asian Journal of Tropical Medicine and Public Health. 1973;4(1):135-137. PMID: 4577922

[40] Bunnag D, Karbwang J, Thanavibul A, Chittamas S. Ratana pongse Y, Chalermrut K, Bangshang KN, Harinasuta T. High dose of primaquine in primaquine resistant vivax malaria. Transactions of the Royal Society of Tropical Medicine and Hygiene. 1994;88: 2 18-219. DOI: 10.1016/0035-9203(94)90305-0

[41] Collins WE, Jeffrey GM. Primaquine resistance in *Plasmodium vivax*. The American Journal Tropical Medicine and Hygiene. 1996;55(3)341-349. DOI: 10.4269/ajtmh.1996.55.243

[42] Fernando D, Rodrigo C, Rajapakse S. Primaquine in vivax malaria: An update and review on management issues. Malaria Journal. 2011;10-15. DOI: 10.1186/1475-2875-10-351

[43] Baird JK. Therapeutic principles of primaquine against relapse of *Plasmodium vivax* malaria. IOP Conf. Series: Earth and Environmental Science 12132455(627081980) 012098. DOI: 10.1088/1755-1315/125/1/012098

[44] Dijanic C, Nickerson J, Shakya S, Dijanic A, Fabbri M. "Relapsing malaria: A case report of Primaquine resistance", *Case Reports in Infectious Diseases*, vol. 2018, Article ID 9720823, 3 Pages. DOI: https://doi.org/10.1155/2018/9720823

[45] Bennett JW, Pybus BS, Yadava A, Tosh A, Jason RN, Sousa C, McCarthy WF, Deye G, Melendez V, Ockenhouse CF. Primaquine failure and cytochrome P-450 2D6 in *Plasmodium vivax* malaria. The New England Journal of Medicine. 2013;369(14):1381-1382. DOI: 10.1056/NEJMc1301936

[46] Baird JK, Louisa M, Noviyanti R, Ekawati L, Elyazar I, Subekti D, Chand K, Gayatri A, Instiaty, Soebianto S, Crenna-Darusallam C, Djoko D, Hasto BD, Meriyenes D, Wesche D, Nelwan EJ, Sutanto I, Sudoyo H, Setiabudy R. Association of Impaired Cytochrome P450 2D6 Activity Genotype and Phenotype With Therapeutic Efficacy of Primaquine Treatment for Latent Plasmodium vivax Malaria. Journal of the American Medical Association Network Open. 2018;1(4):e181449. DOI: 10.1001/jamanetworkopen.2018.1449

[47] Peters W. The evolution of tafenoquine--antimalarial for a new millennium?". Journal of the Royal Society of Medicine. 1999; 92(7):345-352. DOI: 10.1177/014107689909200705

[48] Haston JC, Hwang J, Tan KR. Guidance for Using Tafenoquine for Prevention and Antirelapse Therapy for Malaria — United States. "Morbidity and Mortality Weekly Report. 2019;68 (46): 1062-1068. DOI: doi:10.15585/mmwr.mm6846a4

[49] Quinn JC, McCarthy S. Tafenoquine versus Primaquine to prevent relapse of *Plasmodium vivax* malaria. The New England journal of medicine. 2019 May 9;380(19):1875. DOI: 10.1056/NEJMc1902327

[50] Homewood CA, Warhurst DC, Peters W, Baggaley VC. Lysosomes, pH and the anti-malarial action of chloroquine. Nature. 1972; 235: 50-52. DOI: 10.1038/235050a0

[51] Yayon A, Cabantchik ZI, Ginsburg H. Identification of the acidic compartment of *Plasmodium*

falciparum-infected human erythrocytes as the target of the antimalarial drug chloroquine. European Molecular Biology Organization. 1984;3: 2695-2700. PMCID: PMC557751

[52] Bray PG, Janneh O, Raynes KJ, Mungthin M, Ginsburg H, Ward SA. Cellular uptake of chloroquine is dependent on binding to ferriprotoporphyrin IX and is independent of NHE activity in *Plasmodium falciparum*. Journal of Cell Biology. 1999;145: 363-376. DOI: 10.1083/jcb.145.2.363

[53] Bray PG, Mungthin M, Ridley RG, Ward SA. Access to hematin: The basis of chloroquine resistance. Molecular pharmacology. 1998;54: 170-179. DOI: https://doi.org/10.1124/mol.54.1.170

[54] Ridley RG. Malaria: Dissecting chloroquine resistance. 1998. Current Biology. 1998; 8:8346-8349. DOI: 10.1016/s0960-9822(98)70218-0

[55] Peters W. Resistance in human malaria IV: 4-aminoquinolines and multiple resistance. In: Chemotherapy and Drug Resistance in Malaria. Vol 2. London: Academic Press, 1987:659-786.

[56] Payne D. Spread of chloroquine resistance in *Plasmodium falciparum.* Parasitology Today. 1987;3:241-246. DOI: 10.1016/0169-4758(87)90147-5

[57] Rieckmann KH, Davis DR, Hutton DC. *Plasmodium vivax* resistance to chloroquine? Lancet. 1989;2:1183-1184. DOI: 10.1016/s0140-6736(89)91792-3

[58] Baird JK, Basri H, Purnomo Bangs MJ, Subianto B, Patchen LC. Resistance to chloroquine by *Plasmodium vivax* in Irian Jaya, Indonesia. The American Journal of Tropical Medicine and Hygiene. 1991;44:547-552. DOI: 10.4269/ajtmh.1991.44.547

[59] Phillips EJ, Keystone JS, Kain KC 1996. Failure of combined chloro- quine and high-dose primaquine therapy for *Plasmodium vivax* malaria acquired in Guyana, South America. Clin Infect Dis *23*: 1171-1173.

[60] Price RN, Seidlein LV, Valecha N, Nosten F, Baird JK, White NJ. Global extent of chloroquine-resistant *Plasmodium vivax*: A systematic review and meta-analysis. Lancet Infectious Diseases. 2014;14(10):982-991. DOI: 10.1016/S1473-3099(14)70855-2

[61] Asih PBS, Syafruddin D, Leake J, Sorontou Y, Sadikin M, Sauerwein RW, Vinetz J, Baird JK. Phenotyping clinical resistance to chloroquine in *Plasmodium vivax* in northeastern Papua, Indonesia. International Journal for Parasitology: Drugs and Drug Resistance, 2011;1:28-32. DOI: 10.1016/j.ijpddr.2011.08.001

[62] Suwanarusk R, Chavchich M, Russell B, Jaidee A, Chalfein F, Barends M, et al. Amplification of pvmdr1 associated with multidrug-resistant Plasmodium vivax. J Infect Dis. 2008; 198(10):1558-64. https://doi.org/10.1086/592451 PMID: 18808339; PubMed Central PMCID: PMC4337975

[63] Baird JK, Valecha N, Duparc S, White NJ and Price RN. Diagnosis and treatment of plasmodium vivax malaria. Am. J. Trop. Med. Hyg., 95(Suppl 6), 2016, pp. 35-51 doi:10.4269/ajtmh.16-0171

[64] Ferreira MU, de Sousa TN, Rangel GW, Johansen IC, Corder RM, Ladeia-Andrade S, Gilf JP. Monitoring plasmodium vivax resistance to antimalarials: Persisting challenges and future directions. International Journal Parasitology Drugs and Drug Resistance. 2021;15:9-24.DOI: 10.1016/j.ijpddr.2020.12.001

[65] Price RN, Simpson JA, Nosten F, Luxemburger C, Hkirjaroen L, ter Kuile F, Chongsuphajaisiddhi T,

White NJ. Factors contributing to anemia after uncomplicated falciparum malaria. The American Journal of Tropical Medicine and Hygiene. 2001; 65(5): 614-22. DOI: https://doi.org/10.4269/ajtmh.2001.65.614

[66] Cowman AF, Morry MJ, Biggs BA, Cross GA, Foote SJ. Amino acid changes linked to pyrimethamine resistance in the dihydrofolate reductase-thymidylate synthase gene of *Plasmodium falciparum.* Proceedings of the National Academy of Sciences of the United States of America. 1988;85:9109-9113. DOI: 10.1073/pnas.85.23.9109.

[67] Peterson DS, Walliker D, Wellems TE. Evidence that a point mutation in dihydrofolate reductase-thymidylate synthase confers resistance to pyrimethamine in falciparum malaria. Proceedings of the National Academy of Sciences of the United States of America. 1988;85: 9114-9118. DOI: 10.1073/pnas.85.23.9114

[68] Foote SJ, Galatis D, Cowman AF. Amino acids in the dihydrofolate reductase-thymidylate synthase gene of *Plasmodium falciparum* involved in cycloguanil resistance differ from those involved in pyrimethamine resistance. Proceedings of the National Academy of Sciences of the United States of America. 1990;87: 3014-3017. DOI: 10.1073/pnas.87.8.3014

[69] Amimo F, Lambert B, Magit A, Sacarlal J, Hashizume M. Shibuya K. Plasmodium falciparum resistance to Sulfadoxine-Pyrimethamine in Africa: A systematic analysis of national trend. British Medical Journal Global Health. 2020;5(11):e003217. DOI: 10.1136/bmjgh-2020-003217

[70] Doberstyn EB, Teerakiartkamjorn C, Andre RG, Phintuyothin P and Noeypatimanondh. Treatment of vivax malaria with sulfadoxine-pyrimethamine and with pyrimethamine alone. Transactions of the Royal Society of Tropical Medicine and Hygiene, 1979; 73, 1

[71] Asih,PBS, Marantina SS, Nababan R, Lobo NF, Rozi, mIR, Sumarto W, Dewi RM, Sekartuti, Taufik AS, Mulyanto, Sauerwein RS and Din Syafruddin. Distribution of Plasmodium vivax pvdhfr and pvdhps alleles and their association with sulfadoxine–pyrimethamine treatment outcomes in Indonesia. Malar J 2015;14:365 DOI 10.1186/s12936-015-0903-0

[72] Nakato H, Vivancos R, Hunter PR. A systematic review and meta-analysis of the effectiveness and safety of atovaquone–proguanil (Malarone) for chemoprophylaxis against malaria. Journal of Antimicrobial Chemotherapy. 2007;60(5):929-936. DOI: 10.1093/jac/dkm337

[73] Syafruddin, Siregar JE, Marzuki S. Mutations in the *cytochrome b* gene of *Plasmodium berghei* conferring resistance to atovaquone. Molecular and Biochemical Parasitology. 1999;104:185-194. DOI: 10.1016/s0166-6851(99)00148-6

[74] Korsinczky M, Chen N, Kotecka B, Saul A, Rieckmann K, Cheng Q. Mutations in *Plasmodium falciparum* cytochrome b that are associated with atovaquone resistance are located at a putative drug-binding site. Antimicrobial Agents and Chemotherapy, 2000;44(8):2100-2108. DOI: 10.1128/aac.44.8.2100-2108

[75] Tu Y. The discovery of artemisinin (qinghaosu) and gifts from Chinese medicine. Nature Medicine. 2011;17(10):1217-1220. DOI: 10.1038/nm.2471

[76] Mok S, Ashley EA, Ferreira PE, Zhu L, Lin Z, Yeo T, Chotivanich K, Imwong M, Pukrittayakamee S, Dhorda M, Nguon C, Lim P, Amaratunga C, Suon S, Hien TT, Htut Y,

Faiz MA, Onyamboko MA, Mayxay M, Newton PN, Tripura R, Woodrow CJ, Miotto O, Kwiatkowski DP, Nosten F, Day NPJ, Preiser PR, White NJ, Dondorp AM, Fairhurst RM, Bozdech B. Drug resistance: Population transcriptomics of human malaria parasites reveals the mechanism of artemisinin resistance. Science. 2015 ;347(6220):431-435. DOI: 10.1126/science.1260403

[77] Nosten F, Luxemburger C, ter Kuile FO, Woodrow C, Eh JP, Chongsuphajaisiddhi T, White NJ. Treatment Of Multidrug-Resistant *Plasmodium falcipa*rum Malaria With 3-Day Artesunate-Mefloquine Combination. The Journal of Infectious Diseases. 1994;170(4):971-977. DOI: https: //doi.org/10.1093/infdis/170.4.971

[78] Eastman RT, Fidock DA. Artemisinin-based combination therapies: A vital tool in efforts to eliminate malaria. Nature Reviews Microbiology. 2009;7(12):864-874. DOI: 10.1038/nrmicro2239

[79] Noedl H, Se Y, Schaecher K, Smith BL, Socheat D, Fukuda MM, Artemisinin resistance in Cambodia 1 (ARC1) study consortium. Evidence of artemisinin-resistant malaria in western Cambodia. The New England Journal of Medicine. 2008;359(24):2619-2620. DOI: 10.1056/NEJMc0805011

[80] Dondorp AM, Nosten F, Yi P, Das D, Phyo AP, Tarning J, Lwin KM, Ariey F, Hanpithakpong W, Lee SJ, Ringwald P, Silamut S, Imwong M, Chotivanich K, Lim P, Herdman T, An SS, Yeung S, Pratap Singhasivanon, Nicholas P J Day, Niklas Lindegardh, Socheat D, White NJ. Artemisinin-resistant plasmodium falciparum malaria. The New England Journal of Medicine. 2009;361(5):455-467. DOI: 10.1056/NEJMoa0808859.

[81] Phyo AP, Nkhoma S, Stepniewska S, Ashley EA, Nair S, McGready R, Moo CL, Al-Saai S, Dondorp AM, Lwin KM, Singhasivanon P, Day NPJ, White NJ, Anderson TJM, Nosten F. Emergence of artemisinin-resistant malaria on the western border of Thailand: A longitudinal study. Lancet. 2012 ;379(9830):1960-1966. DOI: 10.1016/S0140-6736(12)60484-X

[82] Hien TT, Thuy-Nhien NY, Phu NH, Boni MF, Thanh NV, Nha-Ca NT, Thai LH, Thai LQ, Toi PV, Thuan PD, Long LT, Dong LT, Merson L, Dolecek C, Stepniewska K, Ringwald P, White NJ, Farrar J, Wolbers M. *In vivo* susceptibility of *Plasmodium falciparum* to artesunate in Binh Phuoc Province Vietnam. Malaria journal. 2012;11:355. DOI: https://doi.org/10.1186/1475-2875-11-355

[83] Kyaw MP, Nyunt MH, Chit K, Aye MM, Aye KH, Aye MM, Lindegardh N, Tarning J, Imwong M, Jacob CG, Rasmussen C, Perin J, Ringwald P, Nyunt MM. Reduced susceptibility of *Plasmodium falciparum* to artesunate in southern Myanmar. PLoS ONE. 2013;8(3):e57689. DOI: 10.1371/journal.pone.0057689

[84] Chotivanich K, Udomsangpetch R, Dondorp A, Williams T, Angus B, Simpson JA, Pukrittayakamee S, Looareesuwan S, Newbold CI, White NJ. The mechanisms of parasite clearance after antimalarial treatment of *Plasmodium falciparum* malaria. Journal Infectious Diseases. 2000; 182(2):629-33. DOI: https://doi.org/10.1086/315718

[85] Buffet PA, Milon G, Brousse V, Correas JM, Dousset B, Couvelard A, Kianmanesh R, Farges O, Sauvanet A, Paye F, Ungeheuer MN, Ottone C, Khun H, Fiette L, Guigon G, Huerre M, Mercereau-Puijalon O, David PH. *Ex vivo* perfusion of human spleens maintains clearing and processing functions. Blood. 2006;107(9):3745-3752. DOI: 10.1182/blood-2005-10-4094

[86] Commons RJ, Simpson JA, Thriemer K, Abreha T, Adam I, Anstey NM, Assefa A, Awab GR, Baird JK, Barber BE, Chu CS, Dahal P, Daher A, Davis TME, Dondorp AM, Grigg MJ, Humphreys GS, Hwang J, Karunajeewa H, Laman M, Lidia K, Moore BR, Mueller I, Nosten F, Pasaribu AP, Pereira DB, Phyo AP, Poespoprodjo JR, Sibley CH, Stepniewska K, Sutanto I, Thwaites G, Hien TT, White NJ, William T, Woodrow CJ, Guerin PJ, Price RN. The efficacy of dihydroartemisinin-piperaquine and artemether-lumefantrine with and without primaquine on *Plasmodium vivax* recurrence: A systematic review and individual patient data meta-analysis. PLoS Medicine. 2019; 16(10): e1002928. DOI: https://doi.org/10.1371/journal.pmed.1002928

[87] Ratcliff A, Siswantoro H, Kenangalem E, Maristela R, Wuwung RM, Laihad F, Ebsworth EP, Anstey NM, Tjitra E, Price RN. Two fixed-dose artemisinin combinations for drug-resistant falciparum and vivax malaria in Papua, Indonesia: an open-label randomised comparison. Lancet. 2007; 369(9563): 757-765. DOI: https://doi.org/10.1016/S0140-6736(07)60160-3

[88] Hasugian AR, Purba HL, Kenangalem E, Wuwung RM, Ebsworth EP, Maristela R, Penttinen PMP, Laihad F, Anstey NM, Tjitra E, Price RN. Dihydroartemisinin-piperaquine versus artesunate-amodiaquine: superior efficacy and posttreatment prophylaxis against multidrug-resistant *Plasmodium falciparum* and *Plasmodium vivax* malaria. Clinical Infectious Diseases. 2007; 44(8): 1067-74. DOI: https://doi.org/10.1086/512677

[89] Smithuis F, Kyaw MK, Phe O, Win T, Aung PP, Oo APP, Naing AL, Nyo MY, Myint NZH, Imwong M, Ashley E, Lee SJ, White NJ. Effectiveness of five artemisinin combination regimens with or without primaquine in uncomplicated falciparum malaria: An open-label randomised trial. Lancet Infectious Diseases. 2010; 10(10): 673-81. DOI: https://doi.org/10.1016/S1473-3099(10)70187-0

[90] Gogtay N, Kannan S, Thatte UM, Olliaro PL, Sinclair D. Artemisinin-based combination therapy for treating uncomplicated *Plasmodium vivax* malaria. Cochrane Database Systematic Review. 2013;10 CD008492. DOI: 10.1002/14651858.CD008492

[91] Miotto O, Sekihara M, Tachibana SI, Yamauchi M, Pearson RD, Amato R, Gonçalves S, Mehra S, Noviyanti R, Marfurt J, Auburn S, Price RN, Mueller I, Ikeda M, Mori T, Hirai M, Tavul L, Hetzel MW, Laman M, Barry AE, Ringwald P, Ohashi J, Hombhanje F, Kwiatkowski DP, Mita T. Emergence of artemisinin-resistant *Plasmodium falciparum* with kelch13 C580Y mutations on the island of New Guinea. PLoS Pathogen. 2020;16(12):e1009133. DOI: 10.1371/journal.ppat.1009133

[92] Asih PBS, Dewi RM, Tuti S, Sadikin M, Sumarto W, Sinaga BN, van der Ven AJAM, Sauerwein RW, Syafruddin D. Efficacy of artemisinin-based combination therapy for treatment of persons with uncomplicated *Plasmodium falciparum* malaria in west Sumba District, East Nusa Tenggara Province, Indonesia, and genotypic profiles of the parasite. The American Journal of Tropical Medicine and Hygiene. 2009;80(6):914-918. PMID: 19478248

[93] Syafruddin D. Evaluation of the parasite clearance day following treatment with artesunate-amodiaquine in subjects uncomplicated *Plasmodium falciparum* malaria in Indonesia. 2012. Technical Report TES Indonesia

[94] Syafruddin D. Efficacy and safety of dihydroartemisinin-piperaquine for the treatment of uncomplicated *Plasmodium falciparum* and *Plasmodium vivax* malaria in 5 sentinel sites in Indonesia . 2016. Technical Report TES Indonesia

[95] Poespoprodjo JR, Kenangalem E, Wafom J, Chandrawati F, Puspitasari AM, Ley B, Trianty L, Korten Z, Surya A, Syafruddin D, Anstey NM, Marfurt J, Noviyanti R, Price RN. Therapeutic Response to Dihydroartemisinin-Piperaquine for *P. falciparum* and *P. vivax* Nine Years after Its Introduction in Southern Papua, Indonesia. The American Society of Tropical Medicine and Hygiene. 2018; 98(3):677-82. DOI: https://doi.org/10.4269/ajtmh.17-0662

[96] Asih PB, Rozi IE, Dewayanti FK, Wangsamuda S, Zulfah S, Robaha M, Hutahaean J, Anggraeni ND, Kusumaningsih M, Mulyani PS, Sariwati E, Basri HH, Bustos MDG, Syafruddin D. fficacy and safety of dihydroartemisinin-piperaquine for the treatment of uncomplicated *Plasmodium falciparum* and *Plasmodium vivax* malaria in Northern Papua and Jambi, Indonesia. 2020; medRXiv. DOI: https://doi.org/10.1101/2020.09.04.20188706

[97] Peterson DS, Milhous WK, Wellems TE. Molecular basis of differential resistance to cycloguanil and pyrimethamine in *Plasmodium falciparum* malaria. Proceedings of the National Academy of Sciences of the United States of America 1990;87: 3018-3022. DOI: 10.1073/pnas.87.8.3018

[98] Triglia T, Wang P, Sims PF, Hyde JE, Cowman AF, 1998. Allelic exchange at the endogenous genomic locus in *Plasmodium falciparum* proves the role of dihydropteroate synthase in sulfadoxine-resistant malaria. European Molecular Biology Organization Journal. 17: 3807-3815. DOI: 10.1093/emboj/17.14.3807

[99] Triglia T, Cowman AF. The mechanism of resistance to sulfa drugs in *Plasmodium falciparum*. Drug Resistance Update. 1999;2: 15-19. DOI: doi: 10.1054/drup.1998.0060

[100] Foote SJ, Thompson JK, Cowman AF, Kemp DJ. Amplification of the multidrug resistance gene in some chloroquine-resistant isolates of *P. falciparum*. Cell 1989;57:921-931. DOI: 10.1128/mcb.11.10.5244

[101] Foote SJ, Kyle DE, Martin RK, Oduola AMJ, Forsyth K, KempDJ, Cowman AF. Several alleles of the multidrug-resistance gene are closely linked to chloroquine resistance in *Plasmodium falciparum*. Nature 1990;345:255-258. DOI: 10.1038/345255a0

[102] Cowman AF, Karcz S, Galatis D, Culvenor JG. A P-glycoprotein homologue of *Plasmodium falciparum* is localized on the digestive vacuole. J Cell Biol 1991;113:1033-1042. DOI: 10.1083/jcb.113.5.1033

[103] Ekong R, Robson KJH, Baker DA, Warhurst DC. Transcripts of the multidrug resistance genes in chloroquine-sensitive and chloroquine-resistant *Plasmodium falciparum*. Parasitology 1993;106:107-115. DOI: 10.1017/s0031182000074904

[104] Peel SA, Bright P, Yount B, Handy J, Baric RS. A strong association between mefloquine and halofantrine resistance and amplification, overexpression, and mutation in the P-glycoprotein gene homologue (pfmdr) of *Plasmodium falciparum* in vitro. Am J Trop Med Hyg 1994;51:648-658. DOI: 10.4269/ajtmh.1994.51.648

[105] Barnes DA, Foote SJ, Galatis D, Kemp DJ, Cowman AF. Selection for high-level chloroquine resistance results indeamplification of thepfmdr1gene and increased sensitivityto mefloquine in *Plasmodium falciparum*. EMBO J 1992;11:3067-3075. PMID: 1353446:

[106] Cowman AF, Galatis D, Thompson JK. Selection for mefloquine resistance in *Plasmodium falciparum* is linked to amplification of the pfmdr1 gene and cross-resistance to halofantrine and quinine. Proc Natl Acad Sci USA 1994;91:1143-1147. DOI: 10.1073/pnas.91.3.1143

[107] Fidock DA, Nomura T, Talley AK, Cooper RA, Dzekunov SM, Ferdig MT, Ursos LM, Sidhu AB, Naude B, Deitsch KW, Su XZ, Wootton JC, Roepe PD, Wellems TE. Mutations in the *P. falciparum* digestive vacuole transmembrane protein PfCRT and evidence for their role in chloroquine resistance. Molecular Cell. 2000; 6: 861-871. DOI: 10.1016/s1097-2765(05)00077-8

[108] Sidhu AB, Verdier-Pinard D, Fidock DA, 2002. Chloroquine resistance in *Plasmodium falciparum* malaria parasites conferred by *pfcrt* mutations. Science. 2002;298: 210-213. DOI: 10.1126/science.1074045

[109] Nomura T, Carlton JM, Baird JK, del Portillo HA, Fryauff DJ, Rathore D, Fidock DA, Su X, Collins WE, McCutchan TF, Wootton JC, Wellems TE. Evidence for different mechanisms of chloroquine resistance in 2 plasmodium species that cause human malaria. The Journal of infectious diseases. 2001;183:1653-1661. DOI: 10.1086/320707

[110] Asih PBS, Sadikin M, Baird JK, Leake J, Sorontou Y, Sauerwein RW, Vinetz J, and, Syafruddin D. Polymorphisms of Pvmdr1 gene associated with Chloroquine Resistance Phenotype among *Plasmodium vivax* isolates in Indonesia. Proceeding International Conges for Parasitology. 2010;199- 204

[111] Melo GC, Monteiro WM, Siqueira AM, Silva SR, Magalhaes BM, Alencar AC, Kuehn A, del Portillo HA, Fernandez-Becerra C, Lacerda MVG. Expression levels of *pvcrt-o* and *pvmdr-1* are associated with chloroquine resistance and severe *Plasmodium vivax* malaria in patients of the Brazilian Amazon. PLoS ONE. 2014;9:e105922. DOI: 10.1371/journal.pone.0105922

[112] Lu F, Lim CS, Nam DH, Kim K, Lin K, Kim TS, Lee HW, Chen JH, Wang Y, Sattabongkot J, Han ET. Genetic polymorphism in *pvmdr1* and *pvcrt-o* genes in relation to *in vitro* drug susceptibility of *Plasmodium vivax* isolates from malaria-endemic countries. Acta Tropica. 2011;117:69-75. DOI: 10.1016/j.actatropica.2010.08.011

[113] Imwong M, Pukrittayakamee S, Pongtavornpinyo W, Nakeesathit S, Nair S, Newton P, Nosten F, AndersonTJC, Dondorp a, Day NPJ, White NJ. Gene amplification of the multidrug resistance 1 gene of *Plasmodium vivax* isolates from Thailand, Laos, and Myanmar. Antimicrobial Agents and Chemotherapy. 2008;52:2657-2659. DOI: 10.1128/AAC.01459-07

[114] Silva SR, Almeida ACG, da Silva GAV, Ramasawmy R, Lopes SCV, Siqueira AM, Costa GL, Sousa TN, Vieira JLF, Lacerda MVG, Monteiro WM, de Melo GC. Chloroquine resistance is associated to multi-copy pvcrt-o gene in *Plasmodium vivax* malaria in the Brazilian Amazon. Malaria Journal. 2018;17:267. DOI: 10.1186/s12936-018-2411-5

[115] Sá JM, Kaslow SR, Barro RRM, Brazeau NF, Parobek CM, Tao D, Salzman RE, Gibson TJ, Velmurugan S, Krause MA, Melendez-Muniz V, Kite WA, Han PK, Eastman RT, Kim A, Kessler EG, Abebe Y, James ER, Chakravarty S, Orr-Gonzalez S, Lambert LE, Engels T, Thomas ML, Fasinu PS, Serre D, Gwadz RW, Walker L, DeConti DK, Mu J, Bailey JA, Sim BKL, Hoffman S, Fay MP, Dinglasan RR, Juliano JJ, Wellems TE. *Plasmodium vivax* chloroquine

resistance links to pvcrt transcription in a genetic cross. Nature Communication. 2019;10:4300. DOI: https://doi.org/10.1038/s41467-019-1225

[116] Ariey F, Witkowski B, Amaratunga C, Beghain J, Langlois AC, Khim N, Kim S, Duru V, Bouchier M, Ma L, Lim P, Leang R, Duong S, Sreng S, Suon S, Chuor CM, Bout DM, Ménard S, Rogers WO, Genton B, Fandeur T, Miotto O, Ringwald P, Bras JL, Berry L, Barale JC, Fairhurst RM, Benoit-Vical F, Mercereau-Puijalon O, Ménard D. A molecular marker of artemisinin-resistant *Plasmodium falciparum* malaria. Nature. 2014;505(7481):50-55. DOI: 10.1038/nature12876

[117] Takala-Harrison S, Clark TG, Jacob CG, Cummings MP, Miotto O, Dondorp AM, Fukuda MM, Nosten F, Noedl H, Imwong M, Bethell D, Se Y, Lon C, Tyner SD, Saunders DL, Socheat D, Ariey F, Phyo AP, Starzengruber P, Fuehrer HP, Swoboda P, Stepniewska K, Flegg J, Arze C, Cerqueira GC, Silva JC, Ricklefs SM, Porcella SF, Stephens RM, Adams M, Kenefic LJ, Campino S, Auburn S, MacInnis B, Kwiatkowski DP, Su X, White NJ, Ringwald P, Plowe CV. Genetic loci associated with delayed clearance of *Plasmodium falciparum* following artemisinin treatment in Southeast Asia. Proceedings of the National Academy of Sciences of the United States of America. 2013;110:240-5. DOI: 10.1073/pnas.1211205110

[118] Miotto O, Amato R, Ashley EA, MacInnis B, Almagro-Garcia J, Amaratunga C, Lim P, Mead D, Oyola SO, Dhorda M, Imwong M, Woodrow C, Manske M, Stalker J, Drury E, Campino S, Amenga-Etego L, Thanh TN, Tran HT, Ringwald P, Bethell D, Nosten F, Phyo AP, Pukrittayakamee S, Chotivanich K, Chuor CM, Nguon C, Suon S, Sreng S, Newton PN, Mayxay N, Khanthavong M, Hongvanthong B, Htut Y, Han KT, Kyaw MP, Faiz MA, Fanello CI, Onyamboko M, Mokuolu OA, Jacob CG, Takala-Harrison S, Plowe CV, Day NP, Dondorp AM, Spencer CAC, McVean G, Fairhurst RM, White NJ, Kwiatkowski DP. Genetic architecture of artemisinin-resistant *Plasmodium falciparum*. Nature Genetics. 2015;47:226-34. DOI: doi: 10.1038/ng.3189

[119] Siddiqui G, Srivastava A, Russell AS, Creek DJ. Multi-omics based identification of specific biochemical changes associated with PfKelch13-mutant artemisinin-resistant *Plasmodium falciparum*. J Infect Dis. 2017; 215(9):1435-1444. doi: 10.1093/infdis/jix156

[120] Mbengue A, Bhattacharjee S, Pandharkar T, Liu H, Estiu G, Stahelin RV, Rizk SS, Njimoh DL, Ryan Y, Chotivanich K, Nguon C, Ghorbal M, Lopez-Rubio J, Pfrender M, Emrich S, Mohandas N, Dondorp A, Wiest O, Haldar K. A molecular mechanism of artemisinin resistance in *Plasmodium falciparum* malaria. Nature. 2015; 520(7549):683-687. doi: 10.1038/nature14412

[121] Tyagi RK, Gleeson PI, Pérignon JL, Olliaro P, Arnold L, Tahar R, Prieur E, Decorsterd L, Pengnon JL, Druilhe P. High-level artemisinin-resistance with quinine co-resistance emerges in *P. falciparum* malaria under in vivo artesunate pressure. BMC Medicine (2018) 16:181 https://doi.org/10.1186/s12916-018-1156-x

[122] Hossain MS, Commons RJ, Douglas NM, Thriemer K, Alemayehu BH, Amaratunga C, Anvikar AR, Ashley EA, Asih PBS, Carrara VI, Lon C D'Alessandro U, Davis TME, Dondorp AM, Edstein MD, Fairhurst RM, Ferreira MU, Hwang J, Janssens B, Karunajeewa H, Kiechel JR, Ladeia-Andrade S, Laman M, Mayxay M, McGready R, Moore BR, Mueller I, Newton PN, Thuy-Nhien NT,

Noedl H, Nosten F, Phyo AP, Poespoprodjo JR, Saunders DL, Smithuis F, Spring MD, Stepniewska K, Suon S, Suputtamongkol Y, Syafruddin D, Tran HT, Valecha N, Herp MV, Vugt MV, White NJ, Guerin PJ, Simpson JA, Price RN. The risk of *Plasmodium vivax* parasitaemia after *P. falciparum* malaria: An individual patient data meta-analysis from the World Wid6 Antimalarial Resistance Network. 2020. PloS Medicine 2020;17(11):e1003393. DOI: 10.1371/journal.pmed.1003393

[123] Li J, Zhang J, Li Q, Hu Y, Ruan Y, Tao Z, Xia H, Qiao J, Meng L, Zeng W, Li C, He X, Zhao L, Siddiqui FA, Miao J, Yang Z, Fang Q, Cui L. Ex vivo susceptibilities of *Plasmodium vivax* isolates from the China-Myanmar border to antimalarial drugs and association with polymorphisms in Pvmdr1 and Pvcrt-o genes. PLoS Neglected Tropical Diseases. 2020;14(6):e0008255. DOI: 10.1371/journal.pntd.0008255.

[124] Brashear AM, Fan Q, Hu Y, Li Y, Zhao Y, Wang Z, Cao Y, Miao J, Barry A, Cui L. Population genomics identifies a distinct *Plasmodium vivax* population on the China-Myanmar border of Southeast Asia. PLoS Neglected Tropical Diseases. 2020;14(8):e0008506. DOI: 10.1371/journal.pntd.0008506.

[125] Wang M, Siddiqui FA, Qi Fan, Luo E, Cao Y, Cui L. Limited genetic diversity in the PvK12 Kelch protein in *Plasmodium vivax* isolates from Southeast Asia. Malaria Journal. 2016;15:537. DOI 10.1186/s12936-016-1583-0.

Chapter 14

rRNA Platform Technology for Drug Discovery Methods for Identifying Ligands That Target Plasmodium RNA Structural Motifs

Harrison Ndung'u Mwangi and Francis Jackim Mulaa

Abstract

Determining the structure of the *P. falciparum* 40s leads to better understanding of the structural basis for its protein-synthesizing roles in the cell. This enables researchers in the field of drug development to run *in silico* ligand screening experiments using the solved *P. falciparum* 40S structure as a target against a library of potential anti-malarial compounds. Drug leads identified through this method can lead to further biochemical and *In vitro* binding studies with the ultimate goal of developing new class of anti-malarial drugs. The use of structure prediction and modeling technologies in this study dramatically reduces the time it takes from target identification to drug lead determination. Furthermore, very many compounds that were previously incapable of being experimentally tested can now be tested *in silico* against the generated structure. Owing to the increasing utility of bioinformatics and three dimensional structural modeling software, one can accurately build physical models solely from sequence data by unwrapping the information therein on probable motif sites capable of being anchored onto available compounds or aptamers.

Keywords: *P. falciparum*, Ribosome, 40S subunit, *In silico*, structure determination, Dynamic simulations, docking

1. Introduction

Ribosomes are cellular organelles found in the cytoplasm and primarily responsible for protein synthesis in the cell. Ribosomes' were first observed as dense particles or granules under an electron microscope [1]. The Eukaryote ribosome is a large complex (about 2.6 MDa) molecular machine composed of rRNAs and proteins [2–4]. In the past few years, a combination of X-ray crystallography, NMR spectroscopy and Cryo-electron microscopy has provided new data on the structure of ribosomes [5]. The Eukaryotic ribosome (80S) comprises of two subunits, a large subunit (60S) and small subunit (40S). The ribosome plays a major role during translation of RNA to the various proteins they code for. The process of translation occurs when the message contained in mRNA is decoded and the respective amino acids synthesized into a growing polypeptide chain which eventually folds into a three dimensional functional structure. Protein synthesis is critical for cell viability, hence highlighting the importance of the ribosome in the cell [6].

1.1 Eukaryotic ribosome

A eukaryote ribosome where Plasmodium species falls is designated as 80S and contains two subunits. The smaller subunit 40s is comprised of 18 s rRNA and 33 proteins whereas the large subunit 60S (**Figure 1**) is comprised of the 28S, 5S and 5.8S rRNA and 49 proteins [7–9].

X-ray crystallography and Cryo-electron microscopy methods have been used to solve the three dimensional structures of the ribosome with or without complexed cofactors examples be tRNA, mRNA among other macro molecules successfully [10]. The very first models of eukaryotic ribosome's at resolution between 6.1 and 15 Å were provided by Cryo-electron microscopy, revealed the location and the shapes of the RNA expansion segments and indicated the position of additional protein moieties [11–13]. Later, a crystalline structure of the complete eukaryotic ribosome from *Saccharomyces cerevisiae* was determined at 4.15 Å and later 3.0 Å resolutions [9, 14]. These structures with more clarity gave more insights on understanding the process of translation which captured the ratcheted states of the ribosome which had been postulated over 40 years [15, 16]. Recently the overall crystal structure of the eukaryotic ribosome of *S. cerevisiae* obtained revealed basic architectural similarity, but the larger assembly compared with the prokaryotic counterpart [14].

In addition this structure shows the E-site, A-site, the ribosomal proteins of both the 60S and the 40S subunits together with the expansion segments which gave more knowledge about eukaryotic protein synthesis process. This followed through earlier studies that were done and showed both interfaces of the 60S and 40S subunits views with numbered bridges [17].

1.2 18S rRNA structure

RNA molecules are polymers of nucleotides comprised of 3′-5′ phosphor-diester linked ribose sugars attached to the four bases, pyrimidines: cytosine and uracil and

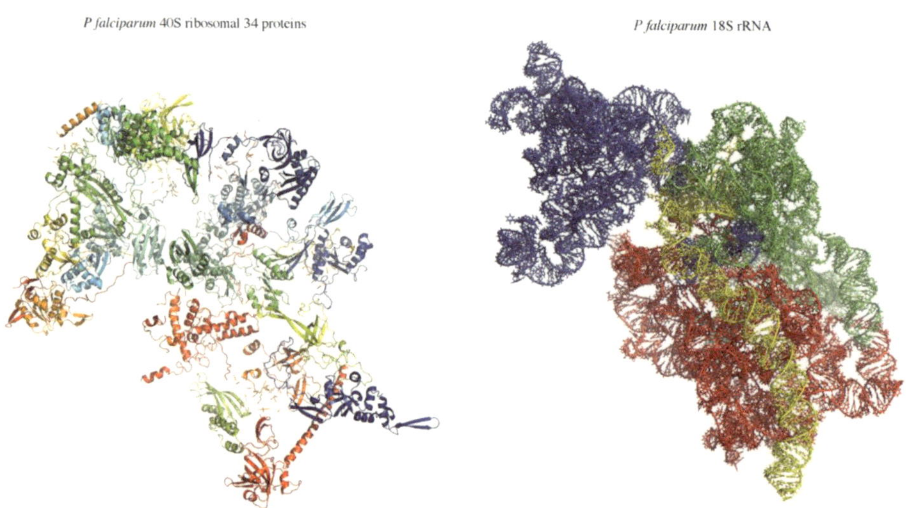

Figure 1.
A graphical presentation of the components of the 40S ribosomal subunit of Plasmodium falciparum.

DOI: http://dx.doi.org/10.5772/intechopen.98776

purines: adenine and guanine in contrast with the DNA [18]. RNA is single stranded containing ribose sugars and uracil base in place of thymine.

While the G-U wobble pair is somewhat different in shape. Base pairing occurs in both DNA and RNA using the hydrogen bonds formed this pairing patterns are governed by Watson and crick rules [19], where adenine complements uracil in RNA (thymine in DNA) and guanine with cytosine in both known as conical base pairing. In places where this pairing does not happen it's known as non-Watson crick structures among these are the sheared GA, GA imino, AU reverse Hoogsteen, and the GU and AC wobble pairs (**Figure 2**) [19, 20]. Determining the RNA secondary structure is the first step of understanding its mechanism of action which is defined by the canonical base paring [21]. The secondary structure of the RNA can adopt elements such as internal loops, mismatches bulges, multi-branched junctions, hairpins and pseudo knots (**Figure 3**).

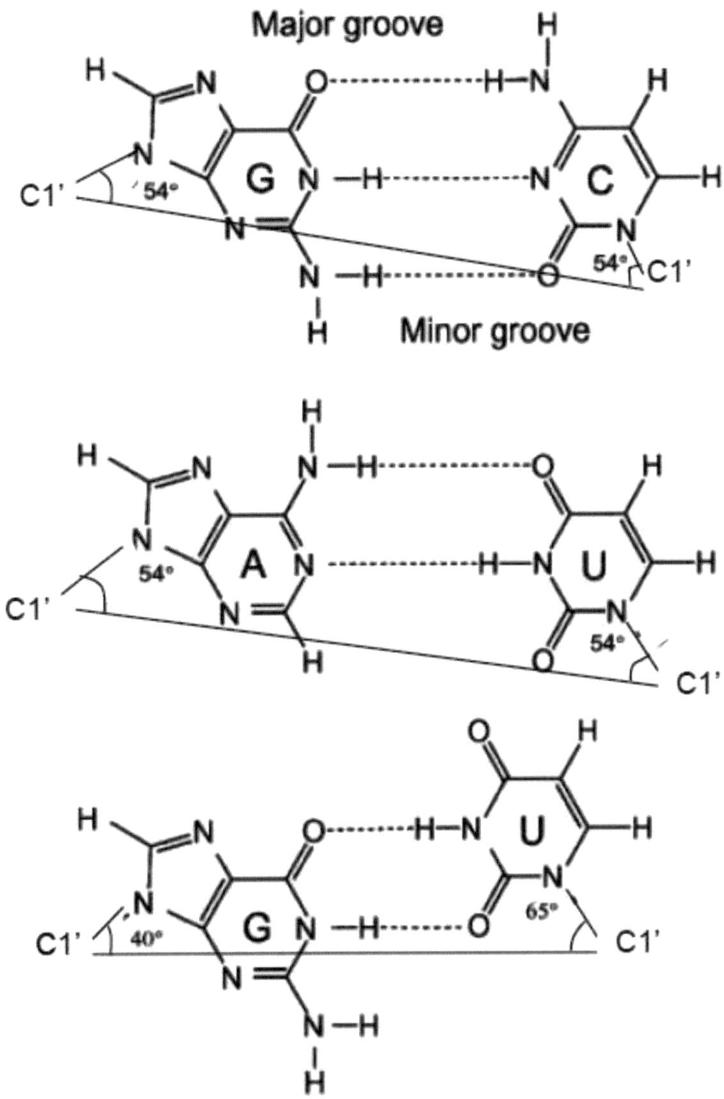

Figure 2.
Watson–Crick G-C and A-U base pairs with a similar angle of ~54. The G-U "wobble base pair" is also shown [9, 18].

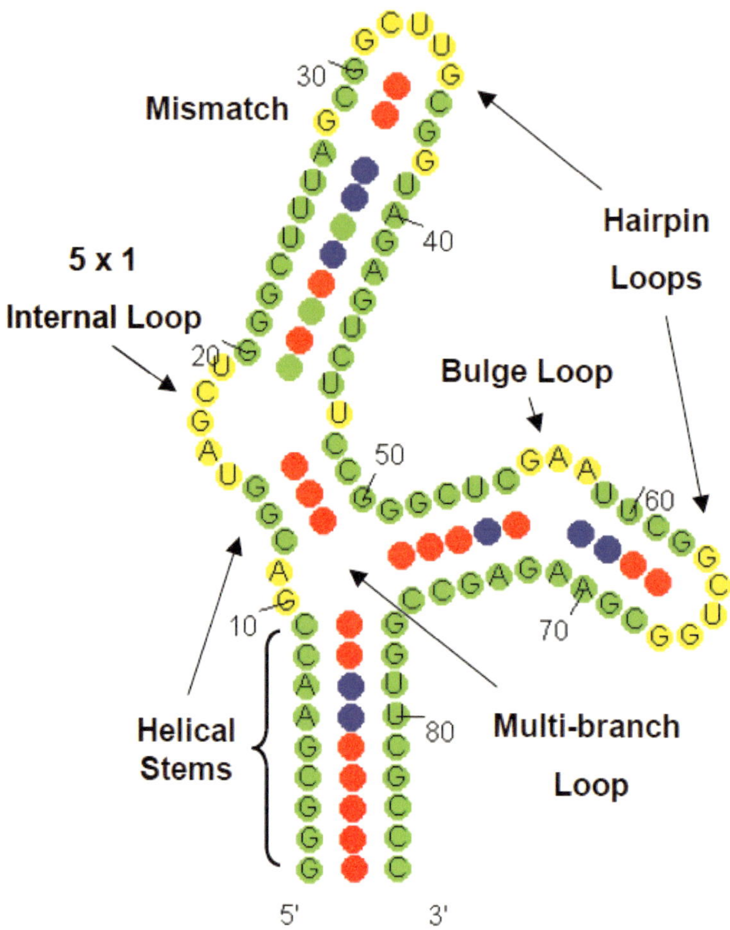

Figure 3.
RNA secondary structure motifs showing representation of Watson crick base paring [9, 18].

Presence of these diverse motifs that can be adopted by the RNA makes it play its functional roles such as recognition, interaction, metal binding and other enzymatic activities [20]. The 18S fold primarily defines the eukaryotic 40S subunit structure which can be divided into features of the small ribosomal subunit including the head, platform, body, beak, shoulder, right foot and left foot (**Figure 4A**) [22]. The secondary structure of the eukaryotic ribosome forms a structure with four major domains which are named according to the region of the sequence from 5′ to the 3′ end. They are 5'major, central, 3'major, and finally 3'minor (**Figure 4B**).

Figure 2 Watson–Crick G-C and A-U base pairs with a similar angle of ~54. The G-U —Wobble base pair|| is also shown [20]. While the G-U wobble pair is somewhat different in shape. **Figure 3** RNA secondary structure motifs showing representation of Watson crick base paring [20].

The 18S rRNA is composed of a region homologous to the prokaryotic 16S rRNA with several eukaryotic specific ESs [23] as shown in **Figure 5**. The ESs helical elements in eukaryotes display variable lengths; however their architecture is found to be preserved [22]. Both segments of ES3 are located on the 5′ domain, ES6 and ES7do form insertions in the central domain, and ES9 and ES12 are found in the 3′ major and 3'minor domain of the 18S RNA, respectively [22].

Eukaryotic 18S rRNA ES6, is the longest consisting of ~250 nucleotides which form five helices that replace the bacterial helix 21. ES6 is inserted between h20

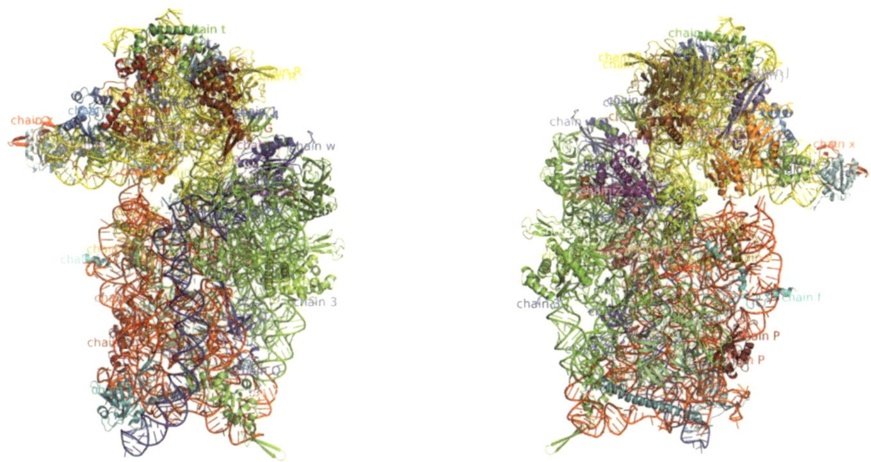

Figure 4.
Architectural tertiary structure of Plasmodium falciparum *40S front and back view. The 18S rRNA is colored differently depending with domains (5'major –red, central-yellow, 3'major-blue and 3'minor- green). Also shown are the 40S ribosomal 34 proteins of* Plasmodium falciparum *interacting with the 18S rRNA to make the total subunit.*

and h22 in the lower back region of the 40S body. A, B, C, and D helices form a large portion of the back of the 40S body and their structure differs considerably from a previous model [24]. C and D Helices are located at an equivalent position to bacterial h21. They stretch across the back of 40S and are buried underneath helix A.ES6B apical loop region is exposed and disordered in the structure, which makes it prone to chemical modification and cleavage by nucleases, as previously observed [25]. The loop region ES3B forms a base pair with helix ES6E loop region which yields to an extended helix which leads to projection from the center of the back toward the left foot of the 40S. Earlier demonstration by computational and biochemical experiments showed this rather unusual quaternary interactions.

The left foot along with ES6E is formed when the ES3B apical region packs against ES3A. ES3 and ES6 quaternary eukaryotic interaction, together with several proteins form a new domain, responsible for more prominent left foot features of the 40S and a broader back. Situated directly below the bleak is helix h16, which is shifted relative to the position in bacteria by as much as 40 Å [25].

In the 40S crystal structure the position of h16 is consistence with those observed in the solution by Cryo-EM of the empty yeast 40S, the 40S-eIF1 or40S-eIF1A complex [26], and the canine and *Thermomyces lanuginosus* 80S [24, 27]. Formation of a connection between the head and the body of the 40S subunit involves h16 upon binding of the initiation factors eIF1 and eIF1A, which might point to a role of this helix in initiation [26].

1.3 RNA as a drug target

The pharmaceutical industries together with the researches have always forecast their efforts more on protein, rather than the nucleic acids as suitable targets of drugs. But the acceleration and advances of studies on the RNA synthesis, structure determination and therapeutic target identification has blown open the question of using RNA as a drug target a very genuine area [28]. In this age due to the wealth of the three dimensional structure of the RNA in various repositories, it is possible they could be used for drug design by observing the target design. It has been a

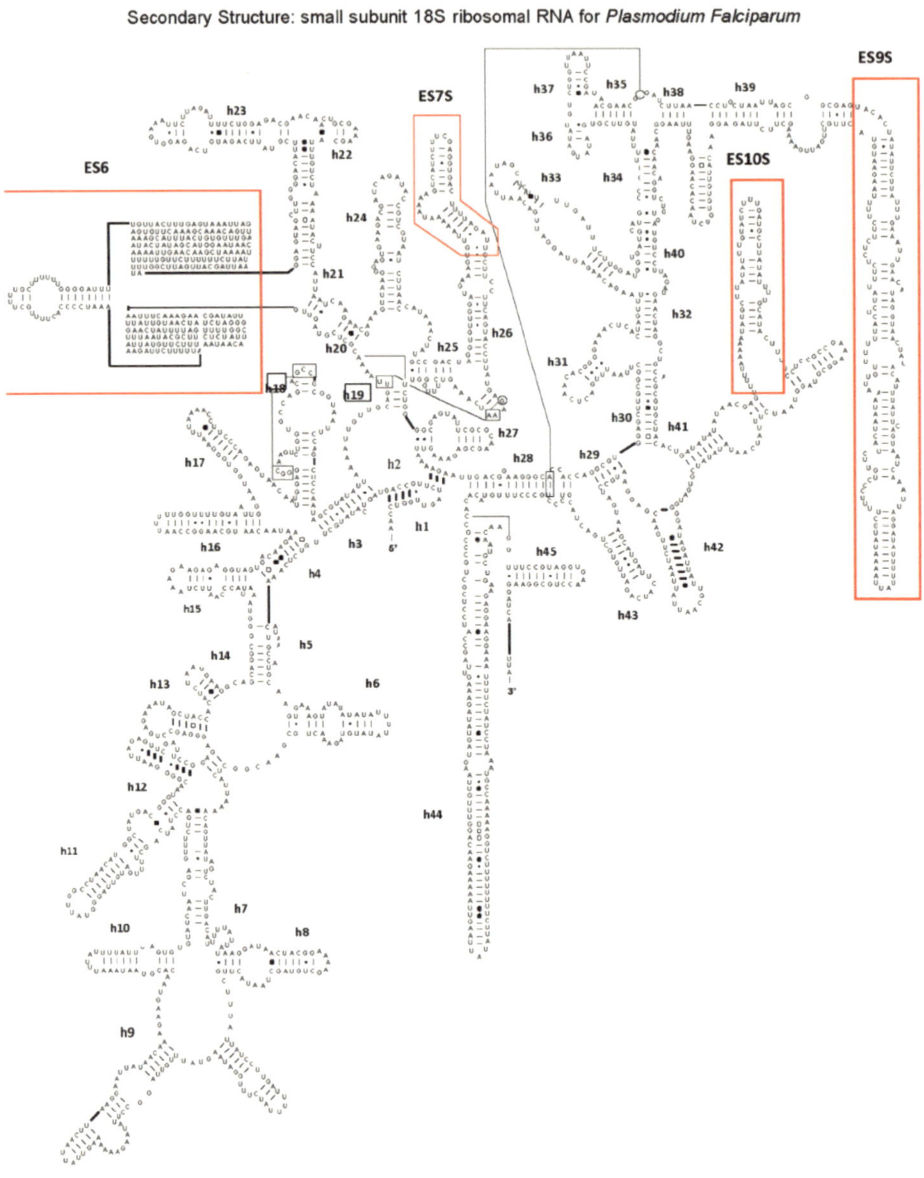

Figure 5.
18S rRNA secondary structure of Plasmodium falciparum *showing the four expansion segment regions (ES) located at the central and 3'major domain [9].*

difficult task in the past to obtain a three-dimensional structure for large RNAs using the crystal and magnetic resonance experimental techniques, which was just restricted to very small fragments [28–30] but newer techniques and more input to the older experimental methods are leading to accurate much larger structures. The RNA on its chemical basis does not show a promising drug target in that it's made up of four different planer bases and negatively charged nucleus [29, 31]. But upon the RNA adopting its conformational architecture, that shows the presence of cavities and pockets which could bind to shape specific rather than sequence specific molecules [31]. The RNA cavities compels the phosphate groups to be in close proximity, that lead to an intensified importance of tightly bound water molecules, electrostatic forces and ions, magnesium divalent ions in particular that can be partly dehydrated [30, 32]. Presence of non-Watson Crick pairs and bulged residues leads the formation of pockets and enlarged grooves that infer function through assembly of existing RNA motifs which are architecturally clearly diverse [30, 33]. The secondary structure of the RNA consist regular double stranded helices that gives it most of its energy content which in turn folds to subsequent three dimensional structure free energy content of between 5-10kcalmol [34]. This gives a Nano molar range binding constant which can be achieved for a small molecule usable to compete with the final step of RNA folding [30, 35]. From the discussed above projections with a number of ways of inserting non Watson crick pairs within helices is very limited leading to the restriction in the number of RNA motifs that are picked as drug target [30]. RNA motifs appear as decreasing size placed one inside the other, with the smaller motif associated with the larger motif [36, 37]. It has been shown that some antibiotics bind structurally in different regions of RNA molecules in the ribosome, such as streptomycin binding to the shallow groove, hygromycin binds to the deep groove of the helix, aminoglycosides at three adenine bulges and macrolides in the tunnel of the nascent polypeptide chain [8, 38–40].

Streptomycin interacts with only phosphate groups of many [40]. In conclusion there are various other ways that ligands interact with the RNA that are not known yet and the growth of a rich three dimensional structural of both RNA and ligands leads to newer technique of drug discovery that may include binding and docking experiments of the structures to obtain newer and stronger intervenes.

2. Methodology

Functional RNA elements have specific RNA sequences and structures that work together as a functional unit. From the perspective of bioinformatics, homology-based searching for both conserved sequences and secondary structures is effective at finding structured RNA motifs [33]. These strategies to determine RNA structures provide the means to investigate the potential of these RNA motifs as drug targets. Although drug development can be accomplished without knowing how a compound works in the cell, hit-to-lead optimization (during which small molecule hits from a high-throughput screen undergo optimization in order to identify promising lead compounds) is greatly facilitated if the target is known [34].

Here, we present a set of in-silico based methods for developing reliable atomic level 3D-models of RNA structures efficiently and cheaply, using sequence information, to accelerate the drug discovery process for plasmodium. Our methodology employs molecular modeling and structure based drug design approach in which we use the 3D experimental ribosome structures information of Plasmodium to identify RNA motifs that could be potential drug targets. Using the information of the rRNA structure and movement we have identified and docked a set of promising anti-infective-like compounds that target biologically functional ribosomal RNA motifs that could be potential drugs against malaria.

2.1 RNA tertiary structure prediction

To determine the spatial structure of RNA, researchers can use experimental techniques, such as bio-crystallography or NMR spectroscopy. However, the experimental techniques, are tiresome, expensive, and require specialized equipment [41]. An alternative to the experimental techniques are computer modeling methods. Although the computer modeling methods are not as accurate as mentioned above experiments, they can be successfully used to investigate the function and mechanism of action of the RNA molecules [42, 43].

Therefore, there is a need for computational methods that can provide reliable models of RNA structures efficiently and cheaply, using only information on a nucleotide sequence [44]. The goal of computational structural bioinformatics is not to replace experimental techniques, but to compliment them especially when the answer for scientific questions are beyond their reach [45]. Unfortunately, despite the fact that computational methods are being continuously improved, they not always predict the correct structures of RNA [44].

The secondary structure determination (or prediction) is often the starting point for the spatial (3D) structure determination of RNA [46]. Methods for predicting tertiary structure of RNA are generally represented in two categories: The first category comprising of the methods that are based on the laws of physics known as ab initio modeling and the second category comprising of the methods based on experimental data.

Methods based on experimental data are further divided to either those that extrapolate knowledge of experimentally solved structures known as de novo modeling and the methods that extrapolate the fragments of already solved structures which include assembly-based methods, comparative or homology modeling and manual building structures based on figments [47–51].

Our methodology focused on using the homology and de novo prediction modeling methods of RNA 3D structure development to produce the 3D structure of the ribosomal RNA (rRNA) of the plasmodium. The implementation was done using ModeRNA [50], RNA123 [20], SimRNA [52, 53]. Any refinement was done by QRNAS software [54].

2.1.1 Modeling of the rRNA model

The ribosomal core model is used as an anchor point for modeling the expansion segments and variable regions. RNA sequences from the structure based sequence alignment were loaded in FASTA format and the cleaned template structure also loaded. The data is submitted for structure modeling as shown by **Figure 6**.

The modeling proceeds by getting a sequence which is obtained from atomic coordinates in one-letter-code, getting a secondary structure by extracting the 2D structure from 3D and return it in the Vienna format and finally analyzing the geometry to check whether the residues of the structure have any unusual features like strange bond and angle values.

2.1.2 Structure evaluation

The WebRASP server is used to compute energy scores for assessing the stability of the modeled RNA structure. The server receives as input a PDB file containing the atomic coordinates of the RNA structure and calculates the energy profile and total energy score of the molecule. The server displays the results graphically and the visualization can be modified by the user. The server relies on RASP [55] for the calculation which is an all-atom knowledge-based potential assessment for scoring of RNA 3D structures based on distance-dependent pairwise atomic interactions.

Further validation is done using MolProbity [56, 57] which is a structure validation server used for all-atom contact analysis. The web service provides broad-spectrum model diagnosis and repair. It evaluates the model quality at both the global and local levels. It relies heavily on the power and sensitivity provided by optimized hydrogen placement and all-atom contact analysis, complemented by updated versions of covalent-geometry and torsion-angle criteria.

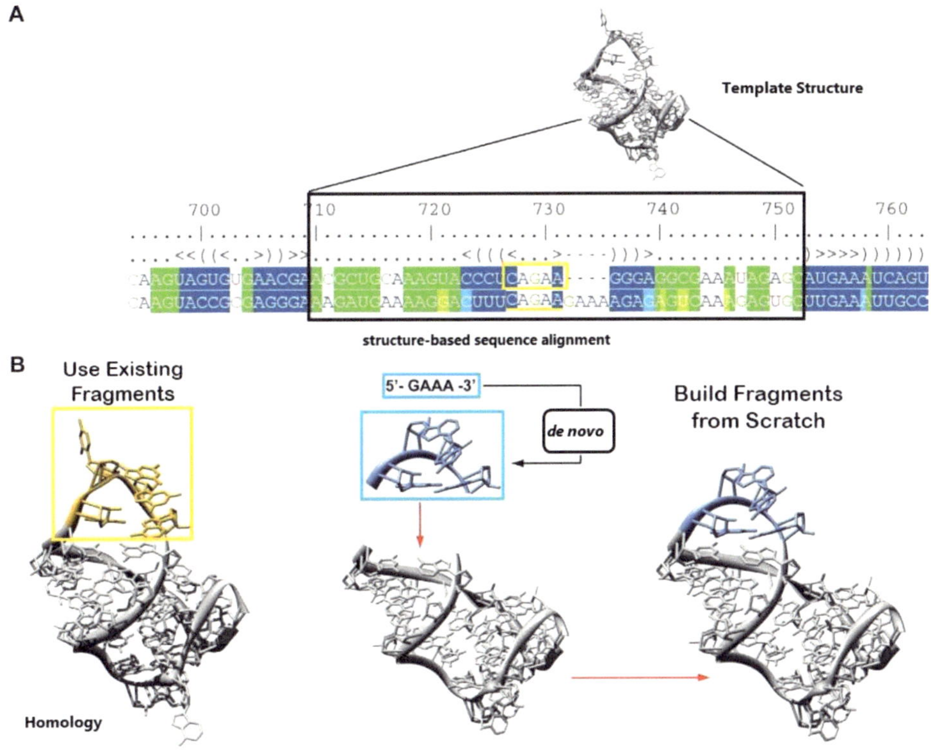

Figure 6.
The schematic diagram of RNA modeling.

2.2 Molecular dynamics simulation

SimRNA [52, 53] was used to analyze conformational landscapes and identify potential alternative structures using the default parameters; 500 simulation steps and 1% of the lowest energy frames of the input subjected to clustering. The software employs a statistical potential to approximate the energy and identifies conformations that correspond to biologically relevant structures.

2.2.1 Visualization and structure analysis

The sequence based and structure-based alignments are visualized using GNU emacs with RALEE [58] and Sublime text3 [59]. The secondary structures are visualized in Varna [60] and xRNA. The 3D model is visualized using USF Chimera [61, 62] and PyMol [63]. Video representations of the model are made using BIOVIA Discovery Studio [64].

2.3 Identification of rRNA motifs

As functional components in three-dimensional conformation of an rRNA, structural motifs provide an easy way to associate the molecular architectures with their biological mechanisms.

One major computational approach for studying RNA structural motifs is to search homologous instances of known motifs by using comparative methods. Traditionally, the motifs are modeled with their 3D geometric features, such as backbone conformations or torsion angles. Although a number of typical tools primarily rely on the 3D atomic coordinates and do perform well for some simple motifs, they may not work for complex ones since the underlying computational methods are too rigid to identify the flexible variations in structures. Using thin formation we integrate pairwise interactions as constraints into the screening for RNA structural motifs besides 3D information, using the FR3D platform [65]. However, as the most critical character of RNAs, the base–base interactions should be used as key factors in the assessment of structural discrepancy directly. Based on this idea, we use RNA Motif Scan to search new motif candidates that share non-canonical base–base interaction patterns with the query [66, 67].

2.4 Structure based molecular docking

Molecular docking is also referred to as small molecular docking is a study of how two or more molecular structures, for instance, drug and catalyst or macromolecule receptor, match along to be a perfect fit [68]. The study employed both the Shape complementarity approach using PatchDock [69].

Shape complementary approach was successful in producing the docking results from compound in the Malaria Pathogen Box.

3. Conclusions

Malaria is a disease spread by the female anopheles mosquito that contains protozoan organisms of the plasmodium genus that actually cause malaria [13]. These thrive in tropical and subtropical areas which predominant in Africa. According to WHO Sub-Saharan Africa carries a disproportionately high share of the global malaria burden.

Malaria is transmitted by the anopheles female mosquito that carries *the P falciparum* that causes malaria. There are about 100 types of plasmodium parasites which can infect a variety of species. Scientist have identified five types that specifically affect humans but of all *P. falciparum* stands out. *P falciparum* found worldwide in tropical and rural ranges, however predominately in Africa. An expected 1 million individuals are killed by this strain each year. The strain can multiply quickly and can adhere to blood vessels in the brain, bringing causing rapid onset of severe malaria including cerebral malaria [9].

The rRNA is a very core component of any cell for the *P falciparum* the 18S rRNA is where we draw our attention to, this is because even after the *P falciparum* undergoes mutation the 18S rRNA of it rarely undergoes any change thus if targeted there will not mutate to resist the drugs. In designing drugs that only attack the rRNA of the *P falciparum* not the proteins therefore we are able to make drugs that are more effective and have a higher efficacy. By docking a large library of compounds into a high-resolution structures of the target receptor 18S rRNA, fewer compounds typically need to be experimentally screened to identify compounds that are active against the target. These rRNA are the most abundant species of RNA in the living cells. They are the largest component of the ribosomes; large RNA-protein particles that form sites for synthesizes proteins and form the bulk of it. rRNAs have evolved as a hub of protein biosynthesis in all living cells performing both catalytic, regulatory and organizational roles [70, 71].

This spurred significant progress in the understanding biology of ribosomes. For example; the translational mechanism of the ribosome and the mode by which the function of the ribosome is altered by antibiotic inhibitors [4, 72]. These results have stimulated new interest in extending our understanding to the more complicated eukaryotic ribosome.

As we begin to get more insights in the working of the prokaryotic ribosomes, the question we are also seeking to answer is "How does the complex eukaryotic ribosome assemble inside living cells? A number of approaches are beginning to address this question. The approaches comprise of a combination of genetic, biochemical, and structural approaches.

Author details

Harrison Ndung'u Mwangi[1,2]* and Francis Jackim Mulaa[1]

1 Department of Biochemistry, University of Nairobi, Nairobi, Kenya

2 HEP Bioinformatics Consultants LTD, Kenya

*Address all correspondence to: harryndungu@gmail.com; mulaa@uonbi.ac.ke

References

[1] Frank J. The Ribosome Comes Alive. Israel Journal of Chemistry. 2010;50(1): 95-98. doi: https://doi.org/10.1002/ijch.201000010.

[2] Garrett R. Mechanics of the ribosome. Nature. 1999;400(6747): 811-812. doi:10.1038/23573.

[3] Noller H, Lancaster L, Zhou J, Mohan S. The ribosome moves: RNA mechanics and translocation. Nature Structural & Molecular Biology. 2017;24:1021-1027. doi:10.1038/nsmb.3505.

[4] Ramakrishnan V. Ribosome Structure and the Mechanism of Translation. Cell. 2002;108(4):557-572. doi:https://doi.org/10.1016/S0092-8674(02)00619-0.

[5] Frank J, Heagle AB, Agrawal RK. Animation of the Dynamical Events of the Elongation Cycle Based on Cryoelectron Microscopy of Functional Complexes of the Ribosome. Journal of Structural Biology. 1999;128(1):15-18. doi: https://doi.org/10.1006/jsbi.1999.4138.

[6] Moore SD, Sauer RT. The tmRNA System for Translational Surveillance and Ribosome Rescue. Annual Review of Biochemistry. 2007;76(1):101-124. doi:10.1146/annurev.biochem.75.103004.142733.

[7] Ben-Shem A, Garreau de Loubresse N, Melnikov S, Jenner L, Yusupova G, Yusupov M. The Structure of the Eukaryotic Ribosome at 3.0 Å Resolution. Science. 2011;334(6062): 1524. doi:10.1126/science.1212642.

[8] Carter AP, Clemons WM, Brodersen DE, Morgan-Warren RJ, Hartsch T, Wimberly BT et al. Crystal Structure of an Initiation Factor Bound to the 30S Ribosomal Subunit. Science. 2001;291(5503):498. doi:10.1126/science.1057766.

[9] Mwangi, Harrison Ndung'u., Peter Wagacha, Peterson Mathenge, Fredrick Sijenyi, and Francis Mulaa. "Structure of the 40S ribosomal subunit of *Plasmodium falciparum* by homology and de novo modeling." *Acta pharmaceutica sinica B* 7, no. 1 (2017): 97-105..

[10] Ban N, Nissen P, Hansen J, Moore PB, Steitz TA. The Complete Atomic Structure of the Large Ribosomal Subunit at 2.4 Å Resolution. Science. 2000;289(5481):905. doi:10.1126/science.289.5481.905.

[11] Spahn CMT, Jan E, Mulder A, Grassucci RA, Sarnow P, Frank J. Cryo-EM Visualization of a Viral Internal Ribosome Entry Site Bound to Human Ribosomes: The IRES Functions as an RNA-Based Translation Factor. Cell. 2004;118(4):465-475. doi:10.1016/j.cell.2004.08.001.

[12] Spahn CMT, Beckmann R, Eswar N, Penczek PA, Sali A, Blobel G et al. Structure of the 80S Ribosome from Saccharomyces cerevisiae—tRNA-Ribosome and Subunit-Subunit Interactions. Cell. 2001;107(3):373-386. doi:https://doi.org/10.1016/S0092-8674(01)00539-6.

[13] Becker T, Bhushan S, Jarasch A, Armache J-P, Funes S, Jossinet F et al. Structure of Monomeric Yeast and Mammalian Sec61 Complexes Interacting with the Translating Ribosome. Science. 2009;326(5958): 1369. doi:10.1126/science.1178535.

[14] Ben-Shem A, Jenner L, Yusupova G, Yusupov M. Crystal Structure of the Eukaryotic Ribosome. Science. 2010;330(6008):1203. doi:10.1126/science.1194294.

[15] Spirin AS. The Second Sir Hans Krebs Lecture. European Journal of Biochemistry. 1969;10(1):20-35.

doi:https://doi.org/10.1111/j.1432-1033.1969.tb00651.x.

[16] Bretscher MS. Polypetide chain termination: An active process. Journal of Molecular Biology. 1968;34(1):131-136. doi:https://doi.org/10.1016/0022-2836(68)90239-8.

[17] Yusupov MM, Yusupova GZ, Baucom A, Lieberman K, Earnest TN, Cate JHD et al. Crystal Structure of the Ribosome at 5.5 Å Resolution. Science. 2001;292(5518):883. doi:10.1126/science.1060089.

[18] Sijenyi, Fredrick, Pirro Saro, Zheng Ouyang, Kelly Damm-Ganamet, Marcus Wood, Jun Jiang, and John SantaLucia. "The RNA folding problems: different levels of sRNA structure prediction." In *RNA 3D structure analysis and prediction*, pp. 91-117. Springer, Berlin, Heidelberg, 2012.

[19] Watson JD, Crick FHC. Molecular Structure of Nucleic Acids: A Structure for Deoxyribose Nucleic Acid. Nature. 1953;171(4356):737-738. doi:10.1038/171737a0.

[20] Sijenyi F, Saro P, Ouyang Z, Damm-Ganamet K, Wood M, Jiang J et al. The RNA Folding Problems: Different Levels of sRNA Structure Prediction. In: Leontis N, Westhof E, editors. RNA 3D Structure Analysis and Prediction. Berlin, Heidelberg: Springer Berlin Heidelberg; 2012. p. 91-117.

[21] Mathews DH, Turner DH. Prediction of RNA secondary structure by free energy minimization. Current Opinion in Structural Biology. 2006;16(3):270-278. doi:https://doi.org/10.1016/j.sbi.2006.05.010.

[22] Rabl J, Leibundgut M, Ataide SF, Haag A, Ban N. Crystal Structure of the Eukaryotic 40S Ribosomal Subunit in Complex with Initiation Factor 1. Science. 2011;331(6018):730. doi:10.1126/science.1198308.

[23] Cannone JJ, Subramanian S, Schnare MN, Collett JR, D'Souza LM, Du Y et al. The comparative RNA web (CRW) site: an online database of comparative sequence and structure information for ribosomal, intron, and other RNAs. BMC Bioinformatics. 2002;3:2-. doi:10.1186/1471-2105-3-2.

[24] Taylor DJ, Devkota B, Huang AD, Topf M, Narayanan E, Sali A et al. Comprehensive Molecular Structure of the Eukaryotic Ribosome. Structure. 2009;17(12):1591-1604. doi:https://doi.org/10.1016/j.str.2009.09.015.

[25] Alkemar G, Nygård O. Secondary structure of two regions in expansion segments ES3 and ES6 with the potential of forming a tertiary interaction in eukaryotic 40S ribosomal subunits. RNA. 2004;10(3):403-411. doi:10.1261/rna.5135204.

[26] Passmore LA, Schmeing TM, Maag D, Applefield DJ, Acker MG, Algire Mikkel A et al. The Eukaryotic Translation Initiation Factors eIF1 and eIF1A Induce an Open Conformation of the 40S Ribosome. Molecular Cell. 2007;26(1):41-50. doi:https://doi.org/10.1016/j.molcel.2007.03.018.

[27] Chandramouli P, Topf M, Ménétret J-F, Eswar N, Cannone JJ, Gutell Robin R et al. Structure of the Mammalian 80S Ribosome at 8.7 Å Resolution. Structure. 2008;16(4):535-548. doi:10.1016/j.str.2008.01.007.

[28] Pearson ND, Prescott CD. RNA as a drug target. Chemistry & Biology. 1997;4(6):409-414. doi:https://doi.org/10.1016/S1074-5521(97)90192-7.

[29] Hermann T, Westhof E. Saccharide–RNA recognition. Biopolymers. 1998; 48(2-3):155-165. doi:https://doi.org/10.1002/(SICI)1097-0282(1998)48:2<155::AID-BIP5>3.0.CO;2-I.

[30] Vicens Q, Westhof E. RNA as a Drug Target: The Case of Aminoglycosides. ChemBioChem. 2003;4(10):1018-1023. doi:https://doi.org/10.1002/cbic.200300684.

[31] Hermann T. Rational ligand design for RNA: the role of static structure and conformational flexibility in target recognition. Biochimie. 2002;84(9):869-875. doi:https://doi.org/10.1016/S0300-9084(02)01460-8.

[32] Velagapudi S, Seedhouse S, Disney M. Structure-Activity Relationships Through Sequencing (StARTS) Defines Optimal and Suboptimal RNA Motif Targets for Small Molecules. Angewandte Chemie (International ed in English). 2010;49:3816-8. doi:10.1002/anie.200907257.

[33] Batey RT, Rambo RP, Doudna JA. Tertiary Motifs in RNA Structure and Folding. Angewandte Chemie International Edition. 1999;38(16):2326-2343. doi:https://doi.org/10.1002/(SICI)1521-3773(19990816)38:16<2326::AID-ANIE2326>3.0.CO;2-3.

[34] Cundliffe E. Antibiotics as probes of ribosomal structure and function. In: Edwards DI, Hiscock DR, editors. Chemotherapeutic Strategy: Proceedings of the Symposium held on June 2-4 1982 at the World Trade Centre, London UK. London: Palgrave Macmillan UK; 1983. p. 65-78.

[35] Thomas JR, Hergenrother PJ. Targeting RNA with Small Molecules. Chemical Reviews. 2008;108(4):1171-1224. doi:10.1021/cr0681546.

[36] Grabow W, Andrews G. On the Nature and Origin of Biological Information: The Curious Case of RNA. Biosystems. 2019;185:104031. doi:10.1016/j.biosystems.2019.104031.

[37] Grabow WW, Zhuang Z, Swank ZN, Shea J-E, Jaeger L. The right angle (RA) motif: a prevalent ribosomal RNA structural pattern found in group I introns. Journal of molecular biology. 2012;424(1-2):54-67. doi:10.1016/j.jmb.2012.09.012.

[38] Brodersen DE, Clemons WMJ, Carter AP, Wimberly BT, Ramakrishnan V. Crystal structure of the 30 S ribosomal subunit from Thermus thermophilus: structure of the proteins and their interactions with 16 S RNA. J Mol Biol. 2002;316(3):725-768. doi:10.1006/jmbi.2001.5359.

[39] Carter AP, Clemons WM, Brodersen DE, Morgan-Warren RJ, Wimberly BT, Ramakrishnan V. Functional insights from the structure of the 30S ribosomal subunit and its interactions with antibiotics. Nature. 2000;407(6802):340-348. doi:10.1038/35030019.

[40] Brodersen DE, Clemons WM, Jr., Carter AP, Morgan-Warren RJ, Wimberly BT, Ramakrishnan V. The Structural Basis for the Action of the Antibiotics Tetracycline, Pactamycin, and Hygromycin B on the 30S Ribosomal Subunit. Cell. 2000; 103(7):1143-1154. doi:10.1016/S0092-8674(00)00216-6.

[41] Hawkins AE, Fabris D. RNA Structure Determination by Structural Probing and Mass Spectrometry: MS3D. In: Leontis N, Westhof E, editors. RNA 3D Structure Analysis and Prediction. Nucleic Acids and Molecular Biology. Berlin, Heidelberg: Springer Berlin Heidelberg; 2012. p. 361-89.

[42] Klostermeier D, Hammann C. Optical spectroscopy and calorimetry. RNA Structure and Folding. 2015.

[43] Ding F, Dokholyan NV. Multiscale Modeling of RNA Structure and Dynamics. In: Leontis N, Westhof E, editors. RNA 3D Structure Analysis and Prediction. Nucleic Acids and Molecular

Biology. Berlin, Heidelberg: Springer Berlin Heidelberg; 2012. p. 167-84.

[44] Šponer J, Lankaš F. Computational Studies of RNA and DNA. Challenges and Advances In Computational Chemistry And Physics. Dordrecht, The Netherlands.: Springer; 2004.

[45] Laing C, Schlick T. Computational approaches to RNA structure prediction, analysis, and design. Curr Opin Struct Biol. 2011;21(3):306-318. doi:10.1016/j.sbi.2011.03.015.

[46] Russell R. Introduction and Overview. In: Russell R, editor. Biophysics of RNA Folding. New York, NY: Springer New York; 2013. p. 1-10.

[47] Flores SC, Jonikas M, Bruns C, Ku JP, Schmidt J, Altman RB. Methods for Building and Refining 3D Models of RNA. In: Leontis N, Westhof E, editors. RNA 3D Structure Analysis and Prediction. Nucleic Acids and Molecular Biology. Berlin, Heidelberg: Springer Berlin Heidelberg; 2012. p. 143-66.

[48] Leontis N, Westhof E. RNA 3D Structure Analysis and Prediction Nucleic Acids and Molecular Biology vol 27. Berlin Heidelberg: pringer-Verlag 2012.

[49] Rother K, Rother M, Boniecki M, Puton T, Tomala K, Łukasz P et al. Template-Based and Template-Free Modeling of RNA 3D Structure: Inspirations from Protein Structure Modeling. In: Leontis N, Westhof E, editors. RNA 3D Structure Analysis and Prediction. Nucleic Acids and Molecular Biology. Berlin, Heidelberg: Springer Berlin Heidelberg; 2012. p. 67-90.

[50] Rother M, Milanowska K, Puton T, Jeleniewicz J, Rother K, Bujnicki JM. ModeRNA server: an online tool for modeling RNA 3D structures. Bioinformatics. 2011;27(17):2441-2442. doi:10.1093/bioinformatics/btr400.

[51] Rother M, Rother K, Puton T, Bujnicki JM. RNA tertiary structure prediction with ModeRNA. Brief Bioinform. 2011;12(6):601-613. doi:10.1093/bib/bbr050.

[52] Boniecki MJ, Lach G, Dawson WK, Tomala K, Lukasz P, Soltysinski T et al. SimRNA: a coarse-grained method for RNA folding simulations and 3D structure prediction. Nucleic Acids Res. 2016;44(7):e63. doi:10.1093/nar/gkv1479.

[53] Magnus M, Boniecki MJ, Dawson W, Bujnicki JM. SimRNAweb: a web server for RNA 3D structure modeling with optional restraints. Nucleic Acids Res. 2016;44(W1):W315-W319. doi:10.1093/nar/gkw279.

[54] Piatkowski P, Kasprzak JM, Kumar D, Magnus M, Chojnowski G, Bujnicki JM. RNA 3D Structure Modeling by Combination of Template-Based Method ModeRNA, Template-Free Folding with SimRNA, and Refinement with QRNAS. RNA Structure Determination: Methods and Protocols. 2016. p. 217-35.

[55] Capriotti E, Norambuena T, Marti-Renom MA, Melo F. All-atom knowledge-based potential for RNA structure prediction and assessment. Bioinformatics. 2011;27(8):1086-1093. doi:10.1093/bioinformatics/btr093.

[56] Chen VB, Arendall WB, 3rd, Headd JJ, Keedy DA, Immormino RM, Kapral GJ et al. MolProbity: all-atom structure validation for macromolecular crystallography. Acta Crystallogr D Biol Crystallogr. 2010;66(Pt 1):12-21. doi:10.1107/S0907444909042073.

[57] Davis IW, Leaver-Fay A, Chen VB, Block JN, Kapral GJ, Wang X et al. MolProbity: all-atom contacts and structure validation for proteins and nucleic acids. Nucleic Acids Res. 2007;35(Web Server issue):W375-83. doi:10.1093/nar/gkm216.

[58] Griffiths-Jones S. RALEE--RNA ALignment editor in Emacs. Bioinformatics. 2005;21(2):257-259. doi:10.1093/bioinformatics/bth489.

[59] Skinner J, Bond W. Sublime Text 3 3.1.1 ed. Darlinghurst NSW 2010, Australia: Sublime HQ Pty Ltd; 2018.

[60] Darty K, Denise A, Ponty Y. VARNA: Interactive drawing and editing of the RNA secondary structure. Bioinformatics. 2009;25(15):1974-1975. doi:10.1093/bioinformatics/btp250.

[61] Yang Z, Lasker K, Schneidman-Duhovny D, Webb B, Huang CC, Pettersen EF et al. UCSF Chimera, MODELLER, and IMP: an integrated modeling system. J Struct Biol. 2012;179(3):269-278. doi:10.1016/j.jsb.2011.09.006.

[62] Pettersen EF, Goddard TD, Huang CC, Couch GS, Greenblatt DM, Meng EC et al. UCSF Chimera--a visualization system for exploratory research and analysis. J Comput Chem. 2004;25(13):1605-1612. doi:10.1002/jcc.20084.

[63] Schrödinger LLC. The PyMOL Molecular Graphics System. 2.1 ed. New York, NY: Schrödinger LLC; 2018.

[64] BIOVIA DS. Discovery Studio Modeling Environment, Release 2017, Dassault Systèmes, 2016. San Diego2016.

[65] Petrov AI, Zirbel CL, Leontis NB. WebFR3D--a server for finding, aligning and analyzing recurrent RNA 3D motifs. Nucleic Acids Res. 2011;39(Web Server issue):W50-5. doi:10.1093/nar/gkr249.

[66] Zhong C, Tang H, Zhang S. RNAMotifScan: automatic identification of RNA structural motifs using secondary structural alignment. Nucleic Acids Res. 2010;38(18):e176. doi:10.1093/nar/gkq672.

[67] Zhong C, Zhang S. RNAMotif ScanX: a graph alignment approach for RNA structural motif identification. RNA. 2015;21(3):333-346. doi:10.1261/rna.044891.114.

[68] Musyoka TM, Kanzi AM, Lobb KA, Tastan Bishop O. Structure Based Docking and Molecular Dynamic Studies of Plasmodial Cysteine Proteases against a South African Natural Compound and its Analogs. Sci Rep. 2016;6:23690. doi:10.1038/srep23690.

[69] Schneidman-Duhovny D, Inbar Y, Nussinov R, Wolfson HJ. PatchDock and SymmDock: servers for rigid and symmetric docking. Nucleic Acids Res. 2005;33(Web Server issue):W363-7. doi:10.1093/nar/gki481.

[70] Noller HF, Green R, Heilek G, Hoffarth V, Hiittenhofer A, Joseph S et al. Structure and function of ribosomal RNA. Biochem Cell Biol. 1995;73:997-1009

[71] Eisen J, Coil D. Fact Sheet: Ribosomal RNA (rRNA), the details In: Lester E, editor. microBEnet: the microbiology of the Built Environment network: microBEnet; 2018.

[72] Mwangi, Harrison N.; Muge, Edward K.; Wagacha, Peter W.; Ndakala, Albert; Mulaa, Francis J. 2021. "Methods for Identifying Microbial Natural Product Compounds that Target Kinetoplastid RNA Structural Motifs by Homology and De Novo Modeled 18S rRNA" *Int.* J. Mol. Sci. 22, no. 9: 4493. https://doi.org/10.3390/ijms22094493

Chapter 15

Malaria: Introductory Concepts, Resistance Issues and Current Medicines

Dejen Nureye

Abstract

Malaria continues to be the main community health problem in numerous nations. Six species of *Plasmodium* are documented as the cause of human malaria infection. Among others, *Plasmodium falciparum* and *Plasmodium vivax* parasites produce an immense challenge in the public health. *Anopheles funestus* and *Anopheles gambiae* are the major transimmiter of the disease (malaria) from one person to another. The disease parasite has a complicated cycle of life that occurs in human and mosquitoes. In general, malaria diagnosis is divided into parasitological and clinical diagnosis. Internationally, the death rate of malaria becomes reduced although few records from Ethiopia describe the presence of raised prevalence of malaria in certain areas. Apart from reduction in incidence and prevalence, transmission of malaria is continued throughout the globe. Hence, its control needs a combined approach comprising treatment with effective antimalarial agents. A lot of novel compounds are under pre-clinical and clinical studies that are triggered by the occurrence of resistance among commonly used antimalarial drugs. In addition to the already known new compounds and targets for drug discovery, scientists from all corner of the world are in search of novel targets and chemical entities.

Keywords: Malaria, *Plasmodium*, antimalarial drugs, resistance, clinical trials, novel compounds

1. Introduction

Malaria itself or a disease looks like malaria has been distinguished before 4,000 years. The term *malaria* was derived from two Italian words "*mala aria*" meaning foul or bad air [1]. This name is originated from the observation that malaria cases were prevalent in areas where there is bad air associated with the accumulation of pools [2]. Malaria is caused by the genus *Plasmodium* (mosquito-borne apicomplexan parasite). At the time of bite by infected female *Anopheline* mosquitoes, this protozoal blood infection become conveying from one person to the next person [3, 4]. According to Miller *et al.* [5], malaria is expressed as a disease caused by repeated life cycle of the *Plasmodium* in the red blood cell. It is also defined as an illness brought by a parasite that lives some of the life in humans and some in mosquitoes [6].

The causative agents for malaria infection are among the genus *Plasmodium*, phyllum *Apicomplexa*, class sporozoa, family *Plasmodidae* and order Haemosporidia

IntechOpen

[7]. *Plasmodium* is considered to be instigated from photosynthetic protozoa, which is known as dinoflagellate. Among more than 200 different *Plasmodium* species, around 14 species are pathogenic to humans [8, 9]. The remaining species affect animals, such as rodents, monkeys and reptiles [10]. Five of the human pathogens, *P. ovale* sub-species (*P. ovale curtisi* and *P. ovale wallikeri*), *P. falciparum, P. vivax* and *P. malariae* are well known etiologic agents for human malaria. Infrequently, we could be naturally or accidentally infected by many simian species including *P. knowlesi*, *P. cynomolgi, P. bastianelli, P. brasilianum*, *P. schwetzi* and *P. inui*. Disease with *P. knowlesi* happens in individuals if an *Anopheles* mosquito previously diseased by a monkey malaria parasite bites humans. Incubation period (the time between the bite of mosquito and developing malaria symptoms) for falciparum, vivax and ovale, and malariae is 12, 14 and 30 days, respectively. But infections by *P. malariae* can exist in the blood for a very long period, may be decades, without ever producing symptoms. A person with asymptomatic (no symptom) *malariae* infection, however, can infect others, either through blood donation or mosquito bites. Incubation period is different for different persons and depends on the amount of the parasite involved [11–13].

Malaria is widely distributed throughout tropical regions in Africa, Asia, Hispaniola (Dominican Republic and Haiti), Central and South America, the Middle East and Oceania. The global prevalence of malaria species differs. *Falciparum* and *vivax* malaria pose the greatest public health challenge. *Falciparum* is mainly prevalent on the African continent and in the World Health Organization (WHO) regions of South East Asia, the eastern Mediterranean and Western Pacific. It is responsible for most deaths from malaria. *Plasmodium* parasites are affected by temperature. The development of *Plasmodium* species become slows as the temperature drops. When the temperature drops below 60°F, *P. vivax* totally stops developing. *P. falciparum* can regrate to develop at a bit elevated temperatures. This effect elaborates why malaria parasites are present in temperate environments. *Vivax* has a wider geographic distribution since it can grow in its vector at lower temperatures, cooler climates and elevated altitudes. However, *vivax* is more common in the Indian subcontinent and Central America. Despite it occurs in over all Africa, the risk of *vivax* infection is relatively low there due to lack of Duffy gene in most people of Africa [6, 14]. But, there is a supporting facts that *vivax* can be transmitted to negative Duffy blood group residents in Africa including Ethiopia [15]. South America and South East Asia have both *falciparum* and *vivax* species. *P. ovale* has an unusual distribution (present in West Africa, New Guinea and Philippines). Although, *malariae* has been wiped out from temperate climates, it persists in African sub-region [16]. *P. knowlesi* occurs in South East Asia with cases widely distributed in Sabah and Sarawak in Malaysian Borneo, and peninsular Malaysia. Cases have been reported from a number of other countries in South East Asia, and in travelers [12].

Mosquitoes of the genera Culex, *Anopheles*, Mansonia and Aedes may act as malaria vectors [16]. Nonetheless, malaria is transmitted mainly via the bite of *Anopheles* mosquitoes, which comprise 537 known species and majority (87%) of them have been formally named [17]. Nearly, 70 of these species are able to transmit *Plasmodium* parasite to human hosts and 41 of 70 are considered to be dominant vector species [1]. *Anopheles gambiae* and *A. funestus* are the most efficient vectors of malaria in the world. They are also the primary vectors of malaria in Africa [18]. In Ethiopia, two primary vectors of Africa and *A. pharoensis* are recognized as the dominant malaria vectors [15].

While some species grow in temperate climates and even continue to exist in the Arctic summer, majority of *anopheline* mosquitoes survive in tropical and subtropical regions. It was believed that *anopheline* mosquitoes are not breed on altitudes higher than 2,000 to 2,500 m. In this geographical boundary, there are a lot of malaria free places as its transmission is extremely reliant on the local environment and epidemiologic situations. *Anopheline* mosquitoes prefer comparatively clean water as their larval habitat (site for egg-laying and development of larvae) though species vary in the quantity of salinity and organic content and amount of sun exposure and temperature they prefer in their breeding sites. For example, city conditions can generate new spaces to mosquito larvae for development. Agricultural activities can also affect breeding site of mosquitoes. While the draining and drying of swamps removes the breeding areas of larvae, water-filled irrigation ditches could provide mosquitoes a new site for breeding. Egg, larva, pupa and adult (imago) are the four developmental phases of *anopheline* mosquitos. Adult males copulate to females in flight to provide adequate sperm for all subsequent egg-laying. To develop the first batch of their eggs, adult females require at least 2 blood meals but one blood meal is enough to develop each successive batch. As development of egg needs around 48 h, blood-seeking is recurring every two to three nights. Under most favorable conditions, the average lifetime of the female (adult) *anopheline* mosquito is equal to or more than three weeks. External factors including temperature, moisture and natural enemies could decrease its prolonged existence. Adult males, in contrast, generally live a few days. If the mean ambient temperature goes beyond 35°C or humidity drops below fifty percent, longevity is drastically decreased, directly affects malaria transmission. In most tropical regions, cases of malaria become increased at the time of rainy season as the rainfall expands breeding grounds. The adult male *anopheline* feeds on nectar, while the adult female feeds primarily upon blood of warm-blooded animals, predominantly mammals. Some female *anopheline* mosquitoes that have a preference toward humans are termed *anthropophagic* (*anthropophilic*). Others who choose animals, such as cattle, are expressed as *zoophagic* (*zoophilic*). The interval over which a mosquito is attracted to its favorite source of blood usually ranges 7–20 m. Many *Anopheles* mosquitoes are either nocturnal (active at night) or crepuscular (active at dusk or dawn). Some are endophagic (feed indoors) while others are exophagic (feed outdoors). After blood feeding, some of them wishs to rest indoors (endophilic) while others intended to rest outdoors (exophilic) [6, 19, 20].

Mentioned earlier, malaria is transmitted from one individual to the next individual via the bite of female *Anopheles* mosquito that has been acquiring the parasite from the first person. The female mosquito needs blood protein for her egg maturation. *Anopheles* mosquitoes are attracted to human by a number of factors (for example heat, odor and exhaled carbon dioxide) and usually bite us between sunset and sunrise [12]. Since *Plasmodum* resides in red blood cells, malaria is also transmitted via donation of blood, transplantation of organ and sharing of needles or syringes contaminated by infected blood. A new born child could also acquire congenital malaria from her/his mother before/during birth [11, 21]. Rarely, accidental nosocomial (hospital acquired) transmission of malaria may occur, for example, where there is a breach in infection control or as a result of a medical procedure [12, 22]. Moreover, transmission of malaria can largely be affected by global warming [23, 24].

Cases of malaria occur in non-endemic areas without an apparent travel history is known as **cryptic malaria**. If the conditions are appropriate for the transmission cycle of *Plasmodium* to be maintained, periodic (sporadic) outbreaks of locally acquired malaria may occur when an imported malaria case happens in a non-endemic district and is bitten by a malaria vector that can transmit parasite to another person. This is called **introduced malaria**. This is generally results in a small cluster of 1 or 2 cases even though larger outbreaks may sometimes occur. If the environmental (climatic) conditions allow, malaria may also occur if a person is bitten with infected mosquito that has been imported to a non-endemic region. This can be occured around airports (**airport malaria**) or from a mosquito that has stowed away in hand luggage (**baggage** or **luggage malaria**) if aircraft have not been disinsected in a well manner [12].

Chills, high fever, malaise, headache, muscle aches and sweating are the most frequently reported symptoms of malaria infection. The current diagnostic methods used for identification of *Plasmodium* species from blood samples are light/fluorescence microscopy (gold standard method), immuno-chromatographic lateral flow assays (RDTs-rapid diagnostic tests), serology tests, and nucleic acid amplification techniques including PCR (polymerase chain reaction) and isothermal amplification [25]. Rolling circle enhanced enzyme activity detection (REEAD) and micromagnetic resonance reflaxometric (MMR) tests are recently developed parasitological methods appropraite for utilization in field detection of malaria infected individuals for population screenings [26].

Around 44% of world population is at risk from malaria [27]. The risk varies according to season, geographic location, activities, type of accommodation, and the use of malaria prevention drugs and bite avoidance measures. Approximately 229,000,000 cases of malaria, most (94%) from the WHO African Region, are taken place globally in 2019. The disease was caused 409,000 deaths worldwide and most (94%) of which are also from the African Region. Most cases of malaria in Africa are resulted from *P. falciparum*. In 2019, global case incidence and mortality rate of malaria was reduced by 57 and 10%, respectively. Malaria continues to strike hardest against children and pregnant women in Africa. Children aged <5 years are the most exposed group affected by malaria, accounted 67% of global malaria deaths in 2019 [28]. In the USA, roughly 1,500–2,000 cases of malaria in recent travelers are reported every year. Pregnant mothers have high vulnerability to *falciparum* malaria. *P. falciparum* malria contributes 8 to 14 percent low birth weight in malaria-endemic areas, which in turn minimize the likelihood of a baby's survival [19].

All travelers visiting malaria endemic regions are at risk of acquiring malaria. Certain travelers including pregnant women, children, older travelers, immunosuppressed individuals, those with an absent or dysfunctional spleen, and those with complex co-morbidities are at high risk for severe disease if they have malaria. As they are peculiarly attractive to mosquitoes and have high risk of developing severe infection with increased risk of death compared to non-pregnant mothers, pregnant women should be advised to stay away from (not travel to) malarious areas. Travelers who lost their spleen or travelers who have severe impairement of spleen are at particular risk of severe malaria and are advised to avoid travel to malarious areas. If travel is essential, antimalarial drugs are advised in both high and low risk areas, together with rigorous bite avoidance and awareness of the need for prompt medical attention if symptoms develop [12].

Malaria endemic regions are classified into stable and unstable malaria transmission areas. In stable regions, for example in most of sub-Saharan African countries, transmission of malaria is year-round with high infection rates. The population, predominantly adults, may therefore develop a degree of immunity with the majority of clinical cases occurring in infants and children. In unstable regions such as India, malaria transmission has a tendency to be seasonal with short epidemics of varying intensity. Transmission of malaria in these unstable regions is less sustained, hence the communities have weak immunity and all age categories may be affected [12]. In addition to health related impacts, there is a severe burden on economic setors in terms of lost days of labor due to the disease. In fact, malaria is considered to take off 1.3 percent from the economic growth and 40 percent from public health costs of some African countries. It also affects developing nations in most aspects including determent of tourism [29].

Malaria is one of the major infectious diseases in Ethiopia [30, 31]. *Falciparum* and *vivax* are the main two species found in Ethiopia, accounting for 60% and 40% of malaria cases, respectively [32]. *Falciparum* has been the major cause of epidemics, and of most malaria deaths [33]. In Ethiopia, the epidemiological pattern of malaria transmission is generally unstable and seasonal; the level of transmission varies from place to place because of differences in altitude and rainfall patterns [32]. Depending on these rainfall patterns, transmission tends to be highly heterogenous geo-spatially within each year as well as between years [34]. Changes have been observed in the epidemiology of malaria through time. Global warming (changes in climate) are likely to lengthen the transmission seasons of important vector-borne diseases like malaria and to alter their geographic range [35]. Previously, malaria was known to occur in areas below 2000 m but currently it has been documented to occur indigenously even in areas above 2400 m, such as Addis Ababa [32]. Months from September to December and June to August are high malaria transmission seasons in Ethiopia. About 30,485,416 Ethiopians are living at high risk places for malaria infection. In 2019, 213 deaths and 904,496 confirmed cases due to malaria were reported by Ethiopian Federal Ministry of Health (FMoH) [25, 28]. Despite decreased malaria occurrence rate and death rate in Ethiopia since 2010 [28], high prevalence was observed in some areas in contrast to high household coverage of control interventions [36, 37]. This increment may be associated with individuals having poor socio-economic status [38]. Ethiopia has achieved only half of the millennium development reduction target of malaria. For this reason, the country must strengthen its malaria control and treatment approaches to attain the sustainable development goals [39].

2. The parasite life cycle

All types of malaria parasite have a similar and complex life cycle (**Figure 1**). The main part of the complexity related with the life cycle of *Plasmodium* is due to the parasite's capability to (a) modifiy its cellular and molecular make up, which is under control by a genome with more than 5,000 genes, and (b) developed in intra-cellular and extra-cellular niches in both mosquito and mammalian host [42]. The life cycle of every *Plasmodium* species infecting humans is distinguished by an exogenous sexual phase (sporogony), in which replication takes place in many *Anopheles* mosquito species, and an endogenous asexual phase (schizogony), which occurs in the vertebrate hosts. The sexual cycle is taken place in the gut and abdominal wall of some species of female mosquito, whereas the asexual cycle that causes the disease symptoms is taken place in the liver and RBCs of the humans [16]. The life cycle within the mosquito takes approximately 8 to 35 days, after which the parasite becomes infective. When the mosquito bites the skin, the sporozoite (motile infectious form of the parasite) will be injected in to human's dermis and then searchs a blood vessel to feed from it. The insect discharges different vasodilators to raise the possibility of finding a vessel. It also salivates into our blood to avoid blood clotting. The destiny of these sporozoites is not clearly illustrated; however they can take one to two hour to exit from the dermis. The trap-like protein of the sporozoites plays a role to exit the dermis (using gliding motility) and enters to the blood-stream. Those sporozoites remained in the skin could be killed and drained by the lymphatics, where a host immune response is activated. After 30 to 60 minutes of the injection, the thread-like shaped sporozoites will be transported to the liver through the vascular system. One single sporozoite in one hepatocyte multiplies into tens of thousands of exoerythrocytic merozoites [6, 43].

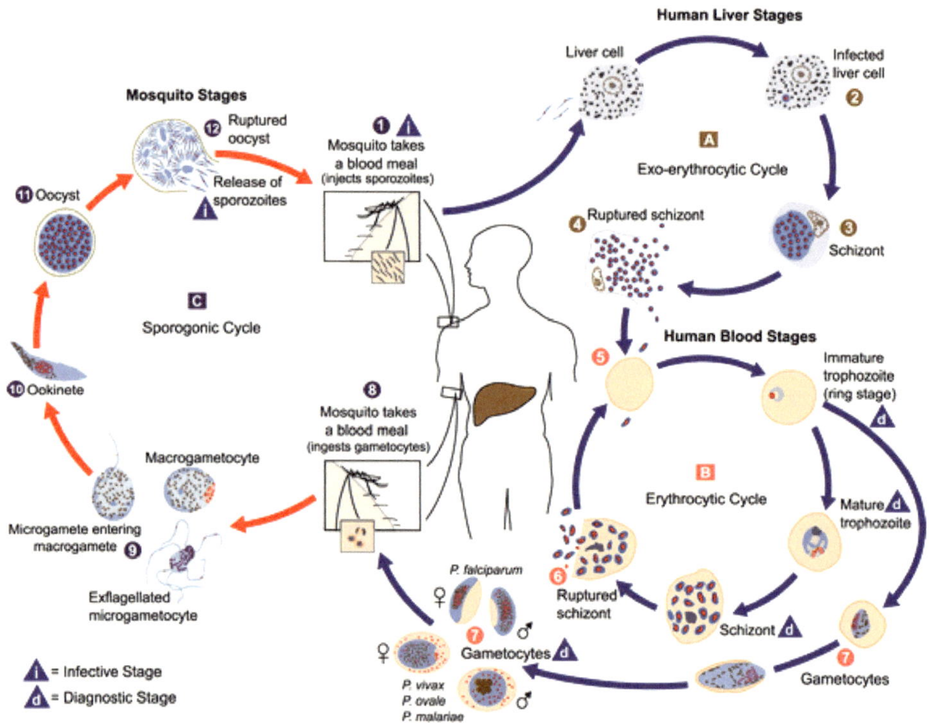

Figure 1.
Life cycle of malaria parasites [40]. The malaria parasite life cycle involves two hosts. During a blood meal, a malaria-infected female Anopheles mosquito inoculates sporozoites into the human host ❶. Sporozoites infect liver cells ❷ and mature into schizonts ❸, which rupture and release merozoites ❹. After this initial replication in the liver (exo-erythrocytic schizogony A), the parasites undergo asexual multiplication in the erythrocytes (erythrocytic schizogony B). Merozoites infect red blood cells ❺. The ring stage trophozoites mature into schizonts, which rupture releasing merozoites. Some parasites differentiate into sexual erythrocytic stages (gametocytes) ❼. The gametocytes, male (microgametocytes) and female (macrogametocytes), are ingested by an Anopheles mosquito during a blood meal ❽. The parasites' multiplication in the mosquito is known as the sporogonic cycle C. While in the mosquito's stomach, the microgametes penetrate the macrogametes generating zygotes ❾. The zygotes in turn become motile and elongated (ookinetes) ❿ which invade the midgut wall of the mosquito where they develop into oocysts ⓫. The oocysts grow, rupture, and release sporozoites ⓬, which make their way to the mosquito's salivary glands. Inoculation of the sporozoites ❶ into a new human host perpetuates the malaria life cycle [41].

Within 7 to 12 days, the sporozoites develop into schizonts and then grow up to thirty thousand merozoites, which burst the liver cells [44]. Alternatively, some of the sporozoite of *vivax* and *ovale* species turn into hypnozoites (dormant form) in the liver for months/years and can cause relapsed malaria [4, 45]. Unusually, the reappearance of *falciparum* malaria was observed in patient's years after departure of an endemic area. This indicates that *falciparum* has a dormant stage although occurs occassionally [46–49]. Then, the asexual erythrocytic cycle begins and the merozoites start invading red blood cell to consume hemoglobin for their growth. The parasites then multiply 10 times every 2 days, destroying RBCs and infecting new cells throughout the body. Inside the host red blood cell, the *Plasmodium* continues its maturity from the early ring stage to late trophozoite. Then, following mitotic divisions, the trophozoite undergoes to the schizont stage, which consists 6–32 merozoites depending on the *Plasmodium* species [50, 51].

The period from acquiring infection through mosquito bite and the first appearance of the trophozoites in RBCs is called "prepatent period". This constant time is the characteristic of every species. It lasts 9 days in falciparum, 11 up to 13 days in vivax, 10 up to 14 days in ovale, 15 days in malariae and 9 up to 12 days in knowlesi.

When the blood schizont bursts, the discharged merozoites maintain the life cycle through invading the neighbor red blood cells until it is brought under control. The rupture of schizonts is accompanied by the manifestation of the malaria febrile paroxysm typically lasting 8–12 h ("Golgi cycle") and characterized by 3 stages. The first stage (cold stage) is manifested by the quick rise of the temperature together with chills (sensation of the extreme cold). The patient desires to cover with the blankets. The second stage (hot stage) is with the temperature peak (may rises to 41°C), skin vasodilatation, myalgia and very severe headache. Patients feel too burning hot and cast their clothes. During the third stage (sweating stage), the patients have profuse sweating and their fever become drops. Then after, the patients may go to sleep due to tiredness. The typical (classical) symptoms which are stated above may not be appeared in some patients [40, 52]. Cyclical fevers are classically occurs soon before or during lysis of RBC (schizonts rupture). This happens every 48 h in tertian malaria (*vivax*, *ovale* and *falciparum*), and every 72 h in *malariae* infection (quartan *malaria*). At the time of this repetitive cycle, some merozoites differentiate into male and female sexual stages, which are called erythrocytic gametocytes (the only stages transmitted to the mosquito vector) with one nucleus and then cleared by drugs or the immune system, or awaiting the arrival of a blood-seeking *Anopheles* mosquito [6, 50].

The time required for the maturation of gametocytes (do not cause disease) are prominently different among different *Plasmodium* species. *P. falciparum* gametocytes require 8 up to 10 days for development into 5 morphologically different phases or stages (I–V) but *vivax* gametocytes take 48 h for maturity and disappear from blood within three days of sexual phase. In *falciparum*, the first identifiable stages of gametocytes are round compact forms having hemozoin. This stage (stage I) and the subsequent growth steps (stage 2–4) are principally absent from the vascular system, but sequestered in deep tissue in which they grow into mature sausage-shaped stage 5 gametocytes and reappeared in the blood and infective for mosquitoes. In diffrent to *falciparum*, matured *vivax* gametocytes are large and round, filling up almost the whole stippled red blood cell with a prominent nucleus. Because of their rapid maturation than *falciparum*, *vivax* gametocytes become exist in vascular system within a week subsequent to inoculation by mosquito and prior to parasite detection by light microscopy. This creates a major challenge in strategies of *vivax* elimination, as infected persons may be infectious prior to parasite detection using microscopy [53].

When a mosquito takes up erythrocytic gametocytes at the time of blood meal, the gametocytes migrate to the mosquito gut. At the midgut of mosquito, matured gametocytes egress from the host cell and differentiate into male and female gametes. The triggering factors for this differentiation are a fall in temperature, raise in pH and increase in xanthurenic acid concentration. Afterward, undergo fertilization (gametogenesis) - the flagellated forms of microgametes/male gametocytes formed by exflagellation penetrate/fertilize the macrogametes/female gametocytes to form a diploid zygote. The zygote develops into motile ookinetes, which penetrate the mosquito midgut and develop into round oocysts. The oocyst development is the longest developmental phase (takes three up to thirty days) and the only extracellular portion of the *Plasmodium* life cycle. The *falciparum* oocysts mature over a period of 11 to 16 days before releasing the infectious sporozoites (**Figure 1**). The sporozoites vigorously get away from the oocyst and only twenty five percent of those released from oocyst travel via the hemocoelomic fluid to the acinal cells of salivary glands, where following residence for a day, they turn into highly infective stage. They are permanently programmed for their trip in the vertebrate host because they totally lost their capability to invade salivary glands again. The chance of a mosquito for acquiring an infection at the time of blood meal is depend on various human, *Plasmodium* and mosquito factors. The maturity of gametocytes in human host is fundamental to the continuation of malaria transmission and represents a potential bottleneck in the life cycle of malaria parasites. Knowing the biology of gametocyte maturity and the human infectious reservoir at both the individual and population level is therefore essential to ablate disease transmission nonetheless, it is remained ambiguous [52, 53].

3. Conventional medicines

Malaria is a serious and potentially life threatening disease. It can lead to fatal outcomes in only few days, thus treatment should be started as soon as possible. According to their chemical structure and activity, the available antimalarial agents are grouped into 5 classes as shown in **Table 1** [54, 55]. The key targets of modern antimalarial agents are asexual blood stages of *Plasmodium* species (**Figure 2**), responsible for the malaria symptoms [56]. The *4- aminoquinolines* are blood schizonticidal agents and their mechanism of action is ascribed to their ability to form drug-heme adducts and accumulation of free heme, which is toxic for the parasite [57]. It is also belived that their mode of action is attributed by their inhibition of hemoglobin endocytosis and digestion or disruption of normal vesicle trafficking [58].

Chloroquine, the prototype anti-malarial drug, is the drug of choice for both treatment and chemoprophylaxis of all malaria parasites except for chloroquine-resistant *Plasmodium* strains. In addition to schizonticidal activity, it is also moderately effective against gametocytes of *vivax, ovale,* and *malariae* but not against those of *falciparum* gametocytes. Chloroquine does not eliminate dormant liver forms of *vivax* and *ovale,* for that reason primaquine must be added for the radical cure of these species. Although almost all strains of *malariae* are susceptible, *falciparum*, *vivax* and even some *ovale* strains have been reported as resistant to chloroquine. It is no longer recommended for prophylaxis against *falciparum* [59]. Although chloroquine is the first-line therapy for *vivax* malaria in majority of endemic countries, resistance is the core problem facing this drug in different parts of the world. In Africa and South America, its resistance to *falciparum* first appeared in 1978 and 1996, respectively [60, 61]. In Ethiopia, chloroquine treatment failure against *falciparum* and *vivax* malaria was reported for the fist time from Debre Zeit in 1995. Then after, chloroquine resistance has abeen detected

Major Classes	Groups	Specific agents
Quinolines	4-aminoquinolines	Chloroquine, amodiaquine and piperaquine
	8-aminoquinolines	Primaquine, and tafenoquine
Arylaminoalcohols	-	Quinine, mefloquine, halofantrine, and lumefantrine
Antifolate compounds	-	Pyrimethamine, proguanil, Dapsone, and sulfadoxine
Artemisinin and its derivatives	First generation	Dihdyroartemisinin, artesunate, arteether, and artemether
	Second generation	Artemisone
Hydroxynapthoquinone	-	Atovaquone

Table 1.
Classification of antimalarial drugs.

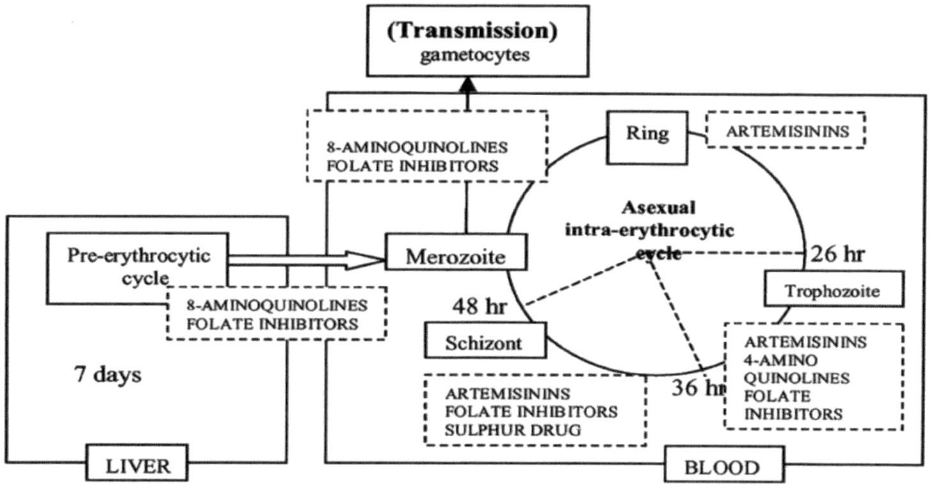

Figure 2.
Plasmodium life cycle with phases targeted by antimalarial drugs. 4-Aminoquinolines target the parasite at the stage where hemoglobin is degraded by parasite protease enzymes. 4-aminoquinolines such as chloroquine and amodiaquine have no effect on the pre-eythrocytic liver stages of parasite development.

in Ethiopia [25, 62]. However, drug resistance to chloroquine can be reversed by certain agents, including verapamil, desipramine, and chlorpheniramine, but the clinical value of resistance-reversing drugs is not established [59].

Amodiaquine is closely related to chloroquine and it probably shares mechanisms of action and resistance with chloroquine. Amodiaquine has been widely used to treat malaria (10 mg base/kg/day for 3 days) because of its low cost, limited toxicity, and, in some areas, effectiveness against chloroquine-resistant strains of *falciparum*. The most important current use is in combination therapy with: (i) sulfadoxine-pyrimethamine (SP) for prophylaxis, and (ii) artesunate [artemisinin-based combination therapy (ACT)] for treatment [13, 59]. **Piperaquine** is a potent and well-tolerated bisquinoline compound thought to act like chloroquine. This lipophilic drug is rapidly absorbed and has an excellent activity on chloroquine-resistant species. Currently, piperaquine combined with dihydroartemisinin (DHA) in co-formulated tablets has shown remarkable efficacy and safety in treating *falciparum* malaria, without visible drug resistance. Piperaquine has a larger half-life (28 days) than amodiaquine (14 days), mefloquine (14 days), and lumefantrine (4 days), leading to a prolonged duration of post-treatment prophylaxis with DHA-piperaquine than with other ACTs; this characteristic is advantageous especially in high transmission areas. DHA-piperaquine (one of the ACTs) is used to treat uncomplicated malaria [59, 63].

Eight-aminoquinolines, tissue schizonticidal agents, are belongs to the only class proven to be effective against the hypnozoites (exoerythrocytic forms) of *vivax* and *ovale* (**Figure 2**). In addition to hypnozoites activity, 8-aminoquinolines can kill gametocytes (the sexual stages of malaria parasites) and consequently block the malaria transmission. Although*falciparum* gametocyte clearance takes days, gametocytes are sterilized within hours; therefore, its effect on oocyst and sporozoite formation (and thus onward transmission of treated infection) precedes its effect on gametocytes carriage. Due to this effect some literatures classify primaquine as sporontocide. The addition of primaquine single dose to ACT is, therefore, recommended by the WHO to reduce gametocyte burden and thus transmission. It has weak activity against the asexual blood stage of *vivax* malaria but with negligible activity against*falciparum* malaria [13].

Primaquine (the prototype drug in 8-aminoquinolines) is indicated for radical cure of *vivax* or *ovale* malaria; for presumptive anti-relapse therapy (terminal prophylaxis- use after the completion of travel to an endemic area to markedly diminish the hypnozoite stages) in population widely exposed to *vivax* or *ovale;* to decrease onward *falciparum* malaria transmission in *falciparum* malaria elimination programmes and in areas threatened by *falciparum* resistance to artemisinins; and as an option for primary (causal and suppressive) prophylaxis against all *Plasmodium* species. Except its use in primary prophylaxis (prevent establishment of infection in the liver by inhibiting the pre-erythrocytic schizogony), primaquine is used in conjunction with an effective blood schizonticide (either ACT or chloroquine) to eradicate erythrocytic stages of *vivax* or *ovale* malaria, and to reduce the possibility of emerging drug resistance [13]. Its mechanism of action is unknown but it is thought to interfere with the cellular respiration of the parasite by means of generating oxygen-free radicals and deregulating the electron transport [64].

Quinine is one of the four antimalarial cinchona alkaloids and has rapid schizonticidal activity against intraerythrocytic malaria parasites. Quinine kills large ring and tropozoite asexual parasites and is gametocidal against *vivax, ovale* and *malariae* but not *falciparum* malaria [65]. Its mechanism of action has not been completely elucidated. The most widely accepted hypothesis is that the drug can inhibit hemozoin crystallization interfering with the heme detoxification process inside the food vacuole (membrane enclosed cell vacuole with a digestive function) [66]. The antimalarial and resistance mechanism of quinine is thought to share similarities to chloroquine.

Mefloquine was first used to treat chloroquine-resistant *falciparum* malaria in Thailand. However, the slow elimination of mefloquine fostered the emergence of drug-resistant parasites [63]. This drug is structurally related to quinine and has two racemic forms, *erythro-* and *threo-*, each composed of a pair of enantiomers, of which the racemic mixture of the *erythro-* enantiomers is the most active against Plasmodia [13]. Mefloquine is a blood schizonticide, active against the erythrocytic stages (15 mg/kg in a single dose) of all malaria parasites. It has more or less the same stage specificity of action as quinine, killing mainly the large ring and trophozoite asexual parasites. It has no significant pre-erythrocytic activity. In combination with artesunate, it can be used to treat uncomplicated malaria [13, 66]. The drug is especially useful as a chemoprophylactic agent for travelers spending weeks, months, or years in areas where *falciparum* and *vivax* infections are endemic due to its slow elimination (delayed half-life), except in clearly defined Thai border regions associated with MDR strains. The mechanism of action is still unknown, probably being different from 4-aminoquinolines. Activity on the parasite seems to be related to the ability of mefloquine to interfere with the transport of hemoglobin from the erythrocyte to the food vacuole. It is also proposed that it inhibits endocytosis of the cytosol by the parasite [13, 63].

Halofantrine hydrochloride is a phenanthrene methanol structurally related to quinine. It is effective against erythrocytic (but not other) stages of all four human malaria species. This synthetic anti-malarial is effective against MDR (including mefloquine resistant) *falciparum* malaria, but its use is limited by irregular absorption and cardiac toxicity. It should not be used for chemoprophylaxis. The mechanism of action by halofantrine is mysterious. It may be similar to that of chloroquine, quinine, and mefloquine; through forming toxic complexes with ferritoporphyrin IX that damage the membrane of the parasite [59, 67].

Antifolates are drugs that target two important enzymes of the folate pathway, namely the Dihydrofolate reductase (DHFR) and dihydropteroate synthase (DHPS). Proguanil and Pyrimethamine target DHFR, whereas sulfadoxine and dapsone act on DHPS. Pyrimethamine and proguanil are active against susceptible strains of all four human malaria species. In *falciparum* malaria sensitive antimalarial drugs, proguanil exhibit activity against both the primary hepatic stages and the asexual blood stages, thus sufficiently controlling the acute attack and usually eradicating the infection. Chloroguanide (proguanil) is also effective in treating acute *vivax* malaria, but relapses may arise after the drug is withdrawn because the latent tissue stages are not affected by this drug. Proguanil therapy does not obliterate gametocytes, but acts as a sporontocide (oocytes in the mosquito gut fail to develop normally) and thus ablate the transmission. It is not actually used alone as resistance to proguanil develops very quickly. Proguanil accentuates the mitochondrial membrane-potential-collapsing action of atovaquone against *falciparum* but displays no such activity by itself. The combination of proguanil and atovaquone is known as Malarone® and it is used as chemoprophylaxis in adults and children ≥11 kg. Atovaquone-proguanil may be considered for the treatment of uncomplicated malaria in travelers (adults and children ≥5 kg) outside malaria-endemic areas. It is highly effective and safe in a 3-day regimen for treating mild-to-moderate attacks of chloroquine- or SP-resistant *falciparum* malaria. The combination of chloroquine (500 mg weekly) and proguanil (200 mg daily) was previously widely used, but with increasing resistance to both agents it is no longer recommended [59, 63].

Pyrimethamine (2, 4-diaminopyrimidines) is a slow-acting blood schizontocide with antimalarial effect ssimilar to proguanil. However, pyrimethamine has greater antimalarial potency. The effectiveness of pyrimethamine against liver stages of *falciparum* is less than that of proguanil, and at therapeutic concentrations, pyrimethamine fails to eradicate hypnozoites of *vivax* and gametocytes of any malaria species. It raises the number of circulating mature infecting gametocytes of *falciparum*, likely leading to increased transmission to mosquitoes during treatment period. Pyrimethamine is typically administered with either a sulfonamide such as sulfadoxine or sulfone such as dapsone to enhance its antifolate activity. Sulfonamides and sulfones are weakly active against erythrocytic schizonts but not against liver stages or gametocytes. They are not used alone as antimalarials but are effective in combination with other agents. Although, no longer recommended due to drug resistance, pyrimethamine was used in synergistic combination with sulfadoxine (Fansidar®) or sulfalene (Metakelfin®) for treatment of uncomplicated malaria and with dapsone for prophylaxis. SP is active predominantly against later development stages of asexual parasites. In the few areas in which it remains effective, SP can be used with artesunate for the treatment of acute uncomplicated malaria. Its resistance is caused by point mutations in DHPS and DHFR [13, 63].

Atovaquone, a highly lipophilic analogue of ubiquinone, is active against all *Plasmodium* species, *Pneumocystis jiroveci* and *Toxoplasma gondii*. It is highly active against asexual blood stage (erythrocytic schizonts) of *falciparum* malaria. This drug (only administered orally) is also effective against liver stages (tissue schizonts) of *falciparum* (allowing prophylaxis to be discontinued only one week after the end of exposure) but not against *vivax* hypnozoites. Since atovaquone is tissue schizonticidal, malarone has an advantage over mefloquine and doxycycline in requiring shorter periods of treatment before and after the period at risk for malaria transmission, but it is more expensive than the other agents. Atovaquone selectively inhibits the parasite mitochondrial electron transport chain at the cytochrome bc1 complex. Selectivity is due to structural differences between the cytochrome b encoded by the parasite mitochondrial DNA and that encoded by the host mitochondrial DNA. Regeneration of ubiquinone (electron acceptor for *Plasmodium* dihydroorotate dehydrogenase [DHODH] enzyme, essential for pyrimidine biosynthesis) is the primary function of mitochondrial electron transport in *falciparum* species. Synergism activity between proguanil and atovaquone is resulted from the capability of non-metabolized proguanil to enhance the mitochondrial toxicity by atovaquone [59, 63, 68].

Artemisinins (endoperoxide sesquiterpene lactone) is a potent and fast acting blood schizonticidal killing all parasite stages, inducing more rapid parasite clearance and fever resolution than any other currently licensed antimalarial drug. Artemisinins have no effect on hepatic stages. They have been reported to reduce gametocytogenesis (young *falciparum* gametocytes), thus reducing transmission of malaria (preventing the spread of resistant strains). However, artemisinin has some pharmacokinetic limitations such as low solubility, poor bioavailability, and short half-life. To overcome some of these problems, semi-synthetic derivatives have been developed. First generation derivatives include the oil-soluble methyl ether, artemether (artemotil [arteether] is a closely related compound); the water soluble hemi-succinate derivative, artesunate; and DHA. Moreover, all active compounds possess a distinctive 1,2,4-trioxane pharmacophore, which is essential for the antimalarial activity since the corresponding acyclic compounds lacking the endoperoxide are biologically inactive [67, 69]. The precise mechanism of action of artemisinin is unclear and still controversial [70]. It has been suggested that the endoperoxide bond undergoes reductive activation by iron^{2+} or iron^{3+}-heme. This redox reaction produces carbon-centered radicals that alkylate target molecules leading to parasite's death [71]. Alternative views suggest that artemisinin inhibits *P. falciparum* encoded sarcoendoplasmic reticulum Ca^{2+}-ATPase (*PfATP6*) [72]. Another proposed mechanism is that artemisinins act as oxidant drugs through oxidation of flavin adenine dinucleotide (FADH2) and parasite flavoenzymes [73].

The standard treatment of malaria employs ACTs to increase treatment efficacy and reduce selection pressure for the emergence of drug resistance. Artemisinins cause a significant reduction of the parasite burden. As such, only 6–8 days of treatment are required to remove the parasites from the blood. Artemisinins do not display significant clinical cross-resistance with other drugs. Artemisinins should not be used for chemoprophylaxis because of their short half-life, which translates into high recrudescence rates. ACTs have lower toxicity and are considered safe to use in children and non-pregnant mothers. However, the widespread distribution of counterfeit (clinically sub-standard) agents that contain small quantities of artemisinin derivative threatens the effective administration of ACTs. The artemisinins and its derivatives generally are not used alone because of their limited ability to eradicate infection completely or its short plasma $t_{1/2}$ translates into substantial treatment failure rates. ACT consists of an artemisinin derivative combined with a long-acting antimalarial drug. To promote patient adherence to treatment by reducing course of therapy from 6 to 8 days to 3 days and to avoid the use of artemisinins as monotherapies due to their brief duration of action, fixed-dose combination formulations into a single tablet are available for all recommended ACTs (artemether + lumefantrine, artesunate + amodiaquine, artesunate + mefloquine, dihydroartemisinin + piperaquine, pyronaridine + artesunate, and artesunate + SP), except for artesunate plus SP. Artesunate-SP is not recommended in many areas owing to unacceptable levels of resistance to sulfadoxine-pyrimethamine. **Lumefantrine** is a fluorene derivative belongs to the group of quinine, halofantrine and mefloquine. This drug is belived to act similar to other members of the group (prevent haem detoxification within the food vacuole of the parasite, thus causing accumulation of the toxic haem complex). Lumefantrine (benflumetol) is formulated with artemether (COARTEM) [13, 63].

The WHO recommends ACT for the treatment of uncomplicated malaria caused by *falciparum* parasite or by chloroquine resistant *vivax*, *ovale, malariae* and *knowlsi*. Quinine plus clindamycin is used for uncomplicated malaria treatment in the first trimester of pregnancy [13]. In Ethiopia, Coartem (artemether-lumefantrine) is suggested as the first-line drug for uncomplicated *falciparum* malaria and chloroquine for other species (*vivax, malariae, ovale* and *knowlesi*) but oral quinine is considered as a second option [62]. Given their rapid and potent activity against even MDR parasites, injectable artesunate becomes the drug of choice for severe malaria globally in infants, children, lactating women and pregnant mothers of all trimester. After one day, the course of therapy should be completed using oral ACT [13]. Quinidine plus tetracycline, doxycycline, or clindamycin is the treatment of choice for severe malaria in the USA [74]. In Ethiopia, injectable artesunate is the drug of choice and intramuscular artemether is an alternative agent. When these 2 drugs are not available, injectable quinine is used to treat severe malaria [62].

Co-resistance of quinine with artesunate-amodiaquine (one of the most widely used ACTs) was fully verified both *in vivo* and *in vitro*. Given the widespread use of ACT worldwide, the suggestion that ART pressure might also favor quinine resistance is of major concern. Undeniably, the present dependence on artemisinins to manage both uncomplicated and complicated malaria, together with absence of possible therapeutic options, leaves decision-makers with very limited alternatives. This would have very bad consequences not only in the therapy of individual cases, but would cripple efforts to conquer malaria globally [75]. According to the current study, DHA-piperaquine is not treating malaria effectively across the eastern Greater Mekong subregion. A highly drug-resistant *falciparum* co-lineage is evolving, acquiring novel resistance mechanisms. So, resistance among artemisinin and its partner drug will continue to evolve, producing *Plasmodium* strains more capable of surviving treatment, which can subsequently spread across a wider geographical area. As a consequence, accelerated *falciparum* malaria elimination in this region is required urgently, to avert further spread and avoid a potential global health emergency. In the dearth of new antimalarial classes to replace the present first-line therapies, the use of existing treatments in the form of triple ACTs, in which an artemisinin is combined with 2 partner agents such as DHA-piperaquine and mefloquine, could be a viable alternative [76].

Despite decades of intense research, no licensed malaria vaccines are available until now [77]. A lot, but a better understanding is required on host immunity and the *Plasmodium* to improve vaccines. In Phase-3 clinical testing, the first proven antiparasite vaccine (a circumsporozoite protein vaccine [RTS, S/AS01]) reduced clinical malaria in children. Nonetheless, young infants do not respond well, and implementation studies with mortality endpoints are awaited. The irradiated *P. falciparum* sporozoites such as PfSPZ, which is closer to pivotal Phase-III trials, can be manufactured and have been shown to prevent infection in some African countries. Most recently, African trials of gamete protein vaccines started and placental malaria vaccines entered human testing. Blood-stage targets of protective antibodies remain unknown, but new proteins implicated in erythrocyte invasion and egress offer promise [78]. Limitations in efficacy, absence of standard predictive biomarkers of protective efficacy and the need to constantly update vaccine formulations due to antigenic polymorphism further underscore the current reliance on chemotherapy [79]. However, the occurrence of resistance (malaria parasites survive and/or multiply despite the proper administration and absorption of an antimalarial medicine in the dose normally recommended) [80] among commonly used drugs is a major problem. Resistance against antimalarial drug results in a global revival of malaria creating a major problem to malaria control. Indiscriminate and widespread utilization of antimalarial agents contributes to *Plasmodium* species to evolve and develop resistance mechanisms [81, 82]. As a result, old and novel chemicals are under per-clinical and clinical studies. Despite the widespread development of resistance and difficulties in poor areas to afford and access effective antimalarial drugs, currently used and potent drugs, such as artemether, chloroquine and quinine, are obtained from plant sources. Hence, it is imperative to focus on traditionally used medicinal plants for the discovery of possible new innovative antimalarial sources for the future.

4. Genetic basis of drug resistance

Resistance to antimalarial compounds occurs because of the parasites selection with genetic mutations such as single nucleotide polymorphisms (SNP) or gene amplifications that confer decreased susceptibility [83]. A number of factors aid the emergence of current antimalarial drug resistance. Some of them, among others, are the mutation rate of *Plasmodium*, the overall parasite load, the strength of drug selected, the treatment compliance, and poor adherence to treatment guidelines. Inappropriate dose, poor pharmacokinetic profile, fake drugs lead to inadequate drug exposure on parasites [84, 85], and poor quality antimalarial (falsified antimalarial without active ingredients) drugs may aid and abet the occurnce of resistance by increasing the risk of hyperparasitaemia, recrudescence, and hypergametocyopaenia [86, 87].

The two malaria parasites (*falciparum* and *vivax*) that cause most of malaria cases of human beings have developed resistance to almost all current antimalarial drugs. The capability of these *Plasmodium* species to develop resistance is mainly due to the large numbers of parasites in the infected individual's bloodstream at the time of the asexual blood stage infection in conjunction with the mutability of their genomes [88]. Now a day, controlling MDR*falciparum* malaria is become a very challenging work for the reason that endogenous allelic exchanges occurred in *falciparum* species have increased the treatment failures and drastically increased the resistance level globally. Since evolution is a continuous process, how we stop the formation of drug resistant mutant alleles is a very concerning question. Usually, high mean parasitemia index is observed in*falciparum* infected persons but *vivax* infection generally exhibits low parasitemia index secondary to its preference to invade reticulocytes rather than erythrocytes [89, 90].

Resistance to chloroquine in*falciparum* is due to point mutations in the gene encoding *pfcrt* (*P. falciparum* chloroquine resistance transporter) and *pfmdr* (*P. falciparum* multidrug resistance protein [P-glycoprotein transporter proteins]), resulting in reduced drug accumulation in the food vacuole [91]. Chloroquine-resistant *vivax* was first reported from Papua New Guinea in 1989. High grade chloroquine-resistant *vivax* is prevalent in areas such as Indonesia and Oceania (considered as chloroquine resistance epicenters) [92]. It is more challenging to detect chloroquine resistance in *vivax* since parasitemia is generally low relative to*falciparum*. In addition, it is not easy to distinguish *vivax* recrudescence from relapses as a result of reactivation of dormant hepatic parasites in endemic settings. Moreover, there is no robust *in vitro* culture system for *vivax*, so confirmation with *in vitro* susceptibility testing is even more challenging for *vivax* than for*falciparum*. Although *pvcrt-o* (*P. vivax* chloroquine resistance transporter-o) is orthologous to *pfcrt*, there is no clear direct association between chloroquine resistance and mutations in *pvcrt-o*. One current study in patients with recurrent *vivax* infections in the Brazilian Amazon found that chloroquine resistance was associated with increased copies of gene encoding *pvcrt-o* [88].

Amodiaquine and its slowly eliminated active metabolite (desethylamodiaquine) are structurally related to chloroquine, this explains the cross resistance observed in the field, where parasites were reported to harbor mutations on *pfcrt* and *pfmdr1* after amodiaquine treatment failure [93]. Therefore, amodiaquine is used in combination therapy with SP for prophylaxis and artesunate for treatment.

DHA-piperaquine (co-formulated tablet) has shown excellent efficacy (without apparent drug resistance) and safety in treating *falciparum* malaria. But now, resistance has been reported from Western Cambodia to be associated with a point mutation of *pfcrt* and amplification of *plasmepsin* 2 and 3 genes in *falciparum* parasites. The *plasmepsin* genes encode aspartic proteases that function as hemoglobinases in the parasitie's digestive vacuole. The mechanism of resistance is not clearly known; however hypothesized that increased hemoglobin digestion due to the amplification decreases the reactive heme species concentrations that piperaquine binds, thereby overcoming the inhibition of heme detoxification by piperaquine [88].

Documents written regarding **quinine** resistance are rare, but isolated cases have been reported from Thailand, North India, East Africa and South America [93]. Resistance mechanisms to quinine appear to be more complex. *In vitro* cross resistance between quinine, other aryl aminoalcohols, and 4-aminoquinolines is observed, suggesting that there may be a common genetic mechanism of resistance among those drugs. Mutations in *pfmdr1* and *pfcrt* have been found to confer decreased susceptibility of the parasite to quinine. Yet, they are not sufficient to bring resistance, implying that there are additional genes involved. A quantitative trait loci analysis done to detect genes associated with quinine resistance in 71 *falciparum* isolates from diverse locations has been identified *pfmdr1*, *pfcrt*, and *pfnhe-1* (*P. falciparum* Na^+/H^+*exchanger-1*). *Pfnhe-1* encodes *falciparum* Na^+/H^+exchanger 1 and is on chromosome 13. M**efloquine** resistance by both *falciparum* and *vivax* was found to be primarily mediated by *mdr1* amplification (increased *mdr1* copy number), rather than through point mutations similar to chloroquine and antifolate drugs. Resistance to **primaquine** in *vivax* is difficult to verify as it is confounded by reinfections in malaria-endemic regions. A research that done whole genome sequencing of *vivax* from known relapses that occurred despite primaquine therapy found polymorphisms in many putative resistance genes. However, there are currently no known genetic markers of primaquine and tafenoquine resistance [88].

In contrast to chloroquine resistance, which took many years to develop, antifolates resistance developed much faster. The genetic mechanism of resistance for antifolates is more straightforward than chloroquine resistance. The reason for resistanc against antifolates is single point-mutations in the genes encoding either DHFR—*pfdhfr* in *falciparum* and *pvdhfr* in *vivax* malaria, or DHPS—*pfdhps* in *falciparum and pvdhps* in *vivax* malaria. *Dhfr* mutations reduce the overall efficacy of the enzyme and result in a fitness cost for *Plasmodium*. Following changes in first-line therapy of malaria from sulfa-drugs to ACTs, a decline in triple and quadruple *dhfr* mutants has been observed in certain regions. Nonetheless, in nations where SP is part of the ACT or SP is used as intermittent preventive therapy (IPT), these mutants remain prevalent. In addition, the persistence of the *Plasmodium* species carrying *dhfr* mutations may be attributed to the use of trimethroprim-sulfamethoxazole for prophylaxis or for treating opportunistic infections in HIV positive individuals. Interestingly, *falciparum* species in Southeast Asia are able to develop a compensatory mutation for the fitness cost incurred by the mutant *dhfr*. A genome scanning study of *falciparum* strains first identified an amplification surrounding GTP-cyclohydrolase 1 (*gch1*), which encodes an enzyme in the folate biosynthesis pathway that is upstream from DHFR and DHPS. The amplification reduces the cost of acquiring the drug-resistance mutations further downstream in the folate synthesis pathway [88]. **Atovaquone** acquires resistance related to a single mutation of cytochrome b gene of the parasite [68].

Artemisinin resistance in *falciparum* has currently been detected in five countries of Greater Mekong sub-region (Cambodia, Lao People's Democratic Republic, Myanmar, Thailand and Viet Nam). These resistant *Plasmodium* strains have the ability of spreading into many world countries including Africa and then they become a global threat for malaria control and treatment [13, 94]. Though different studies associate artemisinin resistance with mutuation in *pfatp6* (*P. falciparum encoded sarcoendoplasmic reticulum* Ca^{2+}*-ATPase6*), *pfmdr1*, *pffd* (*P. falciparum ferredoxin*), *pfarps10* (*apicoplast ribosomal protein s10*), *pfmdr2* or *pfcrt* genes of falciparum, these mutations are thought to represent a background upon which the *kelch13* mutations are especially likely to occur. The genetic mediator(s) of *vivax* resistance against artemisinins is/are not reported till now. Lumefantrine resistance in field isolates has not yet been convincingly demonstrated. However, amplification of the *pfmdr1* gene in *falciparum* and *pvmdr1* in *vivax* has been associated with increased risk of treatment failure of coartem®. Antibacterials such as tetracycline, doxycycline, clindamycin and azithromycin also have antiplasmodial activity although in general their action is slow for malaria treatment. They are recommended only in combination with other antimalarials. Apicoplast ribosomal RNA (23S rRNA) mutation mediated *falciparum* resistance to clindamycin has been found in field isolates. There are no clear markers of doxycycline resistance that have been identified thus far [88, 93].

5. Novel compounds in the pipeline

Mentioned above, the evolving of resistant strains and absence of newer drugs are the limiting aspects in the fight against malaria. These factors prompt the continuing need of studies to bring novel grups of antimalarial compounds, and a re-examination of the present ones. That's why; synthetic peroxides (ozonides) are approved to be viable substitutes of artemisinin. **OZ277** (the first generation ozonide discovered in 2004 and subsequently called **arterolane)** was developed through a collaborative effert between Ranbaxy and MMV (Medicines for Malaria Venture). After a limited phase-3 trials on the combination effects of arterolane and piperaquine, the combined drug has got approval under the trade name **Synriam** in India in 2013, followed by approval in 7 African nations in 2014 [95]. Many new combination treatments, including **azithromycin-chloroquine** [96], **pediatric pyronaridine-artesunate**, **pediatric DHA-piperaquine** [97] and **trimethoprim-sulfamethoxazole** [95], are in phase-3 trials.

A lot of novel chemicals are in phase-II clinical trials (**Table 2**). **Ferroquine (SR97193)** is new organometallic drug completed phase-2 trials in combination with artesunate [98]. Ferroquine retains *in vitro* activity against piperaquine- and chloroquine-resistant *Plasmodium* species. It has a long elimination half-life (16 days). Ferroquine is only moderately effective as single therapy but when combined to artesunate (daily dose of 4/6 mg/kg ferroquine plus 4 mg/kg artesunate for three days); the PCR corrected efficacy at 28 days in treating uncomplicated *falciparum* malaria was 99% [103]. **OZ439** (a synthetic trioxolane) possesses curative and transmission-blocking capacity, and is active against artemisinin-resistant malaria parasites. Much like the current peroxide containing antimalarial agents, the exact mechanism of action of OZ439 has yet to be revealed but it is believed that oxidative stress plays a major role as shown in **Figure 3**. OZ439 [discovered in 2011 by a partnership between Monash University, the University of Nebraska and the Swiss Tropical and Public Health Institute (STPHI)] possesses significantly lower solubility and slightly lower potency than OZ277 [100]. In contrast to other synthetic peroxides and artemisinin derivatives, OZ439 (artefenomel) totally cured mice infected with *P. berghei* at a single oral dose (20 mg/kg) and showed higher prophylactic effect compared to most antimalarial drugs. Next to reports on its safety and pharmacokinetic properties, a combination of artefenomel (fast- and

Class	Name	Activity (Target)	Development Partner	Remark	Ref.
Second-generation peroxide	OZ439 (artefenomel)	Active against blood stage of falciparum and vivax malaria	MMV and Sanofi	Being tested in Phase IIb combination trial with piperaquine, & with ferroquine	[95, 98]
4-aminoquinoline (Organometallic)	SR97193 (ferroquine)	Active against chloroquine-resistant strains	MMV	Currently in combination trial with artesunate	[98]
Synthetic spiroindolone analogue	KAE609 (Cipargamin)	Blood schizonticide for vivax and falciparum	MMV and Novartis	Currently in Phase IIb trials (NCT03334747)	[99, 100]
Second-generation imidazolopiperazine	KAF156	It acts at multiple stages of the parasite life cycle	MMV and Novartis	Now in phase IIb trial in combination with lumefantrine (NCT03167242)	[101, 102]
	DSM265	Long acting agent with blood and liver stage activity and also active against drug resistant parasites	Takeda, MMV and UT Southwestern	Completed human study in combination with OZ439 (NCT02389348).	[100, 101]
Phenothiazine derivative	Methylene blue	Has blood stage activity and also active against mature male and female falciparum gametocytes	University of Heidelberg	Completed Phase-II trial as a combination with primaquine (NCT02851108) in 2017	[103]
3,5-diaryl-2-aminopyridine	MMV048	Has prophylactic and transmission blocking activity	MMV	Currently in Phase IIa clinical trials in Ethiopia	[100]

Table 2.
Promising new antimalarial agents in phase II clinical development.

long-acting drug) with ferroquine was progressed into a phase-2 trials in 2015 to assess the efficacy of a single oral dose in adults and children aimed at replacing the current three doses of artemisinin derivatives. **Artefenomel–ferroquine** has an elimination half-life of 46–62 h. An advantage of this product is that neither of the constituent drugs has been deployed as monotherapy previously [79, 103].

Artemisone (second-generation semi-synthetic artemisinin derivative developed at the Hong Kong University of Science and Technology), a drug in phase-II study, provides a single dose cure in Aotus monkeys infected with *falciparum* malaria at 10 mg/kg when combined with mefloquine 5 mg/kg [104]. Artemisone

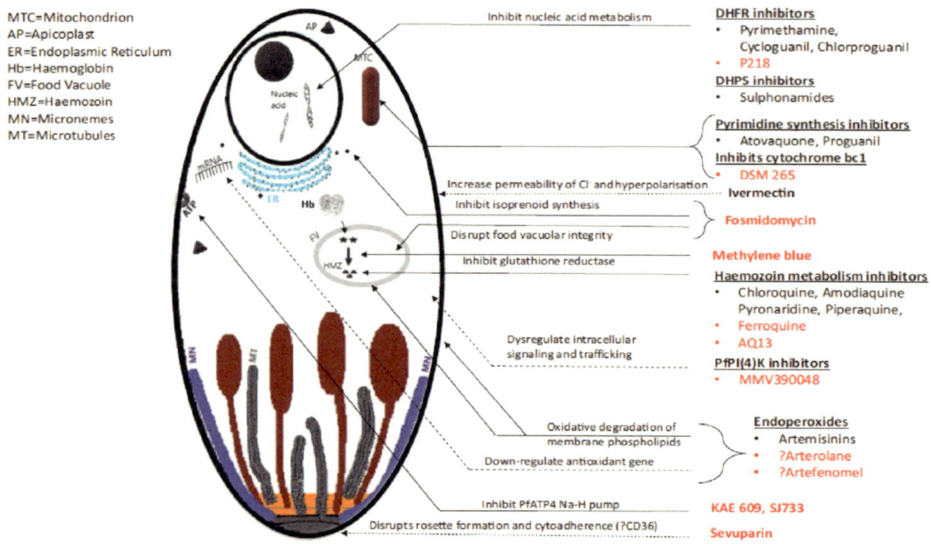

Figure 3.
Schematic representation of intra-erythrocytic trophozoite showing sites of action of newer antimalarials. Agents in red are still in development [100].

has shown to be efficacoiuse as artesunate and possess improved pharmacokinetic properties such as longer half-life and lower neuro- and cytotoxicity than the first generation artemisinins [105]. With the motivation of urgent requirement to develop new artemisinins in combination with new drugs that impart activities toward both intra-erythrocytic asexual and transmissible gametocyte stages, in particular, those of resistant parasites, amino-artemisinins (oxidant drug in which an amino group replaces the oxygen-bearing substituents attached to carbon number 10 of the present clinical artemisinin derivatives DHA, artemether and artesunate) including artemisone and artemiside exhibit potent *in vitro* activities against the asexual erythrocytic stages of *falciparum* malaria. Particularly, these compounds are active against late erythrocytic stage *falciparum* gametocytes, and are highly synergistic in combination with the redox active agent methylene blue. In order to strengthen the selection of best amino-artemisinins for development into novel triple combination treatments also active against artemisinin-resistant *P. falciparum* mutants, new amino-artemisinins were formulated based on the easily accessible and low-priced drug DHA-piperazine. DHA-piperazine was converted into alkyl sulfonamides, aryl sulfonamides, ureas and amides. These derivatives were screened together with the comparator drugs DHA and the amino-artemisinins (until now most active compounds against asexual and sexual erythrocytic stages of *falciparum* and hepatic stage *P. berghei* sporozoites) artemisone and artemiside. Many new amino-artemisinins that contain aryl-urea and -amide groups are found to be potently active against both asexual and late erythrocytic stage gametocytes. Although the activities are superior to those of artemiside and artemisone, the latter (aryl sulfonamide, the aryl urea, and the aryl amides) are more active against the liver stage *P. berghei* sporozoites. In addition, these compounds tend not to display reduced susceptibility against *Plasmodium* species bearing the *Pf* Kelch 13 propeller domain C580Y mutation characteristic of artemisinin-resistant *falciparum* malaria. Thus, the advent of the amino-artemisinins will enable the development of novel combination drugs that by virtue of the amino-artemisinin component itself will possess intrinsic transmission-blocking abilities and may be effective against artemisinin-resistant *falciparum* malaria [106, 107].

Novartis currently has 2 new antimalarial compounds (**KAE609 (Cipargamin)** and **KAF156)** in phase-II clinical testing (**Table 2**) [99]. The occurrence of resistance in artemisinin raises the concern of cross-resistance with arterolane and artefenomel due to chemical similarities between the two groups of compounds. By contrast, cipargamin and KAF156 are structurally unrelated to the artemisinin derivatives. KAE609 has inhibitory effect on *falciparum* cation channel/P-type ATPase-4 transporter (*PfATPase4*) resulting in a build up of Na^+ inside the parasite, leading to cell death. **Cipargamin** was discovered by a partnership between Novartis, the STPHI and the Wellcome Trust. It is equially potent against drug-resistant *Plasmodium* strains and as effective as artesunate against *falciparum* and *vivax* malaria. KAE609 displays a good safety with low cytotoxicity, cardiotoxicity and mutagenic activity. Cipargamin has the ablity to clear parasitaemia quickly in adult individuals (30 mg/day for 3 days) with uncomplicated *falciparum* or *vivax* malaria. This drug is also shows low body clearance, long half-life and excellent bioavailability [100].

KAF156 (identified in 2008 by Novartis and The Scripps Research Institute) is with potential to treat and prevent malaria, and has an elimination half-life of around 48 h. KAF156 is shown to have potent *in vitro* activity against both asexual and sexual blood stages and the pre-erythrocytic liver stages of *Plasmodium* species. In the causal prophylactic rodent malaria model, a single oral dose of 10 mg/kg was shown to be fully protective. KAF156 has also shown transmission blocking activity in the berghei model. A recent phase-2 trial among adults with acute *falciparum/vivax* malaria at five centers in Thailand and Vietnam has showed that KAF156 cleared parasites more rapidly than SP or malarone®, though this rate was slightly slower than artemisinin and DSM265. Additionally, therapeutic responses to treatment by KAF156 suggested effectiveness against *falciparum* and *vivax* infections resistant to each and every one of currently available antimalarials without evident safety concerns. The mode of action of KAF156 is still unclear although mutations have been identified in three genes (*P. falciparum* Cyclic Amine Resistance Locus [*PfCARL*], UDP-galactose and Acetyl-CoA transporters) through culturing of resistant strains [79, 100]. **DSM265** is another compound that complete phase-2a trials (**Table 2**) and inhibit DHODH both in *falciparum* and *vivax* species [104]. It was discovered through collaboration between the University of Texas (UT) Southwestern, the University of Washington, and Monash University. DSM265 has an excellent safety profile, a very low clearance rate and a long half-life in humans. *In vitro* studies suggest a relatively low barrier to resistance selection, so measures to protect this drug, such as matching with a partner with similar elimination kinetics and deploying only as part of a fixed-dose combination will be important [103].

Fosmidomycin, a natural antibacterial drug that inhibit 1-deoxy-D-xylulose 5-phosphate reductoisomerase (an enzyme involved in the synthesis of isoprenoids), is under combination therapy trial with piperaquine (NCT02198807) in phase 2 in order to destroy blood schizonts of uncomplicated *falciparum* malaria [97, 108]. **AQ-13**, a modified chloroquine (differ to chloroquine only in the amine side-chain), last completed phase-II trial (NCT01614964) at the end of 2017 [100], retains activity against chloroquine-resistant strains [109]. The result showed that there are no serious adverse events and the asexual parasites were cleared by day 7 in both groups [79].

Methylene blue, a drug used to treat methaemoglobinemia, acts by inhibiting *falciparum* glutathione reductase and as a result prevents haem polymerization. It is being developed in combination (phase II) with artesunate–amodiaquine as a strategy to protect against emergence of artemisinin resistance secondary to its *falciparum* schizonticidal effect and reduce transmission owing to gametocytocidal activity [110]. **Rosiglitazone**, an anti-diabetic drug, is currently in clinical trials (NCT02694874) as an adjunctive therapy for severe malaria. **Imatinib**, a cancer therapy, is now in phase-2 trials (NCT03697668) as a triple combination with DHA-piperaquine [100]. Polysaccharide heparin analogue **Sevuparin (DF02),** which is taken as an adjunctive therapy, retains the anti-adhesive effects of heparin without the antithrombin properties and has been shown to block merozoite invasion, cytoadherence and rosetting [111]. Sevuparin, a drug treating sickle cell disease, was completed its phase-1/2 trials (NCT01442168) in 2014 as a combination with atovaquone-proguanil [100]. **MMV390048** is an aminopyridine currently in phase-2a trials (NCT02880241) and its target was identified to be lipid *P. falciparum* phosphatidylinositol 4-kinase (*PfPI4K*). This blood schizonticidal drug has destructive activity on multiple stage of the *Plasmodium* with possible efforts for chemoprevention as it inhibits gametocytogenesis and oocyst formation [102, 112]. **Albitiazolium (SAR97276) or bisthiazolium salt**, discovered and developed by Sanofi in 2005, has also reached phase-2 clinical tests (NCT01445938), however further study was terminated in 2012 [100]. It acts mainly by deterring the transport of choline into the parasite [113]. Descoverd in 2012 by a team at the Cape Town University, South Africa, **MMV048** has shown 99.3% reduction in parasitaemia in the *P. berghei* mouse model at a single dose of 30 mg/kg with no signs of parasites after 30 days. This highlights the potential of this compound to act as a single dose therapy. Its target is *PfPI4K*, eukaryotic enzyme that phosphorylates lipids to allow them to regulate intracellular signaling and trafficking. Inhibiting the ATP-binding pocket of *PI4K* (recently revealed as a novel mechanism of action for antimalarial agents) causes disruption in the intracellular distribution of PI4-phosphate (*PI4P*), which inturn results in decreased late-stage development of the parasite. MMV048 is now in phase-2 clinical studies [100].

Quinoline-4-carboxamide **DDD107498** (previously known as **M5717**) is additional treatment panorama that was developed in 2015 by the Drug Discovery Unit (DDU) in Dundee. It is an inhibitor of *P. falciparum* translational elongation factor 2 (*PfeEF2*) with activity against pre-erythrocytic and blood stages as well as mature male and female gametocytes. Henece, it can act as curative and transmission blocking drug. *PfeEF2* is responsible for catalyzing the translocation of mRNA and tRNA. The overall efficacy of drugs that target this elongation factor may be increased due to the expression of *PfeEF2* in multiple stages of the *Plasmodium* life cycle [77, 114]. DDD107498 has shown excellent activity against a number of drug-resistant strains of *Plasmodium* species, and exhibited superior potency than artesunate against *falciparum* and *vivax* in *ex vivo* assays. It has been also demonstrated magnificent pharmacokinetic profiles including better oral bioavailability and long plasma half-life (critical for chemoprevention and single dose therapy) in pre-clinical species. Owing to its *PfeEF2* inhibition and its ability to clear blood stage parasites completely, DDD107498 satisfies the requirements to be a long duration partner and could be used as part of a combination therapy with a fast-acting compounds. In late 2017, DDD107498 was cleared for progression from development to phase-1 clinical tests for volunteers in Australia (NCT03261401) [79, 100].

A dihydroisoquinolone compound **(+)-SJ733**, which inhibits gametocytogenesis and blood schizonts in*falciparum* and *vivax*, is now in human trial. The pre-clinical trials showed that SJ733 (inhibitor of *PfATP4*) worked against *Plasmodium* species that are resistant to current frontline agents. It binds to a malaria parasite protein that serves as a sodium pump to interfere with the protein or to disrupt the malaria parasite's capability to remove excess Na+ from RBCs [115, 116]. When sodium builds up, infected cells become develop rigidity (less flexible) and as a result distroyed by our immune system or get caught in small blood vessels. Currently, around 38 healthy volunteers were recruited as part of the phase-Ia trial in Memphis and phase-Ib test in Brisbane, Australia. In Memphis, about 23 healthy volunteers received increasing doses of the new compound to understand dosing, absorption, safety profile and metabolism. Based on those results, the 15 Australian volunteers received SJ733 after being infected with malaria to understand the antimalarial effectiveness of this novel molecule. No significant SJ733 treatment related side effects were notified in any of the volunteers [117].

Additionally, **CDRI97/78** (fast-acting trioxane first synthesized in 2001 by a team at the Council of Scientific and Industrial Research in India), **ACT-451840** (phenylalanine-based compound developed in 2016 through collaboration between Actelion Pharmaceuticals and the STPHI, **P218** (2,4-diaminopyridine analog and *PfDHFR* inhibitor discovered by BIOTEC Thailand in 2012) and **GSK369796** (N-tert-butyl isoquine developed at the Liverpool School of Tropical Medicine in 2009) are also among componds under/completed phase-1 trials [95, 102]. CDRI97/78 (blood schizonticidal molecule) was well-tolerated in healthy adult volunteers with a half-life of around 12 h. It has shown few and not severe adverse effects. ACT-451840 has the potential to be a fast-acting drug with a long half-life. This agent has shown efficacy against multiple life cycle (asexual and sexual) stages of both*falciparum* and *vivax* malaria, and also harbor additional gametocytocidal activity and, thereby, transmission-blocking properties. The new two step mechanism of action for binding to *PfDHFR* allows P218 to conquer resistance that has emerged after clinical use of pyrimethamine. P218 showed high selectivity to bind malarial than human DHFR, which translates into reduced toxicity. P218 is highly efficacious against*falciparum* and *chabaudi* in mice with ED90 of 1 mg/kg and 0.75 mg/kg, respectively. Along with its high potency and good safety profile, P218 has the potential to be a replacement for pyrimethamine combination with cycloguanil in areas where *PfDHFR* resistance has emerged. P218 has currently completed phase-I trials (NCT02885506). GSK369796 was designed as an alternative to amodiaquine. It completed pre-clinical experments, and was last in phase-I trials in 2008 (NCT00675064) [100].

DM1157, part of a class of compounds known as "reversed chloroquines", was designed to overcome chloroquine-resistant (the parasites expel the drug before it can affect them) strains of*falciparum* malria. Like chloroquine, DM1157 (discovered in 2010 by a research team in Portland State University and further developed by DesignMedix) interferes with the parasite's metabolism, but it also inhibits the parasite's ability to expel the drug. It is currently in Phase I trials (NCT03490162) to evaluate its safety and pharmacokinetics in humans, which is sponsored by the National Institute of Allergy and Infectious Diseases (NIAID). Results of earlier tests in animals suggest that DM1157 could have the same safety and efficacy as chloroquine [100, 118]. Human trials of innovative antimalarial compounds are in the pipeline following Kenyan scientists fruitfully used a derivative from bacteria to kill *Plasmodium* that causes malaria. According to the Kenya Medical Research Institute and its global health partners, the breakthrough could potentially lead to the discovery of new approach for tackling malaria. The promise of a new treatment comes after trials in Burkina Faso found that ivermectin, a conventional drug used for non-malaria parasitic diseases, reduced the transmission rate of malaria. The drug is acted by making the blood of repeatedly treated people lethal to mosquitoes. The experment also revealed that ivermectin can kill *P. falciparum* in mosquitoes that fed on humans who took the drug. As they are more vulnerable, the study is more focused on pregnant women and children and the researchers are getting very encouraging lead compunds. In the near future, latest antimalarial drugs could be in the market if the recent research findings are going ahead. The same bacteria known to kill dangerous pathogens including scabies and river blindness can also be applied in malaria [119].

After identification of a lead compound, optimization of the chemical structure can be started. This step mainly involves examination of the structural activity relationships (SARs) of the compound and optimization of properties such as potency (*in vitro* and *in vivo*), solubility and metabolic stability. The new candidate must also be evaluated for any possible toxicity including cytotoxicity and genotoxicity in pre-clinical trials. **NPC1161B** (the chiral 8-aminoquinoline derivative), developed at the University of Mississippi, was in late preclinical studies for relapse prevention. This compound has a multi-stage activity and there is a development plan to see whether this single enantiomer drug has a more favorable hematological toxicity profile than tafenoquine in Phase-I. **AN13762** (blood schizonticidal), a novel class of benzoxaborole anti-malarial compounds, is emerged in 2017 as the lead compound, showing excellent activity in *in vitro* and *in vivo* (pre-clinical) studies. It has multi-strain efficacy and the ability to act rapidly. It has been shown to be equally potent across a wide range of drug resistant strains. AN13762 has exhibit similar *in vivo* clearance rate when compared to artesunate. The precise mechanism of action for AN13762 remains unknown, though initial studies on hit compound (AN3661) identified the P. *falciparum* cleavage and polyadenylation specificity factor 3 (*PfCPSF3*) as a potential target [100, 103, 120].

Triaminopyrimidine **MMV253** (identified by AstraZeneca in 2015) and an aminomethylphenol **JPC-3210** (active against multidrug resistant falciparum *in vitro*) are long-acting blood schizonticidal agents present in early preclinical experiments [121, 122]. MMV253 (previously AZ13721412) has shown good *in vitro* potency and *in vivo* efficacy. When screened against several mutant resistant strains with different mechanisms of resistance, MMV253 displayed no spontaneous decline in potency which can be attributed to its new mode of action (inhibition of *PfATP4*). Good *in vitro* and *in vivo* correlation was shown with a forecasted human half-life of ~36 h, which is long compared to another fast killing agent (artemisinin, human half-life of 1 h). As of late 2016, Cadila Healthcare pharmaceutical company owns the license for the compound series and is now making further lead development in order to progress the chemical through pre-clinical trials. At the same time that the *Plasmodium* is regulating its Na^+ concentration using *PfATP4*, it also brings in H^+ via the same pathway. To control this increasing concentration of H^+ and maintain an intracellular pH of about 7.3, the *Plasmodium* uses a complementary V-type ATPase transporter to pump out H^+ ion. It was shown that MMV253 has the ability to inhibit the V-type H^+ ATPase as its mechanism of action. **UCT943** (identified in 2016 by a team at the Cape Town University, South Africa in the same campaign as MMV048) is a key compound in a novel class of 2-aminopyrazine antimalarials that has shown single dose curing capability *in vivo* and potential as a clinical candidate. UCT943 (target *PfPI4K*) is potent across multiple life stages of both *falciparum* and *vivax* malaria. UCT943 was in originally in place as a back-up to MMV048, however, due to pre-clinical toxicity, this candidate has been withdrawn [100]. A Mannich base compound, **MK-4815** (2-aminomethyl-3, 5-di-tert-butylphenol), showed potent *in vitro* activity against *falciparum* and hundred percent survival was seen in mice orally treated with 25/12.5/6.25 mg/kg once on the day of infection and then twice daily for an additional 4 days. While comparable volume of distribution at steady state was seen in mice and rhesus monkey, the compound exhibited lower clearance and long plasma half-life in monkeys, indicating the drug possess better pharmacokinetic parameters in the higher species. Although the mechanism of action is still remains unclear, evidences indicate the involvement of the mitochondrial electron transport chain of the *Plasmodium*. Owing to its structural simplicity, effectiveness against MDR *falciparum* strains, good pharmacokinetic profiles and capability to cure acute *P. berghei* infection at a single dose of 50 mg/kg, MK-4815 has a potential as an antiplasmodial agent and of course, is now under additional assessment by MMV as a pre-clinical candidate [79].

In an attempt to identify antiplasmodial agents with new mechanism of action, Kato and his colleagues found a lead compound coded as **BRD7929**. It was shown to target the cytosolic *falciparum* phenylalanyl-tRNA synthetase. This enzyme serves to enable transfer-RNAs deliver the amino acid phenylalanine to nascent proteins during RNA translation and protein synthesis. This bicyclic azetidine showed *in vivo* against *falciparum* and *berghei* infected mice at a single low doses. This molecule was also very potent against the hepatocytic and asexual stages of *falciparum* and exihibited transmission-blocking effect at concentrations that achieved single dose cures of asexual erythrocytic stage infections. Even if BRD7929 showed good (80%) oral bioavailability, improved aqueous solubility and longer half-life in mice (32 h), moderate cytotoxicity was seen thus presenting possible setbacks, which would have to be addressed during further optimization. Nonetheless, the capability of this lead molecule to eliminate blood stage (asexual and sexual) and liver stage parasites suggests that this compound has the potential to cure the disease, provide prophylaxis and block transmission. Currently, a tetraoxane-based antiplasmodial drug candidate, **E209** that can overcome *PfK13* Cys-580-Tyr dependent artemisinin resistance was identified. Further evaluation revealed retention of *in vitro* potency against sensitive and MDR *falciparum* isolates, with no observable cross-resistance with artemisinin. Compound E209 also exhibited equipotent *ex vivo* activity against *vivax* and *falciparum* Indonesian clinical isolates while screening for gametocytocidality showed a transmission reducing profile consistent with the endoperoxides. Equally important *in vivo* studies in *P. berghei* infected mice showed complete parasite clearance with an estimated oral ED_{50} of 4 mg per kg after 3 doses and a 66 percent cure rate following a 30 mg/kg single oral dose. Therefore, this chemical has the potential to use in a superior combination therapies with a partner drug devoid of *in vivo* resistance liabilities hence offers a substantial improvement on the current ACTs and provides an urgently needed alternative agent for malaria treatment and elimination. Moreover, its efficacy against *vivax* and gametocytes indicates the potential of E209 to prevent relapse and block transmission, respectively [79].

SC83288, an amicarbalide derivative developed in 2017 by a team at Heidelberg University, is the only agents in pre-clinical study that are going to treat sever malaria [123]. This new mlecule was shown to be fast-acting and cured *falciparum* infection in a humanized mouse model, with pre-clinical pharmacokinetic and toxicological studies revealing no apparent shortcomings. While the precise mode of action is uknown, *PfATP6* was identified as a putative determinant of resistance to SC83288. However, it has been shown that SC83288 does not directly inhibit this target suggesting *PfATP6* may have a less direct role in its mechanism of action. SC83288 has been evaluated against artemisinins, showing no cross resistance. *Pfmdr*2 has been identified as another possible mechanism of resistance, facilitating the clearance of the drug from the parasite. Its distinct chemotype, ability to rapidly kill parasites, potentially new mechanism of activity and good safety indices than artesunate and quinine support the clinical development of SC83288 as an IV application for the treatment of severe malaria when combined with a slow-acting partner drug. Presently, Heidelberg University Hospital and the German Centre for Infection Research are collaboratively in the process of conducting the regulatory preclinical procedures with the hope of initiating clinical trials in due course [79, 100]. More recently, Miguel-Blanco and his co-workers identified a compound coded as **DDD01034957**. This new antiplasmodial molecule is fast-acting and potent against resistant strains *in vitro*, *in vivo*, and possesses a resistance mechanism linked to the membrane transporter *P. falciparum* ATP-binding cassette-I3

(*PfABCI3*). These finding support further medicinal chemistry lead-optimization of DDD01034957 as a new antimalarial chemical class and provide latest insights to further reduce *in vivo* metabolic clearance [124].

A 4(1*H*)-quinolone derivative **ELQ-300**, structurally engineered from pyridone analogue by Oregon Health and Science University, was potently inhibited blood stages of *falciparum* and *vivax* malaria in clinical field isolates as well as liver stages and transmissible stages of the parasite. ELQ-300 is proved to be highly selective against plasmodial cytochrome bc_1 complexes like atovaquone, suggesting minimized possibility of causing side effects by inhibiting the host enzyme. Similar to atovaquone, it is a slow acting molecule with a delayed parasite reduction ratio, and exhibited strong synergy with proguanil. Mutant selection studies failed to achieve variants, signifying a significantly low susceptibility for resistance. ELQ-300 was extremely potent in *berghei* infected mice with an ED_{50} of 0.016 mg/kg/day and cures the infection by doses as low as 0.1 mg/kg/day, thus owing the capacity to be a combination partner aimed of single dose cure. Further safety assessment indicated that there are no remarkable off target pharmacological activities by this compound. The main obstacle in the clinical development of ELQ-300 is its relatively poor water solubility, which limits the absorption to the extent that only low blood concentrations can be achieved with oral doses. Even though these low blood levels are adequate for treatment, the concentrations remain too low to establish an acceptable safety margin necessary for clinical development. The way forward intended to design bioreversible alkoxycarbonate ester pro-drugs has currently been effectively explored to overcome the physicochemical problems of ELQ-300 and attain bloodstream levels adequate for safety and toxicological studies, as well as getting single dose cures [79]. It is also possible to list **Genz-668764**, **ML238**, **ACT-213615, SAR121** and **TDR84420** within the new chemical entity group [77, 103].

Besides, a **pyrazoleamide 21A092**, which targets sodium channel (ATPase4) like KAE609 and SJ733, is in preclinical discovery phase [125]. **Dantrolene** was identified as a novel inhibitor of plasmodial surface anion channel (PSAC) and it may be a lead compound for antimalarial drug development [126]. **Acridinones** such as **WR249685** and **T3.5**, new class of selective malaria parasite mitochondrial *bc*1 inhibitors, had a great potential to become novel antimalarial drugs [127, 128]. Some antibiotics that have shown potential effects on malaria parasite have been recently studied *in vitro* or *in vivo* intensively. **Macrolide antibiotics** were identified for the first time that they inhibit *in vitro* RBC invasion by merozoite of Plasmodium species. This result directs the development of safe and effective macrolide antibiotics with dual modalities to combat malaria and reduce the parasite's options for resistance. Other antibiotics, such as **quinolones**, **tigecycline**, **co-trimoxazole** or **fusidic acid**, could be used to prevent malaria in the future. Antiadhesion adjunctive therapies, including **levamisole**, are under research in the laboratory [129, 130]. Both *in vitro* and *in vivo* experments showed that an antibacterial and anticancer drug **acriflavine** impairs DNA replication foci formation in *P. berghei* malaria and affects the enzymatic activities of apicoplast specific Gyrase protein. This attention-grabbing work tells us the potential of this old compound to become future antimalarial agent [131]. In another pre-clinical studies, the receptor protein *PfATP6* has been recognized as the common target of curcumin and artemisinin. This reseach was initiated to evaluate the anti-malarial activity of 6 **derivatives of curcumin** based on their binding affinities and correlating the *in silico* docking outcome with the *in vitro* anti-malarial screening results. The *in vitro* results superimpose the results obtained from the *in silico* study thereby encouraging development of promising curcumin leads in the battle against malaria [132]. One approach to discover new biologically active compounds is to combine a steroid skeleton with structural elements endowed with appropriate biological activities.

DOI: http://dx.doi.org/10.5772/intechopen.98725

Recently, Krieg and his co-workers reported on low molecular weight **arylmethyl-amino steroids** with varying constitutions of the basic gonane core and exhibiting excellent antimalarial activity [79]. Moreover, researchers' team has recently discovered thioredoxin enzymes, which are different from the human enzyme but critical for the survival of malaria parasite by balancing the redox state inside the *Plasmodium*. So that, a team is doing experments in collaboration to industry partners to develope novel drugs, which will successfully target this enzyme and kill the parasite without affecting the human host [133]. Although many drugs are in the pipeline, most of them are not able to kill both gametocytes and hypnozoites.

6. Conclusion

Malaria is one of the ancient human diseases and remains an important cause of illness and death among adults as well as children in the world. However, an increasing resistance toward currently available antimalarial drugs is a big obstacle in the fight against malaria. The past instances indicate that resistance to the conventional antimalarial medicines will spread to Africa including Ethiopia. As a result, we are in an urgent need of novel, safe, and effective drugs. Some of the newer compounds possess multi-stage activity and are highly potent in inhibiting the parasite multiplication. Those novel agents that have different structure and new mechanism of action than older drugs could be the game changer in combating malaria. The current breakthroughs will still require long-term financial investments, political will, and scientific endeavor to ensure sustainability and translate to more reduction in global burden of malaria.

List of abbrivations and acronyms

ACT	Artemisinin-based combination therapy
CDC	Center for Disease Prevention and Control
DHA	Dihydroartemisinin
DHFR	Dihydrofolate reductase
DHPS	Dihydropteroate synthase
DHODH	Dihydroorotate dehydrogenase
FMoH	Federal Ministry of Health
MDR	Multi-Drug Resistant
MMV	Medicines for Malaria Venture
NIAID	National Institute of Allergy and Infectious Diseases
RBC	Red Blood Cell
SP	Sulfadoxine-pyrimethamine
UNICEF	United Nations International Children's Emergency Fund
USA	United States of America
WHO	World Health Organization

Author details

Dejen Nureye
Department of Pharmacology and Toxicology, School of Pharmacy, College of Medicine and Health Sciences, Mizan-Tepi University, Mizan-Aman, Southwest, Ethiopia

*Address all correspondence to: dcjenureye@gmail.com

References

[1] Service W, Townson H. The anopheles vector, in Essential Malariology, 4th edition. Gilles H, Warrell D (Ed.). London: Arnold, 2002, 59-84.

[2] Amorosa F, Corbellini G, Coluzzi M. Lessons learned from malaria: Italy's past and sub-Sahara's future. Health and Place, 2005, 11: 65-73.

[3] Carter R, Mendis K. Evolutionary and historical aspects of the burden of malaria. Clin Microbiol Rev., 2002, 15(4):564-594.

[4] Greenwood B, Bojang K, Whitty C, Targett GA. Malaria. Lancet, 2005, 365(9469):1487-1498.

[5] Miller L, Good M, Milon G. Malaria pathogenesis. Science, 1994, 264(5167):1878-1883.

[6] NIAID. Understanding Malaria. Fighting an ancient scourge. No. 07-7139; 2007.

[7] Morrissette S, Sibley D. Cytoskeleton of apicomplexan parasites. Microbiology and Molecular Biology Reviews, 2002, 66(1):21-38.

[8] Chavatte J, Chiron F, Chabaud A et al. [Probable speciations by "host-vector fidelity": 14 species of plasmodium from magpies] [article in French]. Parasite, 2007, 14(1):21-37.

[9] Liu W, Yingying L, Gerald H, Rudicell R, Robertson J, Keele B et al. Origin of human malaria parasite plasmodium falciparum in gorillas. Nature, 2010, 467(7314):420-425.

[10] Gueirard P, Tavares J, Thiberge S, Bernex F, Ishino T, Milon G et al. Development of the malaria parasite in the skill if the mammalian host. Proceedings of the National Academy of Sciences, 2010, 107(43):18640-18645.

[11] Manitoba Health. Communicable Disease Management Protocol-Malaria, November 2001; 2015.

[12] NaTHNaC. Malaria. Travel Health Pro. Available online from: https://travelhealthpro.org.uk; 2020.

[13] WHO. Guidelines for the treatment of malaria, 3rd edition. World Health Organization, Geneva, Switzerland, 2015a.

[14] WHO. World Malaria Report. World Health Organization. Geneva, Switzerland, 2015b.

[15] FMoH. An Epidemiological Profile of Malaria in Ethiopia. Federal Democratic Republic of Ethiopia. Ministry of Health, Addis Ababa, Ethiopia. Version 1.0; 2014.

[16] Solomon L, Okere HC, Daminabo V. Understanding human Malaria: Further review on the literature, Pathogenesis and Disease Control. *Rep Opinion*, 2014, 6(6):55-63.

[17] Harbach R. The phylogeny and classification of anopheles, in Anopheles Mosquitoes-New Insights into Malaria Vectors, Sylvie Manguin (Ed.), Intecth, London, UK; 2013.

[18] CDC. Anopheles Mosquitoes. Center for Disease Control and Prevention. Division of Parasitic Diseases and Malaria, USA; 2015.

[19] CDC. The history of Malaria, an ancient disease. Division of parasitic diseases and Malaria. USA, 2016a.

[20] National Academy of Sciences. 6 The Parasite, the Mosquito, and the Disease. Institute of Medicine. 2004. Saving Lives, Buying Time: Economics of Malaria Drugs in an Age of Resistance. Washington, DC: The National Academies Press, 2019.

[21] Owusu-Ofori A, Parry C, Bates I, et al. Transfusion-transmitted malaria in countries where malaria is endemic: A review of the literature from sub-Saharan Africa. Clin Infect Dis., 2010, 51(10):1192-1198.

[22] Jain SK, Persaud D, Perl TM, et al. Nosocomial malaria and saline flush. Emerging Infectious Diseases, 2005, 11:1097-1099.

[23] Parham P, Christiansen-Jucht C, Pople D, et al. Understanding and Modelling the Impact of Climate Change on Infectious Diseases-Progress and Future Challenges, Climate Change – Socioeconomic Effects, Dr Kherad mand H (Ed), 2011, 43-66.

[24] PMI. President's Malaria initiative Ethiopia, Malaria Operational Plan FY 2014; 2014.

[25] Shibeshi MA, Kifle ZD, Atnafie SA. Antimalarial drug resistance and novel targets for antimalarial drug discovery. Infection and Drug Resistance, 2020, 13:4047-4060.

[26] Kumar S, Renu K. Recently developed new, sensitive, time-effective and cost-effective diagnostic tests of Malaria. Proceeding of Indian National Science Academy, 2015, 81(2):479-483.

[27] RBMP. Evidence for Advocacy: Key Statistics on the Fight against Malaria. Geneva, Switzerland; 2015.

[28] WHO. World Malaria Report. World Health Organization. Geneva, Switzerland, 2020.

[29] Ananya M. Malaria Epidemiology. Reviewed by April Cashin-Garbutt, BA Hons (Cantab) pdf. Available online from: http://www.news-medical.net/health/; 2013.

[30] CDC Global Health-Ethiopia. Centers for Disease Control and Prevention, Center for Global Health. Atlanta, USA, 2016.

[31] Index Mundi. Ethiopia Major infectious diseases. Available online from: https://www.indexmundi.com/ethiopia/major_infectious_diseases.html; 2018.

[32] Alemu A, Abebe G, Tsegaye W, Golassa L. Climatic variables and malaria transmission dynamics in Jimma town, south West Ethiopia. Paras Vect., 2011, 4:30.

[33] Woyessa A, Deressa W, Ali A, Lindtjørn B. Prevalence of malaria infection in Butajira area, south-Central Ethiopia. Malar J., 2012, 11:84.

[34] Jima D, Getachew A, Bilak H, et al. Malaria indicator survey 2007, Ethiopia: Coverage and use of major malaria prevention and control interventions. Malar J., 2010, 9:58.

[35] WHO. Climate change and health. World Health Organization. Geneva, Switzerland, 2018.

[36] Ayalew S, Mamo H, Animut A et al., Assessment of current Malaria status in light of the ongoing control interventions, socio-demographic and environmental variables in Jiga area, Northwest Ethiopia. PLoS One, 2016, 11(1):e0146214.

[37] Yibeltal A, Abeba M, Abebaw B, et al. Prevalence of malaria and associated risk factors among asymptomatic migrant laborers in west Armachiho District, Northwest Ethiopia. Research and Reports in Tropical Medicine, 2018, 9:95-101.

[38] Ayele D, Temesgen T, Henry G, et al. The risk factor indicators of malaria in Ethiopia. Int J Med Med Sci., 2013, 5(7):335-347.

[39] Deribew A, Dejene T, Kebede B, et al. Incidence, prevalence and mortality rates of malaria in Ethiopia from 1990 to 2015: Analysis of the global burden of diseases 2015. Malaria J., 2017, 16:271.

[40] Bhowmik D, Chiranjib B, Navinkanth S, et al. Recent advances in prevention, Treatment and Medication of Malaria. *J Chem Pharm Res.*, 2010, 2(1):83-90.

[41] CDC. Human factors and Malaria. Center for disease prevention and control. Global Health-division of parasitic diseases and Malaria. USA, 2016.

[42] Aly ASI, Vaughan AM, Kappe SHI. Malaria parasite development in the mosquito and infection of the mammalia host. Annu Rev Microbiol., 2009, 63:195-221.

[43] Cowman A, Healer J, Marapana D, Kevin M. Malaria: Biology and disease. Cell, 2016, 167:610-624.

[44] Ricardo T, Parisa K, Katherine A, et al., (2014). Plasmodium life cycle and the pathogenesis of malaria. From innate sensing of malaria parasites. Nat Rev Immunol, 14:744-757.

[45] Walker NF, Nadjim B, Whitty C. Malaria. Medicine, 2010, 38(1):41-46.

[46] Greenwood T, Tomas V, Maria S, et al. Febrile plasmodium falciparum malaria four years after exposure in a man with sickle cell disease. Clin Infect Dis., 2008, 47(4):e39-e41.

[47] Poilane I, Jeantils V, Carbillon L, et al. Pregnancy associated p. falciparum malaria discovered fortuitously: Report of two cases. Gynecol Obstet Fertil., 2009, 37(10):824-826.

[48] Szmitko P, Magdie L, Andrew E, et al. Plamodium falciparum malaria occurring eight years after leaving an endemic area. Diagn Microbiol Infect Dis., 2008, 61(1):105-107.

[49] Theunissen C, Janssens P, Demulder A, et al. Falciparum malaria in patient 9 years after leaving malaria-endemic area. Emerg Infect Dis., 2009, 15(1):115-116.

[50] Jiraprapa W, Salenna E, Huji X, et al. Immunity to asexual blood stage malaria and vaccine approaches. Immunol Cell Biol., 2002, 80:401-414.

[51] UNICEF. Promoting Rational Use of Drugs and Correct Case Management in Basic Health Services. Malaria prevention and treatment. The Prescriber, 2000, No. 18:1-15.

[52] Antinori S, Galimberti L, Milazzo L, Corbellino M. Biology of human Malaria plasmodia including *plasmodium Knowlesi*. Mediterr J Hematol Infect Dis., 2012, 4(1): e2012013.

[53] Meibalan E, Marti M, "Biology of Malaria Transmission," Cold Spring Harbor Laboratory Press, vol. 7, Article ID a025452, 2017. Doi: 10.1101/cshperspect.a025452.

[54] Na-Bangchangb K, Karbwang J. Current status of malaria chemotherapy and the role of pharmacology in antimalarial drug research and development. Fundamental and Clinical Pharmacology, 2009, 23 (4):387-409.

[55] Nicoletta B, Roberta S, Sarah D. Malaria Diagnosis, Therapy, Vaccines, and Vector Control. M. Prato (ed.). *Human and Mosquito Lysozymes*, 2015.

[56] O' Neill PM, Ward SA, Berry NG, et al. A medicinal chemistry perspective on 4-Aminoquinoline antimalarial drugs. Curr Top Med Chem., 2006, 6(5):479-507.

[57] Egan T. Haemozoin formation. Mol Biochem Parasitol., 2008, 157:127-136.

[58] Roberts L, Egan T, Joiner K, et al. Differential effects of quinoline antimalarials on endocytosis in *plasmodium falciparum*. Antimicrob Agents Chemother., 2008, 52(5):1840-1842.

[59] Katzung. Basic and Clinical Pharmacology, 12th edition. The McGraw-Hill Companies, Inc; 2012.

[60] Fogh S, Jepsen S, Effersøe P. Chloroquine-resistant Plasmodium falciparum malaria in Kenya. Trans R Soc Trop Med Hyg, 1979, 73(2):228-229.

[61] Phillips EJ, Keystone JS, Kain KC. Failure of combined chlor-oquine and high-dose primaquine therapy for plasmodium vivax malaria acquired in Guyana, South America. Clin Infect Dis, 1996, 23(5):1171-1173.

[62] FMoH. National Malaria Guidelines 3rd Edition. Federal Democratic Republic of Ethiopia. Ministry of Health, Addis Ababa, Ethiopia, 2012.

[63] Goodman, Gilman's. Chemotherapy of Malaria, in the Pharmacological Basis of Therapeutics, 12th Edition; 2010.

[64] Krungkrai J, Burat D, Kudan S, et al. Mitochondrial oxygen consumption in asexual and sexual blood stages of the human malaria parasite, *Plasmodium falciparum*. *Southeast Asian J Trop Med Public Health*, 1999, 30:636-642.

[65] Achan J, Talisuna A, Erhart A, et al. Quinine, an old anti-malarial drug in a modern world: Role in the treatment of malaria. Malaria J., 2011, 10:144.

[66] Bronner U, Divis P, Farnert A, Singh B. Swedish traveller with *plasmodium knowlesi* malaria after visiting Malaysian Borneo. Malaria J., 2009, 8:15.

[67] Malariasite. Antimalarial Drugs. Available from: http://www.malariasite.com; 2015.

[68] White N, Pukrittayakamee S, Hien T, et al. Malaria. Lancet, 2013, 383:723-735.

[69] Posner GH, Oh CH, Gerena L, et al. Extraordinarily potent antimalarial compounds: New, structurally simple, easily synthesized, tricyclic 1, 2, 4-trioxanes. J Med Chem., 1992, 35:2459-2467.

[70] O'Neill PM, Barton VE, Ward SA. The molecular mechanism of action of artemisinin—The debate continues. Molecules, 2010, 15:1705-1721.

[71] Olliaro PL, Haynes RK, Meunier B, et al. Possible modes of action of the artemisinin-type compounds. Trends Parasitol., 2001, 17:122-126.

[72] Eckstein-Ludwig U, Webb RJ, Van Goethem ID, et al. Artemisinins target the SERCA of *plasmodium falciparum*. Nat., 2003, 424:957-961.

[73] Haynes RK, Cheu KW, Chan HW, et al. Interactions between artemisinins and other antimalarial drugs in relation to the cofactor model—A unifying proposal for drug action. Chem Med Chem., 2012, 7:2204-2226.

[74] CDC. Guidelines for Treatment of Malaria in the United States pdf. Available online from: http://www.cdc.gov/malaria; 2013.

[75] Tyagi RK, Gleeson PJ, Arnold L, Tahar R et al. High-level artemisinin-resistance with quinine co-resistance emerges in P. falciparummalaria under in vivo artesunate pressure. BMC Medicine, 2018, 16:181.

[76] Pluijm RW, Imwong M, Chau NH, et al. Determinants of dihydroartemisinin-piperaquine treatment failure in plasmodium falciparum malaria in Cambodia, Thailand, and Vietnam: A prospective clinical, pharmacological, and genetic study. Lancet Infect Dis, 201; 2019, 19: 952-961.

[77] Nureye D, Assefa S. Old and recent advances in life cycle, pathogenesis, diagnosis, prevention, and treatment of Malaria including perspectives in Ethiopia. The Scientific World Journal, 2020, 2020(1):1-1)17.

[78] Ogundahunsi O, Catteruccia F, Chitnis CE. Eradicating Malaria: Discoveries, challenges, and questions.

Leading Edge Voices. Cell, 2016; 167:595-597.

[79] Okombo J, Chibale K. Recent updates in the discovery and development of novel antimalarial drug candidates. Med chem comm., 2018, 9(3): 437-453.

[80] Popovici J, Pierce-Friedrich L, Kim S, et al. Recrudescence, reinfection, or relapse? A more rigorous framework to assess chloroquine efficacy for plasmodium vivax malaria. J Infect Dis. 2019; 219(2):315-322.

[81] Cowman AF, Crabb BS. Invasion of red blood cells by malaria parasites. Cell, 2006,124(4):755-766.

[82] Lee RS, Waters AP, Brewer JM. A cryptic cycle in haematopoie-tic niches promotes initiation of malaria transmission and evasion of chemotherapy. Nat Commun, 2018; 9.

[83] Kumar S, Bhardwaj T, Prasad D, Singh RK. Drug targets for malaria: Historic to future perspectives. Biomed Pharmacother, 2018, 104:8-27.

[84] Muller O. Challenges for control and elimination in the 21st century. Malaria Afri, 2011, 60:193.

[85] Paget-McNicol S, Saul A. Mutation rates in the dihydrofolate reductase gene of plasmodium falciparum. Parasitology, 2001, 122(5):497-505.

[86] Hall KA, Newton PN, Green MD, et al. Characterization of counterfeit artesunate antimalarial tablets from Southeast Asia. Am J Trop Med Hyg, 2006, 75(5):804-811.

[87] Newton PN, Green MD, Mildenhall DC, et al. Poor quality vital anti-malarials in Africa-an urgent neglected public health priority. Malar J, 2011, 10(1):352.

[88] Cowell AN, Winzeler EA. The genomic architecture of antimalarial drug resistance. Brief Funct Genomics., 2019, 18(5):314-328.

[89] Sidhu ABS, Uhlemann A-C, Valderramos SG, Valderramos J-C, Krishna S, Fidock DA. Decreasing pfmdr1 copy number in plasmodium falciparum malaria heightens susceptibility to meflo-quine, lumefantrine, halofantrine, quinine, and artemisinin. J Infect Dis, 2006, 194(4):528-535.

[90] Tulu AN, Webber RH, Schellenberg JA, Bradley DJ. Failure of chloroquine treatment for malaria in the highlands of Ethiopia. Trans R Soc Trop Med Hyg, 1996, 90(5):556-557.

[91] Bray PG, Martin RE, Tilley L, et al. Defining the role of PfCRT in *plasmodium falciparum* chloroquine resistance. Mol Microbiol., 2005, 56(2):323-333.

[92] Rieckmann K, Davis D, Hutton D. Plasmodium vivax resistance to chloroquine? Lancet. 1989;334(8673):1183-1184.

[93] Aminake MN, Pradel G. Antimalarial drugs resistance in *Plasmodium falciparum* and the currentstrategies to overcome them. Microbial pathogens and strategies for combating them: science, technology and education (A. Méndez-Vilas, Ed.), FORMATEX, 2013, PP. 269-282.

[94] Dondorp AM, Yeung S, White L, et al. Artemisinin resistance: Current status and scenarios for containment. Nature Reviews Microbiology, 2010, 8(4):272-280.

[95] Hemingway J, Shretta R, Wells TN, et al. Tools and strategies for Malaria control and elimination: What do we need to achieve a grand convergence in Malaria? PLoS Biol., 2016, 14(3):e1002380.

[96] Chandra RS, Orazem J, Ubben D, Duparc S, Robbins J, Vandenbroucke P.

Creative solutions to extraordinary challenges in clinical trials: Methodology of a phase III trial of azithromycin and chloroquine fixed-dose combination in pregnant women in Africa. Malar J 2013;12:122.

[97] Bvgh. Malaria Pipelines. *BIO Ventures for Global Health*; 2015.

[98] Marco A, Jutta W, Karine G. Recent advances in malaria drug discovery. Bioorg Med Chem Lett., 2013, 23(10):2829-2843.

[99] Spillman NJ, Kirk K. The malaria parasite cation ATPase PfATP4 and its role in the mechanism of action of a new arsenal of antimalarial drugs. Int J Parasitol Drugs Drug Resist., 2015, 5:149-162.

[100] Tse EG, Korsik1M, Todd MH. The past, present and future of anti-malarial medicines. Malaria J., 2019, 18:93.

[101] Novartis. Backgrounder: Malaria Initiative Pipeline; 2014.

[102] White N, Duong TT, Uthaisil C, et al. Antimalarial activity of KAF156 in falciparum and vivax malaria. N Engl J Med., 2016, 375(12):1152-1160.

[103] Ashley E, Phyo A. Drugs in development for Malaria. Drugs, 2018, 78:861-879.

[104] Phillips MA, Lotharius J, Marsh K, et al. A long-duration dihydroorotate dehydrogenase inhibitors (DRSM265) for prevention and treatment of malaria. *Sci Transl Med*., 2015, 7(296):296ra111.

[105] Haynes RK. From artemisinin to new artemisinin antimalarials: Biosynthesis, extraction, old and new derivatives, stereochemistry and medicinal chemistry requirements. Curr Top Med Chem., 2006, 6:509-537.

[106] Coertzen D, Reader J, van der Watt M, Nondaba SH et al. Artemisone and artemiside are potent panreactive antimalarial agents that also synergize redox imbalance in plasmodium falciparum transmissible gametocyte stages. Antimicrob Agents Chemother, 2018, 62:e02214-e02217.

[107] Wong HN, Padín-Irizarry V, van der Watt ME, Reader J et al. Optimal 10-Aminoartemisinins with potent transmission-blocking capabilities for new artemisinin combination therapies–activities against blood stage P. falciparum including PfKI3 C580Y mutants and liver Stage P. berghei parasites. Front. Chem, 2020, 7:901.

[108] Coleman RE, Clavin AM, Milhous WK. Gametocytocidal and sporontocidal activity of antimalarials against *plasmodium berghei* ANKA in ICR mice and anopheles stephensi mosquitoes. American Journal of Tropical Medicine and Hygiene, 1992, 46:169-182.

[109] Martin S. Antimalarial drugs – What is in use and what is in the pipeline. Archiv Pharm., 2008, 341(3):149-163.

[110] Sulyok M, Ruckle T, Roth A, et al. DSM265 for plasmodium falciparum chemoprophylaxis: A randomised, double blinded, phase 1 trial with controlled human malaria infection. Lancet Infect Dis., 2017, 17(6):636-644.

[111] Leitgeb AM, Charunwatthana P, Rueangveerayut R, et al. Inhibition of merozoite invasion and transient de-sequestration by sevuparin in humans with plasmodium falciparum malaria. PloS One, 2017, 12(12):e0188754.

[112] Chibale K. How Africa is helping expand the global antimalarial drug pipeline. *The conversation*. Available online from: https://theconversation.com/how-africa-is-helping-expand-the-global-antimalarial-drug-pipeline-63527; 2016.

[113] Caldarelli SA, Hamel M, Duckert JF, et al. Disulfide prodrugs of albitiazolium (T3/SAR97276): Synthesis and biological activities. Journal of Medicinal Chemistry, 2012, 55(10):4619-4628.

[114] Clinical Trials. First-in-human trial of single ascending dose, multiple ascending dose and malaria challenge model in healthy subjects NCT03261401. Available online from: https://clinicaltrials.gov/ct2/show/study/NCT03261401?view=results; 2017.

[115] Clinical Trials. First-in-Humans Study of an Oral *Plasmodium falciparum* Plasma Memberane Protein Inhibitor. *St. Jude Children's Research Hospital*. Available online from: https://clinicaltrials.gov/ct2/show/NCT02661373; 2016.

[116] Rutgers University. Promising Malaria Drug to Undergo Clinical Trials. Medical Xpress; 2016. Available from: https://medicalxpress. com/news/2016-03-malaria-drug-clinical-trials.html. [Last accessed on 2020 Sep 05].

[117] Gaur A, Panetta J, Dallas R, et al. St. Jude experimental anti-malarial drug shows promise in first clinical trial. St. Jude Children's Research Hospital. Memphis, Tennessee. Available online from: https://www.stjude.org/media-resources/news-releases/2020-medicine-science news/experimental-anti-malarial-drug-shows-promise-in-first-clinical-trial.html; 2020.

[118] National Institutes of Health. Early Stage Clinical Trial of Antimalarial Drug Begins. U.S. Department of Health & Human Services, News releases; 2018.

[119] Njeru G. Malaria breakthrough as scientists find 'highly effective' way to kill parasite. *The Guardian*. Available online from: https://www.theguardian.com; 2019.

[120] Burrows JN, Duparc S, Gutteridge WE, et al. New developments in antimalarial target candidate and product profiles. Malaria J., 2017, 16(1):26.

[121] Birrell GW, Heffernan GD, Schiehser GA, et al. Characterization of the preclinical pharmacology of the new 2-aminomethylphenol, JPC-3210, for malaria treatment and prevention. *Antimicrob Agents Chemother.*, 2018, 62(4):e01335-e01317.

[122] Fonteilles-Drabek S, Reddy D, Wells TN. Managing intellectual property to develop medicines for the world's poorest. Nat Rev Drug Discov., 2017, 16(4):223-224.

[123] Pegoraro S, Duffey M, Otto TD, Wang Y, Rösemann R, Baumgartner R, et al. SC83288 is a clinical development candidate for the treatment of severe malaria. Nat Commun 2017; 8:14193.

[124] Miguel-Blanco C, Murithi JM, Benavente ED, Angrisano F et al. The antimalarial efcacy and mechanism of resistance of the novel chemotype DDD01034957. Scientifc Reports, 2021, 11:1888.

[125] Jimenez-Diaz MB, Ebert D, Salinas Y, et al. (+)-SJ733, a clinical candidate for malaria that acts through ATP4 to induce rapid host-mediated clearance of Plasmodium. *Proc Natl Acad Sci. USA*, 2014, 111(50):E5455–E5462.

[126] Kang M, Lisk G, Hollinqworth S, et al. Malaria parasites are rapidly killed by Dantrolene derivatives specific for the Plasmodial surface Anion Channel. Mol Pharmacol., 2005, 68(1):34-40.

[127] Beteck R, France J, Richard K, et al. Recent progress in the development of anti-malarial quinolones. Malaria J., 2014, 13:339.

[128] Biagini GA, Fisher N, Berry N, et al., Acridinediones: Selective and potent

inhibitors of the Malaria parasite mitochondrial bc1 complex. Mol Pharmacol., 2008, 73(5):1347-1355.

[129] Gaillard T, Madamet M, Tsombeng F, et al. Antibiotics in malaria therapy: Which antibiotics except tetracyclines and macrolides may be used against malaria?. Malar J., 2016; 15:556.

[130] Wilson DW, Goodman CD, Sleebs BE, et al. Macrolides rapidly inhibit red blood cell invasion by the human malaria parasite, *plasmodium falciparum*. BMC Biol., 2015, 13:52.

[131] Dana S, Dhaneswwar P, Devender D, et al., Potent antimalarial activity of Acriflavine *In vitro* and *In vivo*. ACS Chem Biol., 2014, 9:2366-2373.

[132] Dohutia C, Chetia D, Gogoi K, et al. Molecular docking, synthesis and *in vitro* antimalarial evaluation of certain novel curcumin analogues. Braz J Pharm Sci., 2017; 53(4):e00084.

[133] Lilach S. Parasite' Could Mean more Effective Treatment for Toxoplasmosis and Malaria. An unexpected breakthrough looks promising for finding new drugs to treat two diseases. *The Conversation*; 2018.